ADDITIONAL PRAISE FOR
THE SUBTLE BODY PRACTICE MANUAL

"Everything you need to know and do for self-health—a practical guide from acupressure to Zen, auras to sound and spirit."

C. NORMAN SHEALY, MD, PhD

Author of *From Birth to Bliss—The Power of Conscientious Living*

"While energy is the basis of life, in her important new book Cyndi Dale demonstrates that subtle energy, and the interconnectedness of all life, is the basis of healing. Her comprehensive manual reflects a deep understanding of the subtle body, as well as an inspiration rooted in the healing modalities from many of the world's systems of therapeutic wisdom."

JACK ANGELO

Author of *Distant Healing*

"If I had room for only one book on energy medicine, Cyndi Dale's *The Subtle Body Practice Manual* is the one I would put on my shelf. Complete and comprehensive, it covers everything you could possibly want to know about energy medicine either as a client or as a practitioner. I couldn't put it down."

LINNIE THOMAS

Author of *The Encyclopedia of Energy Medicine*

"We can always count on Cyndi to bring together a plethora of healing systems, then synthesize and present them to us in a practical way. Her hankering to collect and connect shines in this veritable "Energy Healing Wikipedia." There are enough practices for more than a year of healing."

LINDA HOWE

Author of *Healing Through the Akashic Records*

THE
SUBTLE BODY
PRACTICE MANUAL

ALSO BY CYNDI DALE

Books

Advanced Chakra Healing: Cancer; The Four Pathways Approach

Advanced Chakra Healing: Energy Mapping on the Four Pathways

Advanced Chakra Healing: Heart Disease; The Four Pathways Approach

Attracting Prosperity Through the Chakras

Attracting Your Perfect Body Through the Chakra

*Beyond Soul Mates: Open Yourself to Higher Love Through
the Energy of Attraction*

The Complete Book of Chakra Healing (formerly *New Chakra Healing*)

*Energetic Boundaries: How to Stay Protected and Connected
in Work, Love, and Life*

*The Everyday Clairvoyant: Extraordinary Answers to Finding Love,
Destiny and Balance in Your Life*

The Intuition Guidebook: How to Safely and Wisely Use Your Sixth Sense

The Journey After Life: What Happens When We Die

Kundalini: Divine Energy, Divine Life

The Subtle Body: An Encyclopedia of Your Energetic Anatomy

Togetherness: Creating and Deepening Sustainable Love
(with Andrew Wald and Debra Evans)

Audio Programs

Advanced Chakra Wisdom: Insights & Practices for Transforming Your Life

*Energy Clearing: Heal Energetic Wounds, Release Negative Influences,
and Create Healthy Boundaries*

*Healing Across Space & Time: Guided Journeys for Your Past, Future,
and Parallel Lives*

Illuminating the Afterlife: Your Soul's Journey Through the World's Beyond

Video Programs

The Essential Energy Healing Techniques

The Songbird Series

THE
SUBTLE BODY
PRACTICE MANUAL

A Comprehensive Guide to Energy Healing

....

CYNDI DALE

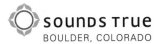

SOUNDS TRUE
BOULDER, COLORADO

Sounds True, Inc.
Boulder, CO 80306

Published 2013

This work is solely for personal growth and education. It should not be
treated as a substitute for professional assistance, therapeutic activities such
as psychotherapy or counseling, or medical advice. In the event of physical
or mental distress, please consult with appropriate health professionals.
The application of protocols and information in this book is the choice of
each reader, who assumes full responsibility for his or her understandings,
interpretations, and results. The author and publisher assume no
responsibility for the actions or choices of any reader.

Cover and book design by Karen Polaski
Illustrations © Richard Wehrman
Printed in the United States of America

Library of Congress Cataloging-in-Publication Data
Dale, Cyndi.
The subtle body practice manual : a comprehensive guide to energy healing /
Cyndi Dale.
      pages cm
Includes bibliographical references and index.
ISBN 978-1-60407-879-4
1. Energy medicine—Handbooks, manuals, etc. 2. Healing—Handbooks,
manuals, etc. I. Title.
RZ421.D352 2013
615.8'51—dc23
                                        2013000543

Ebook ISBN 978-1-62203-049-1
10 9 8 7 6 5 4 3 2 1

This book is dedicated to the healers, sages, and seers who have carried the torch of hope through the centuries.

CONTENTS

INTRODUCTION

We face the extraordinary possibility
of fashioning a health care system
that emphasizes life instead of death,
and unity and oneness instead of
fragmentation, darkness, and isolation.

LARRY DOSSEY, MD

Whether licensed or layperson, we are all healers. Our roles shift and change depending on a myriad of factors, such as our state of health, the health of those around us, the season of our lives, and whether we have chosen healing as a vocation. But at one time or another, each of us takes our turn as healer and self-healer, as practitioner and patient.

Looking deeper, we can observe that we are *all* self-healers *all* the time. Even when we are helping others under the aegis of being a trained practitioner, every training program and each client session is another opportunity to work on ourselves, to detoxify and rebuild in body, mind, and spirit so that we might be clearer conduits for subtle energies.

It was this understanding that led to the writing and publication of *The Subtle Body: An Encyclopedia of Your Energetic Anatomy*, my compendium outlining the subtle energy anatomy. A detailed accounting of the invisible energies that underpin physical reality and our physical bodies, *The Subtle Body* is a comprehensive resource from which healers of all persuasions and experience levels can build a strong knowledge base. It lays a solid foundation for comprehending the intricacies of subtle energy medicine and understanding the modalities and tools that are used around the world to evoke our innate healing abilities.

This book, *The Subtle Body Practice Manual*, is the natural extension of that original resource guide—a hands-on companion about putting subtle energy medicine to work with ease, elegance, and effectiveness. You can use it alone or in conjunction with *The Subtle Body*. *The Subtle Body* provides you with the what, and *The Subtle Body Practice Manual* provides you with the how. And because *The Subtle Body* is so rich with scientific and spiritual research, I have limited such discourse here in *The Subtle Body Practice Manual*. Unless otherwise noted, references to research and scientific data can be found in *The Subtle Body*.

Every day, our human family contends with minor ailments, major illnesses, emotional distress, mental upsets, and sometimes the need for a simple energy boost. There are many ways to address our issues when we get off balance. This book's carefully chosen tools and techniques can be immediately useful to both the self-healer and the experienced healing professional. As healing is the purpose and goal of this information, it is useful to examine what healing really is, especially when it's viewed through the lens of subtle energy practices.

WHAT DOES HEALING MEAN?

"What is the true nature of healing?" is one of the most important questions we can contemplate as practitioners or self-healers working with subtle energy. In effect, all practitioners, whether their approach is conventional or holistic, are energy healers, and so we must all ask this question at some point. The answer will prove to be our North Star, guiding the way through all kinds of terrain along the healing journey (whether that journey is a one-hour session or a years-long partnership between healer and client).

As we venture into the subtler realms, one of the most important distinctions we can make is between healing and curing. To cure is to focus on the eradication of symptoms, whereas to heal is to emphasize and support a person's inherent state of wholeness. The subtle energy practitioner starts from the premise that a person is always whole at the deepest level, no matter what—even if they are missing a limb, wrestling with depression or cancer, or trying to shake off a nasty cold. A practitioner of any type who is focused on curing is likely to place an emphasis on diagnostics and relieving symptoms. A subtle energy practitioner, on the other hand, will work with a person to gain relief—and possibly release— from the *cause* of their symptoms.

Subtle energy healers work to help themselves or others recognize and embrace their innate wholeness, regardless of appearances or even the outcome of treatment. Instead of achieving wholeness, healing is a matter of remembering and recovering the wholeness that already *is*. Whether we are working with others or on ourselves, it is incumbent upon us that we not attempt to make all supposed frailties disappear. Subtle energy tools and techniques are far more effective when we understand that wholeness doesn't equal perfection. I have been fortunate to see with my own eyes the remarkable shifts that can take place—the movement toward wellness—when people feel supported in an environment of compassion and acceptance.

Understanding and believing in wholeness is a deeply optimistic state, one that we may encounter with our podiatrist *or* our reflexologist, and one we seek to acknowledge within ourselves. The trust in our natural ability to return to balance just may be the invisible bridge (the subtle energy bridge) that connects the best of allopathic medicine with the brilliant field of healing that used to be called, not so very long ago, "alternative."

THE BEST OF BOTH WORLDS: COLLABORATIVE AND COMPLEMENTARY METHODS OF HEALING

An acupuncturist steps back and nods his head. "Your problem is caused by an energy block in the liver," he says, pointing out the "stagnant liver chi" in your toe.

A physician peers at the x-ray and nods her head. "See what's going on here?" She points to the picture of the organ just under your ribs. "That's your liver. That's where your issue lies."

Who is right? Is it the acupuncturist, whose perspective of the liver is linked to an intricate flow of energy throughout your body, one that somehow mysteriously involves your toes? Or is it the conventional doctor, who views your liver as a single organ unto itself, one that sits quietly beneath your ribs, minding its own business?

Well, both of them are right. Our organs—in fact, many parts of us—anchor somewhere physically. But they are also energetic, which means that they connect to other parts of ourselves in ways that are hard to measure, see, or prove. The subtle aspects of our organs are part of the energy anatomy that we will explore in part 1, a complex set of the fast-moving energy channels, organs, and fields that compose what I think of as the "you underneath or around yourself," the energies that establish the rules and foundation for physical health and wellbeing. This energy anatomy and its systems are the basis of subtle energy medicine. And while subtle energy practitioners often work with energy systems that transform *sensory* or physical energy into *subtle* energy (and vice versa), one of the subjects of chapter 1, they can also work with concrete systems, like those in the physical body.

Because of our Western cultural conditioning, most people don't typically think of their general practitioner, gynecologist, or dermatologist as subtle energy practitioners. (The doctors may not think of themselves this way either.) Contrary to popular opinion, allopathic medicine—or what we often call Western medicine or conventional medicine—is actually an energy-based practice. Surgery and prescription medicines work on our physical energy systems, while x-rays and ECGs (electrocardiograms) measure the energetic patterns present in our bodies. Since our bodies are made up of energy, any practice or method that involves the body is a subtle energy practice. Subtle energy medicine can't be claimed by holistic practitioners, naturopathic doctors, and "alternative" healers alone. Therefore, we in the helping and healing professions can officially let go of the "us and them," dualistic perspective and join forces. Knowing that all medicine is really subtle energy medicine can result in greater benefits and brighter outcomes for everyone concerned—practitioners, physicians, healers, patients, clients, and those who love them.

When it comes to healing modalities and types of practitioners, there is an overflowing cornucopia of options available. The following is a list of broad categories and how they're typically used:

Allopathic medicine, also known as Western or conventional medicine, is absolutely necessary for critical or chronic care, diagnostic needs, surgery, physical intervention, trauma, physical therapy, prescription medicine, or if you are ever in any doubt about a situation.

Mental health therapy is often essential for treating depression, anxiety, stress, emotional trauma, or abuse.

Meridian-based therapies, such as acupuncture, acupressure, and Eastern massage styles, are ideal for stress or pain, addictions, emotional issues, and broad physical categories like ear, nose, and throat conditions; heart-related issues; muscle problems; common ailments like infections; skin conditions; and more. (See chapter 3.)

Chakra-based therapies aid in physical, emotional, mental, and spiritual issues of all sorts. (See chapter 4.) They are typically recommended as a complement to allopathic care or other subtle energy practices.

Field-based therapies assist in resolving physical, emotional, mental, and spiritual issues of all varieties. They are also recommended for issues involving boundaries, for protection, and for environmental sensitivities. (See chapter 2.) They are typically recommended as an adjunct to allopathic care or other subtle energy practices. Examples include aura clearing and balancing, aromatherapy, and sound healing.

Natural healing supports allopathic care, in addition to balancing body, mind, and soul through low-impact treatments. The use of herbal medicine, supplements, hands-on healing, spiritual healing, homeopathy, aromatherapy, flower essences, Ayurveda, guided imagery, holistic dentistry, diet/nutritional medicine, exercise, and other forms of natural care all bring about healing. (See all chapters in part 3.)

Bodywork reduces stress and alleviates bodily pain from chronic conditions, as well as supporting allopathic care. Massage, chiropractic treatments, osteopathy, colon therapy, and reflexology are all forms of bodywork. (See chapter 12 for specific hands-on healing techniques.)

Certain forms of subtle energy medicine, such as Healing Touch, Reiki, color healing, and sound healing, fall into several categories. For instance, Healing Touch and Reiki use the hands to clear, balance, and energize the energy system, but they also achieve the same results as bodywork. Color and sound healing can effectively calm the nerves and therefore be adjuncts for mental health therapy, but they also shift the energetic field. You'll discover that many types of subtle energy medicine achieve several goals.

There are so many ways that modalities from the different categories can—and do—complement each other. For example, a person going through an extended period of anxiety and depression may work with a massage therapist and a psychiatrist. At one point in their process, they might also add the Emotional Freedom Technique (EFT, see page 15) to their healing plan. A pregnant woman, in addition to seeing her obstetrician-gynecologist (ob-gyn) and midwife, might discover that working with a healer who specializes in aromatherapy (see page 274) and sound healing (see page 287) exponentially increases her energy level and sense of emotional equilibrium.

Undoubtedly, you are someone who mixes and matches some of the best of both worlds yourself. I know that I do. I eat organic, whole foods; walk daily; and utilize my own energy balancing and healing techniques in one way or another just about every day. And I also employ the services of allopathic practitioners and medicines when I deem necessary. I believe it's important to not rely on a single modality. We are complex beings, and our health needs are complex as well. I suggest that you select modalities and therapies as part of an overall wellness plan that supports your highest goals. Because our needs change over time, it's also important to "never say never" or dismiss a modality out of hand—especially allopathic modalities. A broken bone will require allopathic care; homeopathy won't hold that bone in place. Serious depression can be treated in many ways; you don't want to rule out prescription medicine. All medicine is energy medicine and, if properly dispensed, can boost and bolster your health.

TOPICS IN THIS BOOK

This book gives you a wealth of information about subtle energy healing. In part 1, you will learn about energy medicine and the energetic anatomy, which is made of energy fields, channels, and centers. Part 2 prepares you for serving as a subtle energy healer, whether you are a layperson or a well-decorated professional.

Subtle energy practitioners have special considerations that self-healers do not, and we cover these unique concerns in part 2. For instance, in order to build and maintain a thriving practice as a subtle energy healer of any stripe, we must foster trust and confidence with clients and patients. We need to be well informed about modalities other than our own and be whole-heartedly willing to recommend complementary options when a situation calls for it. We must also follow a code of ethics that incorporates the sometimes unusual considerations of working with subtle energy, such as the use of intuition or spiritual energies. I'll give you an array of philosophies and tools that can help you with trust and ethics; using intuition, intention, and prayer; setting energetic boundaries; and even setting up an office and conducting a client session. As well, this section features the tools I have developed over nearly thirty years of subtle energy studies and professional service. These are techniques I couldn't live without. They provide energetic safety and ease when paired with nearly any other subtle energy modality.

The ideas and techniques in part 2 are certainly vital to the subtle energy professional, but they're also applicable to the layperson. Every time we wipe a child's crying eyes and reach for a homeopathic remedy to heal the "owie," we are serving as a subtle energy practitioner. To hand out advice on herbs to our friends is to wear the mantle of subtle energy practitioner. And so we are all beholden to learn as much as we can about subtle energy protocol as well as the methods available for self- and other care.

Part 3 is where the rubber meets the road, featuring hundreds of techniques available to the subtle energy healer for healing body, mind, and soul. This is the how-to reference for your healing work, showcasing techniques from ancient to contemporary times, developed around the world. From homeopathy to gemstone healing, from meditation to using food as medicine, it's all here and ready to be used. This section will not only expand your understanding of the art and science of subtle energy medicine, but will also show you how to apply that understanding using methods and techniques that are practical, accessible, effective, and fun.

MOVING FORWARD WITH THE TORCH

As a subtle energy healer, you are essentially a torch-bearer. If we are all healers—and we all are—we participate in our own Olympic Games, carrying forward and passing on the most important torch of all: that of hope. Only by working with subtle energies, in addition to the physical body, can we shift medicine, healing, and this world out of its current constrictions into the truth of wholeness. Indeed, as a subtle energy healer, you are a bridge between the past and the future, a collaborative healer who values more than the healing process—a healer who values life. As you discover the bounty and the beauty of the methods and tools offered herein, where East meets West and heaven meets earth, you will understand why you have been called to the practice and process of healing. *You* are a light. *Your* light is needed.

PART I
MAKING SUBTLE ENERGY MEDICINE WORK FOR YOU

Albert Einstein, amongst other great scientists, shattered the Newtonian universe by asserting that human beings are not isolated islands unto themselves. We are composed of energy and energy fields, which interconnect us to all things.

Energy is information that moves. This short sentence is hugely complicated. It means that everything about us, even our inaudible thoughts, secret desires, and the pulse of the tiniest atoms within us, communicates onto a grander stage. It also implies that whatever occurs in the known and unknown world around us creates change inside us.

The information covered in part 1 reflects the fact that everything is energy. Subtle energy practitioners are specialists in noticing, tracking, diagnosing, and moving energy—the noticeable and the less concrete energy that composes disease and leads to imbalance, but also is the building block of wellbeing and health.

In part 1, we will explore the tenets of subtle energy medicine, which involves diagnosing and solving problems with energy—in other words, analyzing the information or vibration of energies causing harm, as well as administering information and vibration to restore balance. You will also be introduced to your energetic anatomy, the beautiful kaleidoscope of energetic systems that compose your subtle energy body. These three systems are made of your energy fields, which emanate from and flow around you; energy channels, rivers of light that carry energy through you; and energy centers, bodies of energy with transformational functions.

You can return to the data in part 1 when conducting any of the exercises throughout this book, as this information is the basis of many of the techniques.

1

SUBTLE ENERGY MEDICINE

Miracles . . . rest not so much upon
faces or voices or healing power
coming suddenly near to us from afar
off, but upon our perceptions being
made finer, so that for the moment
our eyes can see and our ears can
hear what is there about us always.

WILLA CATHER

Fundamentally, subtle energy medicine involves the study and application of the body's relationship to electric, magnetic, and electromagnetic fields, as well as light, sound, and other forms of energy. The body produces these energies and also responds to these energies that are in the outer environment. Regardless of the method used, the primary purpose is to change the frequency of the body's energetic fields, channels, and centers, the three main aspects of the energetic anatomy.

In practice, subtle energy medicine is healthcare that detects and analyzes energy imbalances; it is medicine that treats the whole person. The philosophy that underlies subtle energy medicine is based on an ideal of a balanced life—not necessarily one that is perfectly balanced in every moment, but one that values the physical, emotional, mental, relational, financial, creative, and spiritual aspects of life. Generally speaking, people tend to turn to subtle energy medicine when they want complete care, when they want to look at all sides of a problem. Often, they arrive at the office of a subtle energy practitioner when their old methods of addressing a persistent physical-, emotional-, or mental-health challenge are simply not working. In that sense, I would say that individuals often choose to explore subtle energy medicine when they want to feel hopeful again about their health, their happiness, and their future.

These days, the term *energy medicine* is becoming widely known, which signifies the exciting evolution taking place in the vast field of healthcare. Although the term *subtle energy medicine* may sound rather mysterious to some (a rarified form of medicine that's practiced by an exclusive group of secretly trained adepts), the truth is far more accessible and *inclusive*: subtle energy medicine includes *all* forms of medicine, even allopathic medicine. Whether they are MDs with a holistic focus or Reiki practitioners specializing in working with cancer patients, subtle energy practitioners are trained to look for the energetic imbalances that lead to disease and to rebalance our energies to restore our natural state of health.

Many terms are used to refer to healing methods that focus on the subtle energies of the body—or the subtle body as a whole—including *energetic healing, biofield healing, bioenergetic healing, energy work, energy anatomy, vibrational medicine, spiritual healing,* and of course, *subtle energy healing.* Each of these labels refers to subtle energy medicine, which is any practice that analyzes the subtle energies underlying a health condition in order to determine its true cause and to find effective solutions. Some of these practices, such as feng shui, qigong, and chakra healing, you may already be well acquainted with, while some, such as ThetaHealing, assemblage-point balancing, or acu-yoga, may be relatively new to you.

In any case, whether you are exploring the phenomenon of the subtle body for the first time or a practitioner with years of training, getting grounded in the basic science underlying subtle energy medicine will help to put this book's many tools and techniques to use.

ENERGETIC DISTINCTIONS: FROM PHYSICAL TO SUBTLE

There are two kinds of energy: *sensory energy*, which is physical energy, and *subtle energy*, which involves thoughts, feelings, intuition, and other energetic information. Sensory or physical energy moves more slowly than the speed of light and has to obey natural law, or the rules proposed by classical scientists like Isaac Newton. When we're talking about germs "causing" a cold, we're talking about sensory energy. Subtle energy moves at speeds faster than the speed of light. This complex energy follows the rules of quantum physics and may also be thought of as spiritual energy.

Although our primary focus in this book is on the subtle energies, it's important to emphasize the interconnection between the two types of energy. We sometimes need to do something physical to stimulate the subtle energies, but we also need to stimulate the subtle energies to find a physical balance. Chiropractic work is an example of a practice where physical adjustments affect both the physical body and the subtle body. This interconnection can also be seen in acupuncture, herbal medicine, and many other modalities.

In textbooks, energy is usually defined as the source of power that can be used to accomplish work or a goal or to create an effect. Another way to think of it is as vibration that "talks." Why doesn't your orange juice float out of the glass in the morning? The information in the force of gravity tells it to behave. Energy is really just information that carries a message. Subtle energy medicine helps you to crack open the bottle and get to that message, so that you can respond and "tell" it to work for you, not against you.

Most energy hasn't traditionally been measurable, which is why it's called subtle energy. However, the gap between measurable or verifiable and subtle, or putative, energy is swiftly closing. Every day, science adds to our proof and understanding of subtle energy; some of this research is noted in *The Subtle Body*, the source of the scientific information in this book, unless otherwise noted.

INTERCONNECTED VITAL ENERGIES

For the self-healer or subtle energy practitioner, the real question is, how does subtle energy work? The answer can be encapsulated in the word *interconnectivity*, the idea that everything is unified by fields.

The most basic vital energies include electricity, magnetism, and electromagnetic fields. Every cell and organ of our bodies pulses with electricity. This electricity generates magnetic fields, which surround all parts of us, including each of our cells and organs, as well as our entire bodies. *Biofields* or *biomagnetic fields* are terms used to refer to the energy fields of our bodies or of our body as a whole. These magnetic fields combine to create electromagnetic fields, which not only spread out from us, but also connect us to every other living being. Energy is spread between living beings through these fields.

It is known that biofields exist because they have been imaged with newer technology, including Kirlian photography, aura imaging, and gas-discharge visualization. This equipment shows dramatic differences in people's biofields before and after subtle energy treatments. The energy fields of two people can overlap and interconnect, and energy can be transferred from one person to another through the fields that emanate from every part of our body. If you have ever felt like you "sensed someone's vibe," you actually *did*. Not only can we sense someone's vibration, but the frequency or resonance of their thoughts— whether buoyant and happy or heavy and depressed—also can enter our field and directly impact us. Their energy can uplift us or bring us down, and vice versa. Even patterns of disease, which are vibrational and therefore mobile, can transfer from person to person through the subtle biomagnetic fields that comprise all living beings.

For example, one study employed a magnetometer to quantify biomagnetic fields coming from the hands of meditators and of yoga and qigong practitioners. These fields emanating from the practitioners' hands were a thousand times stronger than the strongest human biomagnetic field. The strength of the hands' fields was as strong as the low intensity and frequency fields (between 2 and 50 hertzian) used in medical research labs for speeding the healing of wounded biological tissues. Yet another study, involving what is called a superconducting quantum interference device (SQUID), demonstrated that large frequency-pulsing biomagnetic fields emanated from the hands of therapeutic-touch professionals during treatments.

As noted, these biofields extend far beyond the physical body, and quantum physics explains how one person's field can interact with someone else's thousands of miles away through what's known as *nonlocal reality*. This nonlocal reality isn't simply empty space. It is comprised of a universal field, or zero-point field, of energy that surrounds and links everything and everyone.

A theory called *quantum entanglement* shows how, through this universal field, we can effect change in people we know or have met. According to this theory, two or more objects or particles that have once connected can interrelate and affect each other even when they're separated. The distance between the two people might be small, as demonstrated in a study conducted by the Institute of Heart Math in California, in which one individual's cardiac signal was registered in another's cardiac recording when the people were sitting quietly opposite one another. Yet other studies show that distance doesn't make a difference. Intention, not prior involvement, is enough to create connection through the universal field.

THE INTERCHANGEABILITY OF ENERGY

Because the two types of energies, subtle and physical, are often the same at one level, just occupying different ends of a continuum, they are interchangeable. You can work physically to produce subtle changes. The opposite is also true. The transfer of energy goes both ways—from subtle to physical and physical to subtle.

For example, on the physical-to-subtle spectrum, a traditional Chinese medicine (TCM) practitioner will give someone with a skin rash a series of acupuncture treatments to support the free-flowing movement of chi (life-force energy) along the blocked energy channel that's giving rise to the rash. What is physical (the rash) begins to transfer out of the body when the subtle energy starts to flow, and pretty soon the skin condition is gone.

On the subtle-to-physical level, someone dealing with extreme insomnia might choose to use the Emotional Freedom Techniques (EFT), which involves tapping on key points of the body while verbalizing statements and affirmations. The ability to sleep is restored by this subtle energy practice that alters the energy causing the negative disruptions and disturbances in brain chemistry, restoring the flow of energy facilitating healthy sleep patterns.

All techniques in this book underscore the truth that subtle energy can transform to physical and vice versa.

SENSING SUBTLE ENERGY: MAKING WHAT IS REAL (BUT INVISIBLE) MORE REAL

When we seek to heal ourselves or another, the steering wheel for creating positive outcomes is *intention*. It is intention that will link you with a known or unknown person to provide healing, intention that will help you uncover your own wounded aspects, and intention that will determine the mix of subtle and physical energetic effects in your work.

The following exercises are intended to assist you in recognizing your own and others' energetic fields and work with and in them. Although these are preparatory exercises, they can be used during a healing session for yourself or another.

PALM-TO-PALM: A PARTNERED EXERCISE

Find a partner who is willing to take three to five minutes to help you feel and sense the flow of subtle energy through the hands.

Step 1: Palm-to-palm. Standing up and facing each other, both partners hold up your hands, palms forward, and bring them together, so the palms of your hands are touching. Send energy to each other through your right hands, and receive energy from each other with your left hands. Take approximately thirty seconds to send and receive energy and sense what you feel.

Step 2: One foot apart. Back up so you are about one foot apart. Hold your hands in the same position, toward each other's palms, but do not touch. Taking another thirty seconds to send and receive energy, sense what you feel at this distance.

Step 3: Six feet apart. Back up so you are six feet apart. With your palms still turned directly toward one another, send and receive energy for thirty more seconds, sensing the flow and exchange of energy at this distance.

(Note: At the one-foot and six-foot distances, you are experiencing quantum entanglement in action. Our fields expand, and the sending and receiving of energy isn't contingent upon physically touching someone.)

Step 4: Switching the circuitry. Now start over, but this time send energy with your left hand and receive with your right. See if you get the same or different results. On average, 80 to 90 percent of people send with their right and receive with their left, and about 10 percent do it the other way.

Step 5: Talk about your experience. Did you feel or sense differences at the various distances? If so, what? How did you feel when sending energy? How did you feel when receiving energy? How did you feel when you reversed the flow? Was this reversal more challenging, easier, or comparable? Overall, what did this exercise teach you about energy?

THE LIGHT IN YOUR HANDS: A SOLO EXERCISE

This solo exercise is a simple yet potent way to feel the subtle energy within and around your own body. It is also a method for bringing the healing, balancing, and energizing qualities of color into your body.

Step 1: The energy in your hands. Rub the palms of your hands together for ten seconds, like you're vigorously scrubbing them. Then hold your hands in a vertical position about one inch apart, palms facing each other, but not touching, and feel the energy you have created between your two hands.

Step 2: Flowing red energy. With this energy now flowing, imagine that you are bringing red energy through the back of your heart, into your chest, down your arms, and through your hands. Do you feel a marked difference between your hands?

Step 3: Flowing blue energy. Imagine blue energy streaming in through the back of your heart, streaming into your chest and arms, and through your hands. What sensations do you experience in your hands with this blue energy? Do you experience anything markedly different in your hands with blue versus red? Do you experience sensation anywhere else in your body? (Know that you can practice with any other color, in addition to red and blue.)

Step 4: Making an energy ball. Now return to a neutral zone, dissipating your colored energies. Pat your hands together as if you are gathering energy and make an energy ball (like a snowball of light). Mindfully create this energy ball, seeing how far you can spread your hands before you can no longer sense the energy.

Step 5: Noting your solo experience. What did you experience with each step of this exercise? You may find it helpful to jot down your thoughts in a journal. You can also experiment with doing this exercise at various times of the day and in different physical locations if you want to take the exploration to another level.

YOUR SPIRITUAL FLAME: A SOLO EXERCISE

This simple solo exercise is a relaxing, soothing, and uplifting way to experience the interconnectivity between your heart and your auric field, the part of your biofield that extends out from around your whole physical body. In some systems, this auric field is said to be composed of seven layers; my own preference is to work with a twelve-layer auric field, in which each layer is associated with the chakra that shares its same numerical label. This exercise also offers a way to *see* your energy field with your eyes and can be used for any self-healing endeavor.

1. You want to be as relaxed as possible, so you might want to sit in a comfortable chair or lie on your bed. Find a private place with low or soft lights—a candle in the corner, light seeping under your door, or the moon or streetlights shining through your bedroom window will suffice. As your eyes become accustomed to the relative dark, hold out your hands and gaze at them. Your eyes should be glazed; you might want to actually peer just beyond your hands and keep your hands in your peripheral vision.

2. Now move your fingertips so both hands are touching, finger to finger. Breathe deeply, sensing the spiritual flame inside your heart. Consciously invite this flame to emanate from your heart, down your arms, through your hands, and into your fingertips.

3. After you can feel the exchange of this spirit flame between your fingertips, examine the outside rim of both hands. You might see a white, hazy, rather dim corona of light.

4. Now move your fingertips slightly apart and gaze at the electrical charge that continues to connect them. If you want, consciously send this energetic

electricity between your fingertips and then move it over your skin, up and down your fingers, and over your hands. What happens? Can you perceive a shift in the hazy white you previously perceived?

5. You can play with this energy as long as you desire. When you are done, gently release your fingers from their position and draw the energy back into your heart. Breathe deeply and return to everyday consciousness.

2

FIELDS OF HEALING
THE ENERGY AROUND YOU

> [T]he Force is what gives a Jedi
> his power. It's an energy field
> created by all living things.
> It surrounds us, penetrates us.
> It binds the galaxy together.
>
> STAR WARS

Each one of us, along with the world we inhabit, is made up of both measurable and subtle energy fields that create and sustain life. Whether they're obvious to or hidden from our senses, all fields interact to create beneficial and harmful effects on living organisms.

The primary differences between physical and subtle fields are often simply the speed of the information and vibration involved. At some extraordinary level, both slow and fast fields, or both sensory and subtle, can be perceived as the same fields—one flowing into another, one creating and sustaining the other. Within the division of material and subtle energy lies yet another subdivision: that of form versus thought. Certain fields are managed by pure form, while others are managed by our thoughts, and yet others by our physical heart. At some level, however, everything affects everything. For instance, our heart affects our thoughts, and our thoughts affect our heart. In order to work with fields to ensure health and happiness, we must distinguish the functions of our various fields.

PHYSICAL AND SUBTLE FIELDS: THE DISTINCTION BETWEEN VERITABLE AND PUTATIVE FIELDS

There are many different kinds of fields, each of which fall into one of two categories: *veritable*, which can be measured, and *putative*, which cannot be measured.

The veritable, or measurable, energy fields are physical in nature and include sound and electromagnetic forces, such as visible light, magnetism, monochromatic radiation, and rays from the electromagnetic spectrum. Our body produces or is affected by all these energies.

Putative energy fields are also called *biofields* or *subtle fields*. Although not separate from mechanical or measurable fields, they occupy a space and run at frequencies that cannot be perceived except through their effects. They are connected to the body by energy channels known as the meridians and the nadis and energy bodies known as the chakras, all of which are able to convert or transfer the fast-moving frequencies (often referred to as chi and prana) into the slower and mechanical, or veritable, fields and forces (electricity, magnetism, and sound, among others). These energy channels and bodies (described in greater detail in chapters 3 and 4) act like antennae, receiving and sending information via the energy fields and also transforming this information so it can be used by the body.

The human body is affected by and creates both types of energy fields—measurable and subtle. The heart, for example, serves as the electrical center of the human body. Its electrical activity shapes the formation of the biofields that surround the body because it emits thousands of times more electricity and magnetism than do the other organs.

Human and personal biofields also interconnect with greater fields that work in two directions:

- Receiving and drawing energy from us
- Providing energy to us

The amazing fact that both we and the world are composed of fields is an invitation to see ourselves as intimately interconnected with and part of the greater world, rather than as self-contained and self-sustaining.

FROM FIELDS TO WAVES TO ATOMS: A QUANTUM TRAJECTORY

To establish a useful knowledge base for understanding the subtle fields, it is important to understand the veritable (measurable) fields, along with the electromagnetic and sound fields that generate and sustain them. (For an in-depth study of each, I recommend referencing *The Subtle Body*, chapters 18 through 27.)

LIFE-SUSTAINING FIELDS

The chief field that generates and perpetuates life is the electromagnetic spectrum, usually perceived as light. Each part of the electromagnetic spectrum

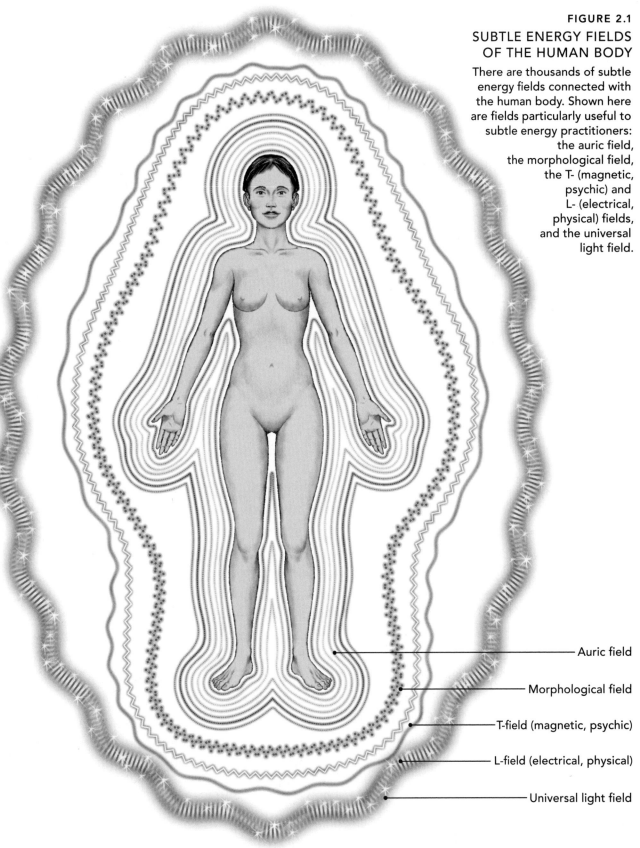

FIGURE 2.1

SUBTLE ENERGY FIELDS
OF THE HUMAN BODY

There are thousands of subtle
energy fields connected with
the human body. Shown here
are fields particularly useful to
subtle energy practitioners:
the auric field,
the morphological field,
the T- (magnetic,
psychic) and
L- (electrical,
physical) fields,
and the universal
light field.

Auric field

Morphological field

T-field (magnetic, psychic)

L-field (electrical, physical)

Universal light field

manifests as radiation that vibrates at a specific rate and therefore is called electromagnetic radiation. Our bodies require a specific amount of each part of this spectrum for optimal physical, emotional, and mental health. We can become ill or imbalanced if we're exposed to too much or too little of any particular part from the spectrum. The other category of life-sustaining fields is sound fields, also called sound or sonic waves.

WAVES

Both the electromagnetic spectrum and sound fields include light waves and mechanical waves.

Light waves. Electromagnetic radiation is described as a stream of photons, wave particles that are the basis of light. These are massless particles that travel at the speed of light. Each contains a bundle of energy and, therefore, information. (Energy *is* information.) The only difference between the types of electromagnetic radiation is the amount of energy found in the photons. Radio waves have photons with the lowest measurable energies, while gamma rays have the most energy. It is important to understand this flow of photons because photons actually compose the physical body, creating a gigantic field referred to as the Field of Light.

The electromagnetic spectrum is understood in terms of low and high energy, wavelength, and frequency. The terms *low energy* and *high energy* simply describe the information or energy of the photons. This energy is measured in electron volts. Wavelength is a way to measure the distance between two points on a wave. Frequency is the number of times that waves cycle per unit of time.

The basic premise of physical electromagnetism is this: electricity generates magnetism. Most classical understandings of electromagnetism depend on the fact that when electricity or charged electrons flow in a current, they create a magnetic field. These forces together compose electromagnetism.

Mechanical waves. Sound waves are considered mechanical waves. They are an important set of waves that both affect us as human beings and emanate from us. They are defined as disturbances that transport energy through a medium via the mechanism of particle interaction—meaning that sound waves are generated by some sort of interaction. In other words, they cannot move unless they are moved. Sound waves run at specific vibrations and penetrate all of existence. Our beating hearts create sound, as do the oceans and the planets in the sky. We can hear some of these sounds and not others, but that does not mean that the inaudible sounds do not affect us. These and other mechanical waves affect us either positively or negatively.

ATOMS

All matter, including the human cell, is created from atoms. Atoms are composed of protons and neutrons, which create the weight within an atom; electrons, which carry charge; and positrons, which represent the anti-electrons and link the atom with its anti-self. Each of these atomic units moves at its own speed and, when combined with other units, creates a certain oscillation or vibration for the atom—and that is what we know as *a field*. In other words, motion produces pressure, and this pressure creates waves that move in a non-ending flow in all directions.

As a practitioner of subtle energy medicine, when you work with the fields generated by a group of atoms (or even a single atom), you can potentially determine the health or the needs of those atomic structures, thus promoting healing.

ENERGY FIELDS OF THE EARTH

Although our primary focus in this chapter is on the energy fields of the human being, an informed subtle energy practitioner will have a comprehensive understanding of the various earth fields, which impact every area of our lives, including our health.

The earth is surrounded by a great magnetic field. This field is generated by the motions of molten metals in the earth's core, but is also affected by radiation that flows from the sun and other sources in the solar system. The resulting magnetosphere extends thousands of miles into space.

We are electromagnetic beings and, as such, are energetically linked within and by this field. Hundreds of clinical studies suggest that the magnetosphere, as well as other natural energies, affects our health, positively or negatively. For instance, several studies, including one based on thirteen years of research in South Africa, suggest a link between geomagnetic storms, caused by large solar flares, and clinical depression. Yet other studies reveal a connection between these storms, which increase radiation in the magnetosphere, and higher suicide rates.[1] Erratic electromagnetic earth energies can potentially cause cancer, heart problems, mental imbalance, insomnia, attention deficit hyperactivity disorder (ADHD), autoimmune deficiencies, and more.[2] Such research has led to new healthcare treatments—including those that use magnets, minerals, oxygen therapy, electricity, and even dietary changes—to establish balance in human energy bodies unbalanced by earth fields.

VERITABLE (MEASURABLE) EARTH FIELDS

Following is a brief overview of the veritable, or measurable, earth fields, including electromagnetic fields and others called *bioenergetically active fields*, or fields that create natural signals that powerfully affect bioenergetic (biological and energetic) beings, such as humans.

Sometimes known as geopathic fields, the fields or energies within the earth's main electrogmagnetic field, or magnetosphere, include:

- Radio waves
- Microwaves
- Infrared radiation
- Visible light
- Ultraviolet radiation
- X-rays
- Gamma rays
- T-rays (terahertz radiation)

The earth's bioenergetically active fields are:

Schumann waves, a basic waveform created by the ionosphere surrounding the earth. These waves vibrate to the primary harmonic of 7.83 hertzian, the same frequency present in the main control centers of the human brain. This frequency also correlates to the high-theta brain wave, which healers such as William Bengston, PhD, author of *The Energy Cure,* suggest opens us into the brain state necessary to perform energy healing.[3]

Geomagnetic waves, or vibrations emanating from the sixty-four trace elements in the earth's crust that influence the earth's magnetic field. The same elements exist in the red blood cells of humans. Some scientists believe that similarity is part of the reason that geomagnetic forces affect humans.

Solar waves, or wavelengths produced by the sun, including acoustic or sound waves, electromagnetic radiation, and gravity waves. Many studies show that we are affected by this solar output.

Sound waves, which are scientifically defined as vibrations that pass through an object or a material. The waves are actually created when the sound hits a barrier and the collision creates a vibration. We hear sounds when the sound hits an object and the surrounding air vibrates. In turn, the vibrating air causes our eardrum (or other parts of our body) to vibrate, and the brain interprets these vibrations as sound. We are highly affected by sound waves, adversely and beneficially. (See chapter 21.)

Serving as the bridge between the earth's veritable and subtle fields are *scalar waves.* Followers of researcher Nikola Tesla assert that these longitudinal waves go faster than the speed of light, thus providing the mechanism for instant communication.

SUBTLE EARTH FIELDS

The earth's subtle fields are:

Ley lines, electromagnetic energy lines on or in the earth. Some people believe these lines are human-made, created by human-built stone formations that result in stored power. Other people believe ley lines are innate tracks of energy in the earth; they are most intense at the places they intersect, so people naturally build at these points to take advantage of the earth's power.

The Hartmann grid, a network of naturally occurring charged lines in the earth that run north to south at a distance about two meters apart and east to west about two and one-half meters apart. They can send energy upward as high as 600 feet. Alternate lines are typically positively and negatively charged, and energetic difficulties arise at the intersections. Between these geometric lines are neutral zones.

The Benker Cubical System, comprising energy lines spaced about ten meters apart, so that they look like square blocks stacked on top of each other. They are magnetically aligned north to south and east to west. These walls of energy are polarized alternatively. Intersections are considered harmful to the human immune system.

The Curry grid, which is based on the idea that the earth is covered with a mystic force field. The grid is composed of lines of energy that crisscross at regular distances. The intersections produce spots of radiation that can be either beneficial or harmful and that can be detected by dowsing or divining. The lines are approximately three meters apart, diagonal to the poles, and run east to west.

Black lines, or naturally generated earth energies that do not form a gridlike network and are most likely localized collections of deadly energies. They can be curved or straight. Also called black streams, they are sometimes considered to be caused by subterranean running water and geological fault lines. Their power is intensified during solar storms and lightning strikes, as well as by other factors. Their toxic and poisonous effect can spread through steel construction, such as girders, and they can even flow upward into the upper levels of a building.

THE VIVAXIS: CONNECTING HUMAN BEINGS TO THE EARTH

Between the human energy fields and the earth's energy fields is a special energetic link called the Vivaxis. In her book *The Vivaxis Connection*, Judy Jacka describes it as a point or a sphere of energy that links a person with their birthplace (the place on earth where the person's mother spent the last few weeks of her pregnancy). No matter how far away the person may move from this place, the Vivaxis continues to link them to this place. Formed from magnetic waves, the Vivaxis operates like an invisible, two-way umbilical cord, connecting us to the earth throughout our bodies. Planetary and earth energies influence our bodies through the Vivaxis, even determining the flow of prana through the nadis.[4] (For more information, including a technique for working with the Vivaxis, see chapter 13.)

ENERGY FIELDS OF THE HUMAN BODY

Just as the earth has both measurable and subtle fields, so do you and I. In this section, you will learn about the subtle human fields that are most applicable to the practitioner of subtle energy medicine.

First, it is important to know that these fields, while seemingly surrounding the human body, also *interpenetrate* it. Fields do not stop at the skin. They are energies that move through all the body's mediums—including the skin and bodily tissue. In all likelihood, these subtle fields determine the nature and health of our entire being. They interact not only with our chakras and meridians, but like all veritable and subtle earth fields, they also respond to everything inside and outside of us, often passing energy from our so-called inside to our outside, and vice versa. In fact, science is confirming that illness and healing can be detected in the subtle fields before they manifest in the physical body.

Every cell in the body and every thought generates a field. Every energy body, meridian, and chakra pulses its own field.

THE UNIVERSAL LIGHT FIELD

The *universal light field*, also called a zero-point field, consists of photons or units of light that regulate every living thing. Our DNA is made of light, and we are surrounded by a field of light, forming a microcosm and macrocosm that dance together. Essentially, we are "frozen light," or biophoton machines. Through the zero-point field, we are interconnected in a nonlocal reality that permeates the cosmos. A nonlocal reality is one that is unmediated, unmitigated, and immediate. This means that events can occur through unknown forces, that the strength of an event is not dependent upon the proximity of the forces, and that changes can occur instantly, despite distance between the force, the event, and us. Many physicists have concluded that reality is indeed nonlocal in nature, as two particles, once in contact, can be separated and yet interact even at great distances.

L-FIELDS AND T-FIELDS

L-fields are life fields, subtle physical fields that are measured electrically. T-fields are thought fields. Each provides a blueprint and design for a different side of reality. They represent the dualistic nature of life as we know it—the yin and yang of Oriental philosophy, the Shakti and Brahma of the Hindu religion. They also represent electrical and magnetic frequencies, the two sides of matter that combine to create the electromagnetic radiation that constantly bathes and nurtures us.

MORPHOGENETIC FIELDS

In biology, a *morphogenetic field* is a subtle field connecting a group of cells that creates specific body structures or organs. For example, a cardiac field becomes heart tissue. Morphogenetic fields (also known as morphological fields) allow an exchange between like-minded species and transfer information from one generation to another. These penetrate the aura as well as the electrical system of the body.

THE ETHERIC FIELDS

Because the word *etheric* is often used as a substitute for the terms *subtle* or *auric*, a slightly expanded description is in order. There are actually independent etheric fields around every vibrating unit of life, from a cell to a plant to a person.

The term *etheric* is a derivative of the word *ether*, which has been considered a medium that permeates space, transmitting transverse waves of energy. Transverse waves are those that pass through only materials in which the particles are closely connected. (Water waves and light waves are examples of transverse waves.)

When associated with the entirety of the auric field, the etheric field surrounds the whole body and serves as a blueprint for the physical human body.

As a separate energy body, the etheric body links the physical body with other subtle bodies and, thus, serves as a matrix for physical growth. Barbara Ann Brennan, the acclaimed teacher and contemporary expert on the aura, suggests that the etheric body exists before the cells grow. Other research asserts that the same is true of the auric field, indicating that it permeates every particle of the physical body and acts as a matrix for it. Kim Bong Han, PhD, whose research is outlined in *The Subtle Body*, links the etheric body and the meridians, suggesting that the meridians are an interface between the etheric body and the physical body. The etheric body creates the meridians, which in turn form the physical body. There is also an etheric field for the soul.

Each of our etheric fields regulates various mental, emotional, spiritual, or physical functions. The following list of independent etheric fields is based on the work of Barbara Ann Brennan and other researchers and clinicians. While these are separate etheric fields, they all affect the human body.

Physical field: Lowest in frequency. Regulates the human body. Sometimes called the gross field.

Emotional field: Regulates the human emotional state.

Mental field: Processes ideas, thoughts, and beliefs.

GEOPATHIC STRESS

GEOPATHIC STRESS REFERS to the harmful effects of natural and artificial fields and of radiation from veritable and subtle fields. The existence of geopathic stress is supported by scientific research, which has validated that constant or extreme exposure to geopathic stressors can result in mild to severe consequences in living beings exposed to them.

Geopathic stress can be the cause of mild to severe maladies, including:

- Body aches and pains
- Irritability and anxiety
- Chronic fatigue
- Insomnia
- Cardiovascular disorders
- Infertility and miscarriage
- Learning challenges
- Behavior problems in children
- Cancer
- Autoimmune disorders

There are two types of measurable field stressors, or sources of natural field pollution. The first is electromagnetic radiation; the others are the earth and sky. On earth, geopathic stress occurs primarily at the crossing points of the earth's natural energy lines, but it also occurs because of radiation caused by subterranean running water, certain mineral concentrations, underground cavities, and fault lines. These are natural energies, but they are not beneficial to people or living beings over long periods of time. There are also fields of energy emanating from space, and these, too, can disturb our body's electromagnetic system.

As human beings, we can be affected by the following types of natural field pollution:

Electromagnetic spectrum pollution, or overexposure to static electric fields, magnetic fields, extremely low frequency (ELF) radiation, radio frequencies, visible light, ultraviolet light, gamma rays, infrared light, microwaves, and x-rays;

Astral field: A nexus between the physical and spiritual realms. Free of time and space.

Etheric template: Exists only on the spiritual plane and holds the highest ideals for existence.

Celestial field: Accesses universal energies and serves as a template for the etheric fields.

Causal field: Also called the ketheric field. Enables access to divine wisdom.

THE AURIC FIELD

The human energy field is primarily composed of the aura, a set of energy bands that graduate in frequency and color as they move outward from the body. Each

---

Pollution from natural physical fields, or overexposure to solar stress, geomagnetic fields, geopathic stress, and the Vivaxis;

Pollution from natural subtle fields, or overexposure to black lines and the lines of the Hartmann grid, the Benker Cubical System, and the Curry grid.

What has led to our current level of geopathic stress? Why are we seeing so many illnesses as a result of field stress? There are two reasons that stand out.

A decrease in the magnetic field. First, the earth's natural magnetic field has decreased in potency over time. About 4,000 years ago, it generated between two and three gauss, but now has an intensity of about only one-half gauss, signifying a reduction of nearly 80 percent. On a microscopic level, the decline in the earth's magnetic field reduces the level of charge in subatomic particles, lessening the overall charge of atoms. Living bodies depend upon charged atoms and molecules to be superconductive, or to support the proper flow of nutrients and messages along the nervous system and through the fluid systems of the body. Not only does the human primary nervous system, including the brain and central nervous system, require this ionic balancing, but so does the secondary nervous system, which likely interacts with the meridians and nadis. Insufficient magnetic input, therefore, adversely affects a human's subtle bodies and fields.

Artificial radiation. Second, artificially produced radiation can cause considerable harm to living organisms, and we are bombarding the planet with a plethora of human-generated electrical and magnetic fields, as well as oceanic amounts of radio waves, microwaves, and other radiations.

of these auric fields opens to different energy planes and energy bodies and also partners with a chakra, thus enabling an exchange of information between the worlds outside and inside of the body.

Some esoteric specialists believe there are seven layers to the aura; others assert there are eight or nine. I work with a twelve-chakra and twelve-auric-layer system that will frequently be featured throughout this book.

Scientists have been investigating and confirming the existence of the aura, the field that surrounds our entire body, for over a hundred years, adding to the knowledge our ancestors already possessed. The aura has been known by many names in many cultures. Christian artists depicted Jesus and other figures as surrounded by coronas of light. The Vedic scriptures and the teachings of the Rosicrucians, Tibetan and Indian Buddhists, and many Native American tribes describe the field in detail. Even Pythagoras discussed the field, which the Greeks perceived as a luminous body.

So what *is* the auric field? Scientists such as James Oschman, author of *Energy Medicine*, consider it to be an unbounded biomagnetic field that surrounds the body. "Unbounded" means that our auric field, composed of up to twelve layers, extends outward from the physical body indefinitely.

There are indications that the auric field is actually made of both electromagnetic radiation (specifically magnetism) and an antimatter that allows a shift of energy between this world and others. This antimatter is what makes healing through the use of intention possible. When a practitioner transmits healing energy based on intention, whether through hands-on or distance healing, that energy is delivered, like an instant message sent through the Internet, to another individual's energy field.

The next two chapters will further connect the dots between the three primary elements of the subtle body—the fields, the meridians, and the chakras. Additionally, the chapters in part 3 offer a wealth of subtle energy tools and techniques for maintaining or restoring balance and health to the fields. Of special note are the following chapters: chapters 12 and 13 (hands-on and distance-healing modalities), chapter 23 (sacred geometry, shapes, symbols, and numbers), and chapters 21 and 22 (sound and color healing), all of which contain resources that are highly effective for working with the human subtle energy fields.

3

CHANNELS OF HEALING
MERIDIAN MAGIC

Beyond my body
my veins are invisible.

ANTONIO PORCHIA
Voices

Acupuncture, acupressure, Chinese herbs, qigong, tai chi, tui na massage—as a healing practitioner, you may be well versed in the use of some of these methods and tools or are perhaps eager to begin learning about them. As cornerstones of traditional Chinese medicine, one of the oldest forms of medicine, all of these treatment modalities and practices have something in common: each is a meridian-based therapy that assists in the delivery of chi, the subtle energy required for life.

No matter what type of subtle energy modality you specialize in, knowledge of the meridians—what they are, what they do, and how to work with them—will add to the depth and effectiveness of your work. In other words, you don't have to be an acupuncturist to benefit from understanding the meridians and the principles that underlie them.

MERIDIAN THERAPY: A WHOLE-BEING APPROACH

Meridians are the channels of energy that provide structure for the body as an energetic system. They are the channels that provide nourishment to the subtle energy body in the form of *chi,* one of the Chinese terms for life energy. Sometimes they are described as energy highways that interconnect the physical universe outside of us with the living tissue inside of us.

Over five thousand years ago, the discovery of these subtle energy channels by the Chinese gave rise to a complex and highly evolved medical system, based less on anatomy than on holism, the perception that a person is a whole being, not a collection of parts. The basic tenet of meridian therapy is that you must treat the root cause of a presenting problem—body, mind, spirit, and emotions—rather than only the symptoms. The ancient Chinese pictured a person as a circle rather than an assemblage of units. But this circle does not encompass only the individual. Each person—each living organism—is connected to, and therefore interconnected by, a universal matrix of energy. What is "in here" is essentially connected to everything "out there."

Traditional meridian therapy draws upon *the five-phase theory* (sometimes called the *five-elements theory*)—a complex and cumulative explanation of meridian-based therapies. In contrast to the ideas behind allopathic medicine, the five-phase theory describes the relationship between all things, rather than outlining independent factors. In addition to expressing that everything reduces to five basic elements, it asserts four major ideas:

- Yin and yang (or polar opposites)
- The internal and external sources of disease
- The cyclical order of life (revealed in the cycles of the seasons)
- The existence of channels of energy that distribute the chi—the meridians

In essence, the five-phase theory explains the self as an energy being.

Having outgrown the perception of being an esoteric healing system or simple folk medicine, traditional Chinese medicine and meridian-based systems are now becoming integrated into Western healthcare systems. Extensive research has verified that the meridians are transporters of chemical, electrical, and etheric energies. Just as the meridians are energetic in nature, so are they physical in nature and in influence. Just as we are physical, so are we energetic.

In that sense, the traditional Chinese medicine (TCM) approach to healing exemplifies subtle energy medicine. It is based upon an understanding that illness is an energetic disturbance or imbalance and that healing is a process of restoring energetic balance. While fully acknowledging the most obvious physical symptoms, it also looks past them to discover the disharmony in the subtle channels that may precede illness.

In addition to the comprehensive body of information pertaining to the channels and five-phase theory contained in *The Subtle Body* encyclopedia, there is no shortage of in-depth information pertaining to this brilliant system of healing. The rest of this chapter is designed to be a quick-reference guide; the basic information it contains is based on my experience as someone who has extensively studied and researched these topics and as a practitioner who integrates the principles into my own work. I've taken care to include exercises and techniques that are powerful yet easy to administer, such as the use of certain acupressure points, qigong techniques, and the Emotional Freedom Techniques (EFT). I've abstained from sharing processes that need to be delivered by a licensed acupuncturist, such as needling, or the use of needles in acupoints, and cupping, or the use of special cups to clear chi blockages. Information such as the "Three Treasures" included in this chapter is referenced in relation to healing work as well. Whether you are looking up what bodily functions the Bladder meridian governs, which organs are most impacted by worry and sadness, which disharmonies are related to the Liver meridian, or what time of day the Heart meridian is most active (11 a.m. to 1 p.m., by the way), this chapter will be a highly useful reference. I have found that even if a subtle energy practitioner does not employ meridian-based therapies for self or other healing, it is imperative to understand the basic concepts, including the science verifying the existence of the meridians. Being lucid in these ideas can help you make use of all available alternative therapies yourself and understand the types of meridian therapies a client might be using.

THE MAJOR MERIDIANS AND VESSELS

There are twelve major meridians and several secondary ones, which are sometimes referred to as vessels. Here we will focus on the twelve major meridians and the two most important vessels.

There are several different abbreviation systems that represent the meridians in "shorthand." This is one commonly used system:

Lung (LU)

Large Intestine (LI)

Stomach (ST)

Spleen (SP)

Heart (HE)

Small Intestine (SI)

Bladder (BL)

Kidney (KI)

Pericardium (PC)

Triple Warmer or Burner (TB)

Gallbladder (GB)

Liver (LR)

Conception Vessel (CV) or Ren Mai

Governor Vessel (GV) or Du Mai

Each of the major meridians governs certain functions of the body. Disharmony, or the disruption of the flow of energy through a particular meridian, results in particular symptoms.

Lung meridian. The Lung meridian regulates chi throughout the body, as well as regulating breathing and many water channels, such as the Kidney and

Bladder meridians, which control the distribution of fluids in the body. Symptoms of disharmony include distension of or a full sensation in the chest, asthma, allergies, coughing, panting, belching, restlessness, cold limbs and hot palms, shortness of breath, skin issues, and overall fatigue.

Large Intestine meridian. The Large Intestine meridian rules elimination and communicates with the lungs to regulate the transportation functions of the body. For instance, it carries waste out of the body and absorbs water before the waste leaves. Problems with this meridian often underlie diseases that affect the head, face, and throat. Disharmony is indicated by toothaches; runny noses and nosebleeds; swelling of the neck; yellow eyes; dry mouth and excessive thirst; a sore throat; pain in the shoulders, arms, and index fingers; as well as intestinal cramping, diarrhea, constipation, and dysentery.

Stomach meridian. The Stomach meridian works closely with the Spleen meridian to energetically support the body's digestion and absorption functions. Together, the two meridians are called *the acquired foundation*, in that they lay the foundation of digestive health for the body. The Stomach meridian assures that the chi, which can be energetically packaged as nutrients, thoughts, or emotions, descends or is passed into the internal system of the body so it can be utilized. If it ascends instead of descends, the result can include nausea and vomiting. Diseases involving the Stomach meridian typically produce gastric disturbances, toothaches, and mental issues (such as obsessively "going over" the same issues), as well as problems that appear on or near the path of the meridian (such as on the front of the shin for the Stomach meridian and other localities) as shown in figures 3.1 and 3.2. Irregularities in this meridian can appear as stomachaches, mouth sores, digestive disturbances, fluid in the abdomen, hunger, nausea, vomiting, thirst, mouth distortion, edema, neck swelling, a sore throat, shuddering, yawning, and a gray forehead. Mental dysfunctions include antisocial and phobic behavior.

Spleen meridian. The spleen is a vital immune organ and essential for transforming food into chi and blood. It does this by changing the essence of food, which is subtle as well as physical, and also working with the Stomach meridian to eventually incorporate the nutrients and chi of food into the blood. It is also considered to house thoughts and to govern the quality of thought available to the mind. Symptoms of disharmony include a distended abdomen, loss of appetite, hepatitis, bleeding disorders, menstrual disorders, loose stools, diarrhea, flatulence, anorexia, stiffness, swollen or stiff knees or thighs, and pain at the root of the tongue.

Heart meridian. The heart governs the blood and the pulse, as well as the mind and spirit. As might be expected, problems with the Heart meridian usually result in heart problems. Disharmony is indicated by a dry throat, heart pain and palpitations, and thirst. Other symptoms include pain in the chest or along the inner side of the forearm, heat in the palms, yellow eyes, insomnia, and pain or cold along the meridian pathway.

Small Intestine meridian. The Small Intestine meridian separates the pure from the impure, including pure and impure foods, fluids, thoughts, and beliefs. Problems in the Small Intestine meridian usually create diseases of the neck, ears, eyes, throat, head, and small intestine, as well as certain mental illnesses. Symptoms of disharmony can include fevers; sore throats; a swollen chin or lower cheek; a stiff neck; a fixed head stance; hearing problems or deafness; yellow eyes; severe pain of the shoulder, lower jaw, upper arm, elbow, and forearm; and intestinal disorders, including irritable bowel syndrome.

Bladder meridian. The Bladder meridian is in charge of storing and eliminating fluid waste. It receives chi from the Kidney meridian and uses it to transform fluids for elimination. Dysfunction of the Bladder meridian leads to bladder problems and symptoms such as urinary disorders and incontinence. It can also lead to problems in the head, including headaches, protruding eyeballs, a runny nose, nasal congestion, neck tension, yellow eyes, tearing, and nosebleeds. Lower-body issues include pain along the spine, buttocks, and calf muscles, lumbar pain, unbendable hip joints, groin issues, and tight muscles around the knee and in the calves.

Kidney meridian. According to classical sources, kidneys "grasp the chi." They are the residence of yin and yang. They also rule the bones, teeth, and adrenal glands. Lack of energetic and physical nourishment results in problems such as swelling, diarrhea, and constipation. Other symptoms of disharmony in the Kidney meridian include backaches, ear problems, anorexia, restlessness, insomnia, weak vision, lack of energy, constant fear, dry tongue and hot mouth, spinal and thigh pain, immovable lower limbs, cold, drowsiness, and painful and hot soles of the feet.

Pericardium meridian. The pericardium is a bag that contains the heart, protecting it from foreign invasions, so it's fitting that the Pericardium meridian works closely with the Heart meridian. This meridian governs the blood and the mind (along with the Heart meridian), thus affecting blood and circulation, as well as personal relationships. Disharmony in the Pericardium meridian is caused by disharmony within heart and blood functions. The most common problems are chest, heart, and breast problems, and symptoms can include chest discomfort, tachycardia or other arrhythmias, swelling in the armpit, a red face, spasms of the elbow and arm, and mania. Note: The heart stores *shen*, spiritual energy or mental energy affecting the soul. Many mental or emotional problems relate to an imbalance in shen, so the Pericardium is an important meridian for any symptoms related to mental illness. The Pericardium protects the heart from disturbances, including overwhelming emotions, which can lead to physical and mental imbalances. Specific shen points, listed in classical TCM and acupuncture manuals, can be used to protect the heart from the excessive emotions that can flow in from the other meridians. (For more on shen, see "The Three Treasures" on page 43 of this chapter. See also "Acupressure to Create Calm: A Shen Pericardium Point" on page 41.)

Triple Warmer (Burner) meridian. The Triple Warmer is not represented by a physical organ. Rather, it is important because of its job, which is to circulate liquid energy throughout the organs. The Triple Warmer distributes a special chi called *source chi*, which is produced by the kidneys. It governs the relationship between all the various organs, allocating chi between them. As its name implies, the Triple Warmer comprises three parts:

> **The Upper Warmer or Burner,** which distributes chi from the diaphragm upward and is most commonly associated with lungs and heart (respiration);

> **The Middle Warmer or Burner,** which delivers chi to bodily areas between the diaphragm and navel and is associated with stomach, spleen, liver, and gallbladder (digestion and assimilation);

> **The Lower Warmer or Burner,** which transports chi below the navel and is associated with reproduction and elimination.

Problems with the Triple Warmer typically manifest as water retention, a stiff neck, and ailments with the ears, eyes, chest, and throat. Symptoms include those related to water imbalance, such as swelling, urinary incontinence and difficulties, and tinnitus (ringing in the ear).

Gallbladder meridian. The Gallbladder meridian runs the gallbladder, which makes and stores bile. On an energetic basis, this meridian governs decision-making. It is closely connected to the liver; therefore, disharmony with the Gallbladder meridian can be shown as liver issues, including bitterness in the mouth, jaundice, and nausea. Other symptoms include frequent sighing, headaches, pain in the jaw and outer corner of the eyes, swelling in the glands, mental illness, indecisiveness, fever, and pain along the meridian.

Liver meridian. To some Chinese practitioners, the liver is considered the "second heart" of the body. This meridian assures the flow of emotions, chi, and blood; controls the body's immune response, as well as its sinews (tendons, ligaments, and skeletal muscles); absorbs what is indigestible; and is associated with the eyes. Liver meridian issues most frequently appear as problems in the liver and genital systems. Symptoms can include dizziness, high blood pressure, hernias, a distended lower abdomen in women, nausea, watery stools with undigested food, allergies, incontinence, muscle spasms, the retention of urine, eye problems, and moodiness or anger.

Conception vessel (Ren Mai). The Conception vessel distributes chi to the major organs and maintains the proper balance of chi and blood within the body. The Conception vessel runs down the front of the body, starting just below the eyes. It circles around the mouth to the chest and abdomen before landing at the perineum. Problems with this vessel include uneasiness, hernias, and abdominal issues.

Governor vessel (Du Mai). Like the Conception vessel, the Governor vessel transports chi to the major organs and balances the chi and blood in the body. The Governor vessel starts at the perineum and travels to the coccyx before making its way to the back of the head. Flowing over the head, it then travels down the front of the face to stop at the canines in the upper jaw. Disharmony in this vessel can cause symptoms such as stiffness and scoliosis.

Figures 3.1 and 3.2 show the paths of all fourteen meridians through the body. For maps of the individual meridians and their major acupoints, see pages 187 to 201 of *The Subtle Body*.

ACUPOINTS

The acupoints are the entryways to the meridians. They are also called *acupuncture points* and *meridian points*. Four to five hundred acupoints have been identified in the human body. (The numbers vary according to the healing system being used.) Each of the points has a particular effect on the different channels and organs in the body. These points are described and pictured in numerous books on traditional Chinese medicine (though their names and purposes differ slightly from system to system). Please see chapter 12, "Hands-On Healing," for a description of the primary ten acupoints and key exercises and techniques that use them for healing and rebalancing.

HOW DO MERIDIANS AND ACUPOINTS FUNCTION?

Meridians are pathways for many different types of physical and subtle energies. While invisible to the naked eye, they are circuits of positive and negative energies, as well as bodily fluids. The energies within the circuits can be measured by various methods. Used in acupuncture, the acupoints display unique and

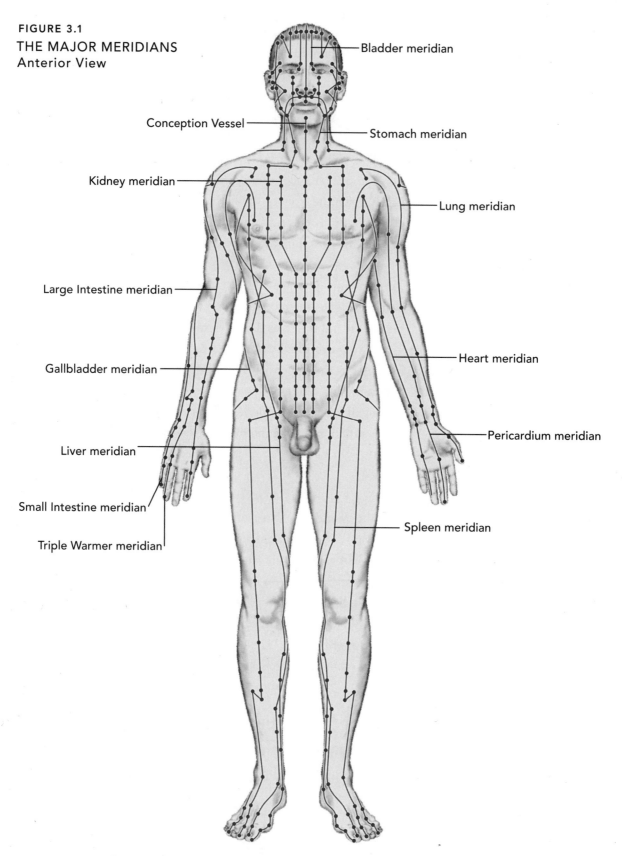

FIGURE 3.1
THE MAJOR MERIDIANS
Anterior View

Bladder meridian

Conception Vessel

Stomach meridian

Kidney meridian

Lung meridian

Large Intestine meridian

Heart meridian

Gallbladder meridian

Pericardium meridian

Liver meridian

Small Intestine meridian

Triple Warmer meridian

Spleen meridian

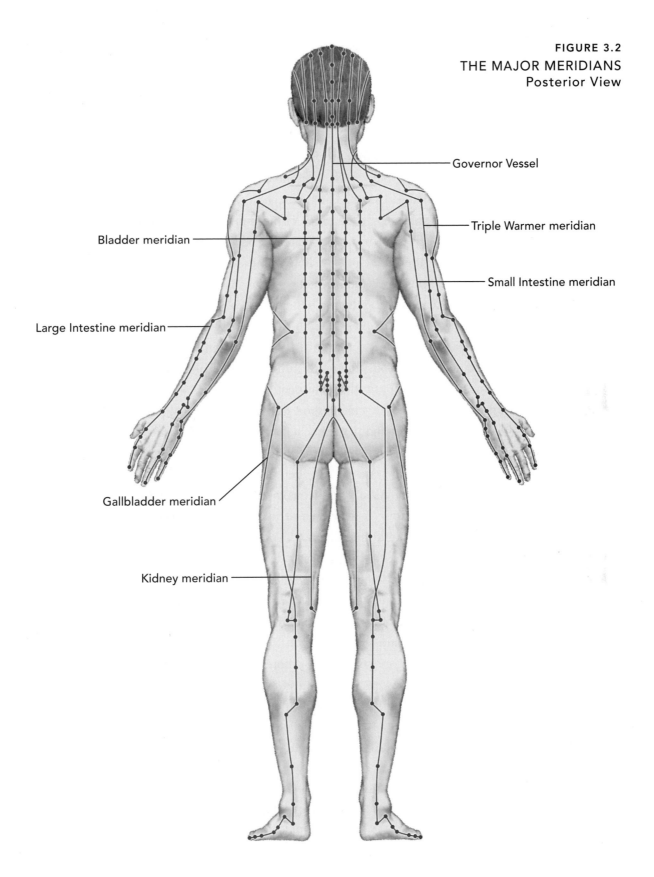

FIGURE 3.2

THE MAJOR MERIDIANS
Posterior View

Governor Vessel

Triple Warmer meridian

Small Intestine meridian

Bladder meridian

Large Intestine meridian

Gallbladder meridian

Kidney meridian

scientifically viable electrical characteristics that distinguish them from the surrounding skin. Electromagnetic in nature, these acupoints can be found by hand, through testing with microelectrical voltage meters, and through the use of applied kinesiology, or muscle testing, which tests the body's reactions to substances, situations, and ideas.

Scientific research supports five different but interrelated theories about how meridians and acupoints work to promote healing.

Biomechanical theory. The biomechanical explanation centers on research that seeks to validate the existence of the meridians. Studies that involve tracking the meridian system with radioactive tracers and identifying the location of acupoints on the motor nerves show that the meridians are part of the body's mechanical framework and interact with the anatomical system.

Bioelectromagnetic theory. Based upon the premise that the human body is an electrical-magnetic phenomenon, this theory focuses on the fact that the body is composed of electrical currents. Polarized electrically generated fields exist in and around the body, including around each of our cells, and are associated with a network of circuits that continually send minute amounts of direct current through the body. The cells responsible for this conduction, called *perineural cells,* are located around nerve fibers. The resulting current is highly influenced by external electromagnetic fields. Within this context, acupuncture points act like amplifiers of the current and the meridians, the conduction vessels for the electricity, or the chi. Working the acupoints smooths the flow of the bioelectricity in beneficial ways. A great deal of research explains how this physiological reality makes acupoint stimulation effective.

Standing wave theory. In 1986, two researchers, Fritz-Albert Popp and Changlin Zhang, teamed up to create a model called the *standing wave superposition hypothesis.* In short, they portrayed the overall meridian system as a holographic image of the body represented in the ears and the feet. This theory also sought to explain the interconnectivity of the acupoints through a process called *superposing,* in which two or more similar waves combine to find a third and more complex one. When these two waves are in rhythm, the resulting wave is more powerful and beneficial than when they are arrhythmic. According to the Zhang-Popp theory, the waves from acupuncture points and the meridians create these beneficial waves and improve our health.

Connective tissue theory. This theory is based on the existence of cytoskeletal structures in every cell in the body. These structures, in effect, form connective tissue. Nuclear magnetic resonance has shown that our muscles are organized in liquid-crystalline-like structures that change drastically when exposed to electromagnetic fields. This alteration occurs because connective tissue carries static electric charges and is influenced by pH, salt concentration, and the dielectric constant of the solvent composing the liquid crystal, such as the lipids of cellular membranes, DNA, and proteins, especially cytoskeletal proteins, such as those found in connective tissue. Many scientists now believe that the meridians lie within this liquid network, or that the meridians simply stimulate the network's responsiveness. In other words, this liquid network carries the electromagnetic responses elicited from acupuncture.

Ductal theory. Research by Professor Kim Bong Han suggests that the meridians are a series of ducts, or tubes, that carry chi. He discovered that the meridians are formed after the initial merging of the sperm and ova. They then develop and spread throughout the developing body in utero.

Secondary electrical system theory. An ever-increasing number of scientists are proposing that the meridian system is part of a secondary electrical system—one that might include, but is also different from, the established circulatory and central nervous systems.

Western science already acknowledges how electricity—and therefore information—flows through the neurons that comprise the central nervous system (the spine and the brain). Through his research, respected Swedish radiologist Björn Nordenström has discovered that electricity also "feeds" a second, separate but interrelated electrical system. This secondary system works between our

ACUPRESSURE TO CREATE CALM: A Shen Pericardium Point

SHEN IS MENTAL or spirit energy; there are shen points on every meridian. The sixth point of the Pericardium meridian, PC 6 or Nei Guan, is a perfect point to press to create calm when you feel disruptive emotions. This point calms the heart, settles the shen or emotions, and relieves pain. It alleviates stomach aches, nausea, vomiting, motion sickness, palpitations, chest constrictions, insomnia, irritability, hypertension, and mental disorders, as well as pain in the elbow and the arm.

To locate PC 6, put your index, middle, and ring fingers together on one hand. Now lay these fingers on the wrist on the inside of your opposite arm; position your ring finger directly over the crease between your hand and wrist, and your index finger will naturally be positioned across the two most prominent tendons in your wrist. PC 6 lies right between these tendons, right near your index finger. The point might feel tender.

Use the tip of your thumb to massage this point while supporting your wrist and lower arm with the fingers of the same hand. Move your thumb in a tiny circular motion for two to three minutes.

connective tissue and the cardiovascular system. The main idea is that electricity is created by the flow of blood within the arteries and the veins, turning our blood vessels into cables surrounded by electromagnetic fields. When cells are damaged, the flow of current to or from an injured area changes, creating electrical effects that stimulate repair. Basically, these fields form a "closed loop," or continuously circulating system of energy and electricity that interacts with our connective tissue.

Nordenström's model suggests that the electrical forces flowing in this secondary system are comparable to chi and that the negative and positive poles of the electrical energy are equivalent to yin and yang. The channels of the flow are quite possibly the meridians.

FIVE-PHASE THEORY

As mentioned, traditional Chinese medicine is based on the five-phase or five-element theory *(wu-hsing)*. The essence of the five-phase theory is the flow of vital life-force energy. Chi flows through the meridians in perfect balance, unless disturbed by internal or external forces that disrupt the elemental units of life.

Five-phase theory can be summarized by the following five statements:

- There are five elements in nature: earth, metal, water, wood, and fire.
- Each element is represented by a certain color.
- The human body is made of these natural, elemental materials.
- These elements move through the human body and its organs in a seasonal cycle.
- Proper treatment of the body involves working with the correct element and its cyclical timing.

The five elements represent energies that succeed each other in a continuous five-phase cycle. The Chinese did not emphasize the elements themselves, but the movement between them. Together these movements make up chi, the vital force.

Each element is associated with a particular bodily system as well as an internal organ. Each organ is either yin or yang. The organs and elements generate each other in a particular pattern.

wood	*feeds*	fire
fire	*creates*	earth
earth	*bears*	metal
metal	*collects*	water
water	*nourishes*	wood

Elements also govern or destroy each other. These degenerative actions are often called overcoming interactions, as they involve one element being overcome or changed by another.

wood	*parts*	earth
earth	*takes in*	water
water	*quenches*	fire
fire	*melts*	metal
metal	*chops*	wood

Understanding this cycle is the key to creating balance within the system. A practitioner diagnoses which elements might need to be generated or decreased and whether the balance of yin and yang is disrupted, and then figures treatment accordingly.

See chapter 14 on the power of qigong and tai chi, most versions of which incorporate the ideas behind the five-phase theory, and chapter 19 on the five-phase theory and food.

THE THREE TREASURES

The Three Treasures, sometimes called the Three Jewels, are keystones in traditional Chinese medicine. From the Taoist perspective, these Three Treasures are like three faces of the same essential substance, the force of life. The Three Treasures are:

Jing, the basic or nutritive physical essence as represented in sperm, among other substances
Chi, the life force connected with air, vapor, breath, and spirit
Shen, the spiritual essence linked with the soul and supernaturalism

Most often, jing is related to body energy, chi to mind energy, and shen to spiritual energy, or the type of mental energy affecting soul issues. These three energies cycle: jing serves as the foundation for life and procreation; chi animates the body's performance; and shen mirrors the state of the soul. One of the many ways that Taoists propose to blend these essential energies is to use physical chi to nourish our jing, or sexual or inherited energy. We then employ jing to enhance our chi, raising it to a higher or more refined level. At this point, we use this refined or more mental chi to build up our shen, our spiritual self. We now reunite our shen with the Tao or the All.

Several techniques in this book, including the exercise in this chapter, "Acupressure to Create Calm: A Shen Pericardium Point," involve working with shen.

Chi is addressed in several exercises, and both chi and shen are addressed in other sections, including "Food and Emotions in Traditional Chinese Medicine: The Five-Phase Approach to Soothing Heart and Mind" in chapter 19. When doing healing work, I often link the presenting problem or issue with one of the Three Treasures, then adapt my work to the appropriate depth. Here's my own cheat sheet to issues matching each of these energies.

Jing issues. Family patterns, inherited and genetic issues, raw sexual problems, growth, development, fertility issues. This is the densest of the three energies. Examine causal issues related to heritage; past-life reasons one might exhibit an inborn characteristic; and DNA-related concerns. For healing, also support the natural aging and maturation processes, as well as lifestyle habits, such as proper diet and sleep.

Chi issues. The focus if we are affected by issues related to movement and activity, our ability to truly "live life." Every phenomenon in the universe is a manifestation of chi, so look to tracking the path of the chi if energy is blocked, stagnant, or stuck. Will need to follow the flow of energy in the body to search for blocks, find pathological factors entering or leaving the body, evaluate the production and transformation of bodily fluids, and evaluate your ability to retain nutrients and warmth, whether from physical substances or even emotional sources.

Shen issues. These are by far the subtlest Treasure-related issues and beg us to examine our assumptive beliefs about our relationship with self and Spirit. Shen issues often manifest as anxiety, depression, or restlessness. Shen can be strengthened by examining psychological problems, by meditation, and by spiritual forms of exercise, such as qigong.

THE SEVEN EMOTIONS AND THE ORGANS

Traditional Chinese medicine practitioners understand that emotions affect physiology. Therefore, they typically assess and treat the emotions, especially in relation to the meridians that they impact. In Chinese medicine, strong emotions are considered the major internal cause of disease. While emotions are normal responses to our external environment, when they are uncontrolled or repressed, they damage our organs and organ systems and open the door to disease by causing yin-yang imbalances, disturbing the flow of the blood and chi, and blocking the meridians, especially those related to a specific type of emotion. In the West, we separate thought from feeling, but in the East, the two are not divided. Emotions are actually thoughts combined with feelings. The thoughts steer our feelings, and the feelings themselves create the chemical, attitudinal, and even electrical environment that impacts specific organs and meridians.

Excessive **joy** consumes Heart meridian energy, leading to deficient Heart energy. It also relaxes the heart, so the heart cannot function effectively. The result can be feelings of agitation, insomnia, palpitations, overexcitement, and mania.

Excessive **anger** consumes Liver meridian energy, leading to deficient Liver energy. It also rises to the head, creating headaches, high blood pressure, and potentially strokes. It also results in feelings of rage, resentment, and frustration.

Excessive **grief and sorrow (sadness)** burn up Lung meridian energy, leading to deficient Lung energy, and also cause abdominal pain and swelling. Common symptoms include crying, tightness in the chest, and lung problems.

Excessive **thought or worry,** also called pensiveness, consumes Spleen meridian energy, leading to deficient Spleen energy, and causes congestion in the spleen. Resulting symptoms include excessive mental stimulation, to the point of fatigue and lethargy.

Fright scatters the chi and disturbs the energy of the Gallbladder meridian. Fright, rather than fear, is caused by things that are startling in present time. It causes indecisiveness, confusion, and lack of courage, and can eventually cause damage to Kidney meridian energy if the frightening situation becomes chronic, such as in the case of long-term abuse.

Long-term **fear** consumes Kidney meridian energy, leading to deficient Kidney energy. Fear also forces Kidney energy downward, causing lower-body problems and kidney conditions. Shock creates chaos in the kidneys, impairing their efficiency. You might be aware that you are living in fear, and that awareness can eventually create depression or restlessness.

Note: In most Traditional Chinese medicine systems, grief and sorrow are considered separate emotions, both affecting the lungs. When added to the feelings of joy, fright, anger, thought or worry, and fear, the result is seven emotions. In other systems, worry and thought (pensiveness) are considered separate emotions.

STEPS FOR ORGANIC EMOTIONAL HEALING

Refer to chapter 17, "Healing with the Ancients," for a meditative exercise to heal the emotions and organs. The following is a process that can be used to resume balance on all levels when you've pinpointed a strong emotional response.

Step 1: Label the overwhelming emotion. Refer to the list of meridian-based emotions. Which of the basic emotions seems to be consuming you? If you're confused, breathe into the part of your body experiencing the greatest tension. Under this tension lies the overpowering emotion.

Step 2: Track this emotion to a meridian. Look up the functions of this meridian to see how the emotional disturbance is affecting you physically, mentally, emotionally, and even spiritually.

Step 3: Identify the lie creating this tension. What are you subconsciously telling yourself that is creating an emotional disturbance? Close your eyes and ask to perceive or see an image that explains an event in the past that might still be affecting you. Based on this experience, what belief do you hold as true? How does this belief seem to protect you from further trauma? Can you find the lie or untruth in this belief?

Step 4. Substitute a truth for the lie. You have been stuck in a reactive mode, which has led to emotional imbalance. What belief would restore balance to your life? Can you frame a higher truth by creating a positive affirmation? Form this affirmation by starting the sentence with an "I" and selecting an active verb, such as, "I am now acknowledging that I am loved" or "I am decisive in selecting people who are kind to me."

THE BODY CLOCK AND CHI CYCLES

In traditional Chinese medicine, *the body clock* provides important feedback for diagnosing and treating chi imbalances. And if you know when a particular organ is at its most or least active state, you can support it through a myriad of techniques, including traditional treatments, proper foods, exercises, breathing, emotional focus, and practices such as qigong, which features organ-specific movements.

Chi moves through each meridian for two hours during a twenty-four-hour day, so for two hours of the day, each meridian achieves its optimum performance.

Each meridian is also considered either yin or yang. Yin meridians move the chi up the body, and yang meridians, down the body. The yin meridians are inhibitory, static, and calming, while the yang meridians are excitatory, dynamic, and activating. When combined, these energies create a unified energy, the one that originated in the universe and continues to flow through it—and us, through our meridians.

The meridians partner as yin/yang pairs in two different ways. In both cases, the complementary meridians are often both treated as they support each other synergistically. The first treatment approach is through organ relationships. For instance, the lung (yin) and large intestines (yang) are paired meridians, as are the stomach (yang) and spleen (yin). You will notice that these meridians are right next to each other on the body clock (shown below) and share an element in common. Symptoms appear during peak, or active hours, if a meridian is processing excessive energy. Symptoms of deficient energy are obvious during the outgoing or sedate wave of chi. Practitioners strengthen the chi of a meridian just after it peaks and reduce an overabundance of chi right before the peak period. The peak, most active times for the meridians are outlined on the list below. Their sedate times are exactly twelve hours later.

For example, the Spleen meridian, which is yin, is at its most active between 9 a.m. and 11 a.m.; the Triple Warmer, which is yang, is at its most active between 9 p.m. and 11 p.m. Thus, the body clock is broken into two-hour cycles:

Lungs	3 a.m. to 5 a.m.	Yin	Metal
Large Intestine	5 a.m. to 7 a.m.	Yang	Metal
Stomach	7 a.m. to 9 a.m.	Yang	Earth
Spleen	9 a.m. to 11 a.m.	Yin	Earth
Heart	11 a.m. to 1 p.m.	Yin	Fire
Small Intestine	1 p.m. to 3 p.m.	Yang	Fire
Bladder	3 p.m. to 5 p.m.	Yang	Water
Kidney	5 p.m. to 7 p.m.	Yin	Water
Pericardium	7 p.m. to 9 p.m.	Yin	Fire
Triple Warmer (Burner)	9 p.m. to 11 p.m.	Yang	Fire
Gallbladder	11 p.m. to 1 a.m.	Yang	Wood
Liver	1 a.m. to 3 a.m.	Yin	Wood

Yet another way to make use of the body clock is to work with the polar opposites, the second main approach to yin/yang partnering. While one meridian is at its peak for two hours, the one opposite it by 12 hours is at its lowest ebb. These paired meridians link with different elements as well as the opposite yin/yang differentiation. In general, if a meridian is "off," its polar opposite will also require assistance. Typically one will be over-energized and the other will be under-energized.

There are several ways to make use of the body clock. The first is to live in alignment with the flow of our chi. For instance, the Kidney meridian, a source of life energy, is active between 5 and 7 p.m., making this an ideal time to exercise and take advantage of the available energy. We might want to eat breakfast between 7 and 9 a.m., when our Stomach meridian is able to promote digestion. However, it might serve you to arise between 5 and 7 a.m., when the Large Intestine is most powerful; at that time of day, we can release the toxins from yesterday through an early morning bowel movement and be cleansed for a new day. Why not get ready for bed when the Pericardium is going to help us unwind, between 7 and 9 p.m.?

It's also helpful to use the body clock to track symptoms, especially chronic problems, to the originating meridian and to treat that meridian, as well as its polar opposite. Do you wake up every night at 3 a.m.? Your Lung meridian might be triggering unresolved issues of grief, which would be beneficial to address in the daytime hours. Since the lungs are responsive to deep breathing, you can also assist yourself with mindful meditation at this wee hour of the morning. Another common awakening time is between 1 and 3 a.m. Many insomniacs lie sleepless during these hours, which is governed by the Liver meridian. We can assist ourselves by focusing on our frustrations and anger, but also taking herbs and eating foods that bolster our Liver meridian's health.

I recommend that you continually refer to the body clock, no matter which exercises you are performing in the practice manual, to get a better idea of which meridians might be most effective to work with.

4

BODIES OF HEALING
THE CHAKRAS

> The chakra system, in fact, is part of
> the ancient and lost mysteries. And,
> in the end, the chakra system in our
> bodies is how we find our way back
> to the most ancient mystery of all—
> God, the Oneness, the Omniscient.
>
> ROSALYN L. BRUYERE
> Wheels of Light

Imagine walking into a medical clinic for an examination, but instead of stripping off your clothes and putting on a paper gown, you step behind what looks like a human-sized television screen.

The clinician on the other side of the screen tells you he is turning on the machine. Suddenly, instead of standing behind a screen, you are inside a huge box that reminds you of an elevator. You hear a soft hum, and then you are surrounded by multicolored, swirling lights.

After a few minutes, the friendly voice says, "Thank you, you can step out now." You do. The colors disappear, the box disintegrates, and once again you are standing behind a garden-variety screen, which you step around to take a chair in front of your doctor. A table separates the two of you.

"Let's see what we have," he says, as he presses a button.

Various holographic images appear atop the table, all pictures of you in 3-D. The doctor doesn't point at your organs; instead, he's examining swirling prisms of light that emanate from the holographic figure.

"Hmmm," he says. "See that dark spot?" He points to the vortex spinning out of your image's hip area. "That's your first chakra," he says. "Looks like you have a block. We'd better figure out if it's still in the subtle sphere or already causing a physical problem."

What is the physician of the future examining? Your *chakras*. He's evaluating your condition based on the coloration, shape, spin, and speed of these energy centers that govern specific physical, emotional, mental, and spiritual concerns of the body. While we may not yet have machines that can take pictures of the chakras, some subtle energy practitioners can evaluate these ultrasonic organs and help you improve your health and wellbeing by working with them.

WHAT IS A CHAKRA?

Chakras are subtle energy organs that manage the flow of energy related to all parts of our lives; they are our personal power centers. They are similar to the physical organs in the body, such as our heart or liver, except that they operate at a higher frequency—one that is not visible to the human eye or measurable by current scientific means. Each of the chakras is paired with a particular layer in *the auric field*, the set of twelve energy bands involved in the subtle exchange of information between the worlds outside and inside of the body (see chapter 2 for a review of the auric field).

The significance of the chakras in the realm of subtle energy healing cannot be overstated. They negotiate both physical and subtle energies, transforming one into the other and back again; therefore, they communicate both sensory and psychic information. Because each chakra runs on a different frequency or vibratory level, they are different colors, and each takes in, interprets, and sends out information or energy that matches its own vibratory level. They also store any and all received information so it is available for time eternal. Thus, they are the basic reason that energy medicine works.

There are hundreds, and possibly thousands, of energetic systems that are used throughout the world, many of which include the chakras and other energy bodies. Here we will focus primarily on the seven-chakra system of the ancient Hindus, as it is the system most widely used by subtle energy practitioners and esoteric physicians. (See the sidebar "Energy Bodies from Other Cultures" for an overview of other energetic systems.) We will also briefly review five additional chakras (chakras 8 through 12) that contribute significantly to our physical wellbeing, personal development, and spiritual growth. (See *The Subtle Body* for comprehensive information on the chakras.)

THE CHAKRAS AND KUNDALINI ENERGY

In Sanskrit, the word *chakra* means "spinning wheel of light." The chakras are whirling rainbow vortexes that come from our spine and swirl around in front of and behind the body, as well as above and below the body. To understand the function and power of the chakras, it is important to view them in their broader context. The Hindu system of the ancient Vedics includes numerous subtle energy bodies and channels.

The chakras, the circular energies of light that regulate the physical body and await spiritual activation.

The nadis, subtle energy streams or conduits that interact with the chakras and the physical body. They convey *prana*, or subtle energy, to cleanse the physical body and invite an energy known as the kundalini upward through the chakras. Many esoteric professionals, as well as scientific researchers, believe the nadis and the meridians are the same.

The koshas, the five sheaths of energy that contain or hold the spirit or essential self. Each of these veils lifts as a person evolves physically, mentally, spiritually, and energetically.

Dozens of other energy bodies contain the human and spiritual dimensions. Many of these additional bodies are described in *The Subtle Body* and other works.

The profound energetic force that unifies these independent bodies is known as *kundalini* energy. Kundalini energy lies within our root chakra (first chakra), so it is often depicted as a coiled serpent resting at the base of the spine. It is divine energy that becomes manifest when it moves—rising through the denseness of the

SCIENTIFIC VALIDATION OF THE CHAKRAS

VALERIE HUNT, EdD, as professor of kinesiology (the study of human movement) at the University of California in Los Angeles, is a pioneer in the field of research that is validating the existence of the chakras. For over twenty years, Hunt has been engaged in measuring human electromagnetic output under different conditions. Using an electromyograph, an instrument that measures the electrical activity of the muscles, she discovered that the physical body emanated radiation at sites typically associated with the chakras. In addition, she discovered that certain levels of consciousness were linked to specific frequencies.

For example, when people in her studies were thinking of daily situations, their energy fields measured frequencies in the range of 250 hertz (Hz). This is the same frequency as the heart field. When psychic individuals had their energy fields tested on the electromyograph, their frequency ranged in a band from 400 to 800 Hz. Trance channelers fell into the 800 to 900 Hz range, and mystics, connected continually to their higher self, registered an energy field above 900 Hz.

For in-depth information on chakra-based research, see *The Subtle Body*.

physical body, awakening the subtle body, and merging and unifying our internal feminine and masculine energies in the realization of supreme consciousness.

In scientific terms, the L-fields and T-fields that we discussed in chapter 2 form unified frequencies that mirror the activity and flow of kundalini. We are all made of the "male" and the "female," the electrical and the magnetic. As we integrate these innate forces, we find balance, harmony, and healing of body, mind, and spirit.

THE SEVEN HINDU CHAKRAS

According to Hindu philosophy, the chakras are subtle energy bodies located within the spinal cord and housed within the innermost core of the *Sushumna nadi*. This core is called the *Brahma nadi*, the carrier of spiritual energy. The nadis carry subtle energy throughout the body and are, as stated above, critical allies in the rising of the kundalini energy.

The core of the Sushumna nadi is considered a spiritual energy body, not a material energy body; therefore, the chakras are most often referred to as subtle in nature. Some Hindu systems, however, connect the chakras with the gross nerve plexuses, which are outside of the spine. In these systems, the chakras are considered physical as well as subtle and are considered the foundation of all existence, psychologically and physically.

Subtle energy medicine is largely based on chakra work, as chakras govern significant aspects of our lives. Several chakra-focused techniques are included throughout the rest of the book. You will be learning practices for uncovering the causes of a problem via the chakras, using color and sound to balance your chakras, and more.

The following descriptions cover several significant details about your chakras. The meaning of the chakra's Sanskrit name provides a clue to the chakra's purpose. Its mission is the overall job relegated to that particular chakra; knowing the mission of each chakra can help you quickly diagnose which chakra you might want to work through.

The emotional focus refers to the types of emotions (feelings and beliefs) managed through this energy center; like the meridians discussed in the last chapter, every chakra hosts a different set of emotions. By figuring out which emotions are troubling you or someone else, you can pinpoint the chakra to work on.

A chakra's "spiritual concern" covers two focuses: the spiritual perception afforded when looking at life through the lens of that chakra and the innate psychic ability frontloaded into that chakra. Each chakra provides a unique psychic glimpse into reality, the subject of a further discussion in chapter 6.

Each chakra corresponds with and connects to a particular location within the physical body. Every chakra is also related to a specific endocrine organ. If you're wondering where to focus healing for a chakra, you can always work through the related endocrine gland. You'll also learn which of the physical organs are affected by each chakra. This knowledge will help you zoom your healing into the chakra that matches physical symptoms.

Finally, each chakra relates to a specific frequency-based color and sound. In chapter 22, you'll find ways to clear a chakra, and therefore life challenges, by using color, and in chapter 21, you'll discover ways to blend sound and color for healing.

THE FIRST CHAKRA: MULADHARA

Meaning of name: *Muladhara* combines *mul*, or "base," and *adhara*, or "support." The name reflects this chakra's ultimate purpose: to serve as our basis in physical life. This chakra is often called the *root chakra*.

Mission: Security and survival

Emotional focus: Primal feelings

Spiritual concern: Deserving to exist; physical sympathy, ability to sense physical energy

Location: At the base of the spine, between the anus and genitals

Endocrine gland: Adrenals

Physical organs and functions governed: Genital organs and adrenals; bones and skeletal structure; coccygeal vertebrae; some kidney, bladder, and excretory functions; skin

Color: Red

Sound: *Lam*

SECOND CHAKRA: SVADHISTHANA

Meaning of name: "Dwelling place of the self," from *sva*, "self" or "prana," and *adhisthana*, or "dwelling place." Also means "six-petaled."

Mission: Feelings and creativity

Emotional focus: All feelings

Spiritual concern: Ability to express feelings; psychic capability of feeling sympathy, through which you can sense others' feelings

Location: Lower abdomen, between navel and genitals

Endocrine gland: Ovaries in women and testes in men

Physical organs and functions governed: Part of kidney system; intestines; some aspects of reproductive system, including the womb; bladder; prostate; sacral vertebrae and nerve plexus; the neurotransmitters determining emotional responses to stimuli

Color: Orange
Sound: *Vam*

THIRD CHAKRA: MANIPURA

Meaning of name: "City of gems"—*mani* means "jewel or gem," *pura* means "dwelling place," and *nabhi* means "navel"
Mission: Mentality, power, and success
Emotional focus: Fears, doubt, and other feelings affecting self-esteem
Spiritual concern: Empowerment; psychic ability to perform clairsentience or "clear sensing" of mental information
Location: Between the navel and the base of the sternum
Endocrine gland: Pancreas
Physical organs and functions governed: Pancreatic system; all digestive organs in the stomach area, including the liver, spleen, gallbladder, stomach, pancreas, and parts of kidney system; lumbar vertebrae and solar plexus–based nerve plexus; some authorities say muscles and the immune and nervous systems
Color: Yellow
Sound: *Ram*

FOURTH CHAKRA: ANAHATA

Meaning of name: "Heart lotus"—*Hrit* means "heart," and *pankaja*, "lotus." Also means "twelve-petaled": *dvadash* is "twelve," and *dala* means "petals"
Mission: Relationships and healing
Emotional focus: Emotions in relationship; all feelings related to love, such as gratitude and appreciation
Spiritual concern: Connection to the Divine
Location: In the physical body, the center of the chest, the heart
Endocrine gland: Heart
Physical organs and functions governed: Heart and lungs, circulatory and oxygenation systems, breasts, lumbar and thoracic vertebrae, cardiac nerve plexus; some authorities say the thymus gland
Color: Green
Sound: *Yam*

FIFTH CHAKRA: VISHUDDHA

Meaning of name: "Pure" or "throat lotus"—*kanth* means "throat," while *padma* means "lotus." Also "sixteen-petaled": *shodash* equates to "sixteen," and *dala* means "petals"

Mission: Communication and guidance

Emotional focus: Expression of all emotions, especially in relation to self-responsibility

Spiritual concern: Sharing divine guidance; psychic ability of clairaudience or "clear hearing"

Location: Throat

Endocrine gland: Thyroid

Physical organs and functions governed: Thyroid and parathyroid glands, larynx and laryngeal nerve plexus; mouth and auditory systems (vocal cords, mouth, throat, ears); lymph and the lymphatic system; thoracic vertebrae

Color of chakra: Blue

Sound of element: *Ham*

SIXTH CHAKRA: AJNA

Meaning of name: "Command"

Mission: Perception and sight (insight, hindsight, future sight)

Emotional focus: Feelings related to self-acceptance, such as self-love and self-awareness

Spiritual concern: Visioning

Location: Above and between the eyebrows

Endocrine gland: Pituitary

Physical organs and functions governed: Pituitary gland, medulla plexus and parts of hypothalamus; olfactory and visual systems, the left eye in particular; memory storage; some aspects of the ears and sinuses

Color: Purple or indigo

Sound: *Om*

SEVENTH OR CROWN CHAKRA: SAHASRARA

Meaning of name: "Void," "dwelling place without support," "thousand-petaled"

Mission: Purpose and spirituality

Emotional focus: Related to spiritual nature

Spiritual concern: Oneness with Divine; psychic gift of prophecy or ability to sense divine plans

Location: Top of the head

Endocrine gland: Pineal

Physical organs and functions governed: Pineal gland, upper skull and cerebral cortex, parts of the hypothalamus, higher learning and cognitive brain systems, parts of immune system, the right eye

Symbol: The thousand-petaled lotus
Color: White; also seen as violet or gold
Sound: *Visarga* (a breathing sound)

THE TWELVE-CHAKRA SYSTEM

One contemporary chakra system is the twelve-chakra system, which I developed and describe in detail in several other books.[1] It is based on the classical Hindu chakra system, but includes an additional five chakras that are located outside of the physical body. While these additional chakras have yet to be measured or recorded, I discovered them through my work as an energy healer. The additional chakras are found above the head, below the feet, and around the body. Having developed an understanding of these additional energy centers, I now make frequent use of them.

Many other chakra systems include chakras beyond the Hindu seven. The Narayana system, a yoga derivative, works with nine chakras, as does the chakra system expounded upon in the *Yogaranjopanishad*, while the Waidika system, a Layayoga method, outlines eleven major chakras. Some schools add an eighth chakra, the Bindu or the Soma, to the typical seven. Many esoteric practitioners locate chakras beyond the physical body, as do some of the more traditional systems. In yogic tradition, it is important to remember that the seventh chakra is located *above* the top of the head, not *at* the top of the head. Other traditions place a chakra underneath the feet, as David Furlong describes in his book

ENERGY BODIES FROM OTHER CULTURES

WESTERN TRADITION FREQUENTLY attributes the chakra system to the Hindus. The truth is that chakra systems have emerged from all corners of the globe—and endured through time. Many of these cross-cultural systems are described in *The Subtle Body*, including those from the Jewish Kabbalah, mystical Christianity, and countries such as Egypt, Africa, and Tibet. *The Subtle Body* also explores chakra constellations from the ancient Mayan, Cherokee, and Inca healing traditions.

In this practice manual, there are several exercises for working with the energy bodies in ways that you might not have considered before now—exercises that are both wonderfully effective and easy to do. For example, in chapter 17, "Healing with the Ancients," there is a brief exercise called "The Luminous Golden Threads" that offers a nature-based approach to chakra healing; it is based on the subtle energy medicine of the Incas, in which chakras are known as *pukios*, and the power of the elements can help us to clear away our troubles.

Working with Earth Energies, as does crystal-energy healer Katrina Raphaell.[2] Nearly all systems recognize secondary or minor chakras.

The twelve-chakra system features the traditional seven, plus these additional chakras.

Eighth chakra: Located just above the head. This chakra is seen as housing several additional energy bodies, including the Akashic Records, which is a record of everything ever seen and done; the Shadow Records, that which was unseen as pertaining to the Akashic Records; and the Book of Life, which reflects the positive aspect of all events. This chakra is colored black or silver and connects with the body through the thymus gland.

Ninth chakra: Located one and a half feet above the head. This chakra contains the "seat of the soul," the spiritual genetics that generate physical reality, such as the physical genes. It also carries the soul purpose and the symbols that sustain the uniqueness of a soul. It is gold and links with the diaphragm.

Tenth chakra: Located a foot and a half under the feet. This is the grounding chakra, because it opens to elemental energy and passes it into the body through the feet. It holds personal soul history as well as stories and energies from one's heritage. It connects a person thoroughly to nature and the natural world. It is brown or earth toned and correlates to the center of the bones.

Eleventh chakra: Surrounds the body, but is concentrated around the hands and the feet. This energy center helps individuals command and transmute physical and supernatural forces. Through it, one can seize command of external energies and direct them for good. It is extraordinary for producing instant change inside and outside of the body. It is rose in color and relates to our connective tissue.

Twelfth chakra: Surrounding the eleventh chakra and the entirety of the body, this energy center represents the outer bounds of the human self. It connects to the body through thirty secondary chakras, which are described in my *Complete Book of Chakra Healing.*

Note: Just outside of the twelfth chakra is *the energy egg,* a three-layer sheath that regulates the linkage between the spiritual realms and the physical body.

WORKING WITH THE CHAKRAS

Each chakra is a prism that regulates a specific set of physical, emotional, mental, and spiritual concerns. This means that we can use them to diagnose problems and create a healing plan for a variety of issues. Understanding the chakras, we can:

- Use physical symptoms to clarify the emotional, mental, and spiritual components of an illness.
- Trace our emotional issues back to the development of a certain part of our body or to the age at which the issues originated. Emotions are the language of the body. If we can reexperience the feeling component and the physical reactions attached to a debilitating situation, we can reprogram self-destructive beliefs and chart a whole new course.
- Isolate the mental or spiritual beliefs affecting us, thereby healing our emotional or physical issues.
- Awaken repressed memories, including in utero and past-life memories, for the purpose of understanding, clearing, and healing. By getting to the root cause of an issue, we can unlock the energy blocks it might be causing.
- Become knowledgeable parents to our own children, supporting them through each development stage.
- Better parent our own inner child, that natural self within each of us waiting for his or her chance at life.
- Make appropriate and wise decisions by pinpointing our current development stage.
- Better understand where, how, and why we get "stuck"—in harmful habits, cycles, and even addictions.

In working with the chakras, we are searching for two points of awareness. First, we want to identify and acknowledge our positive traits, which might be in need of recognition or revitalization. All too often, we bury some of our best qualities beneath a deluge of conflict and misperceptions. Our second goal is to uncover, understand, and change self-destructive beliefs, patterns, and programs.

CHAKRA STRUCTURE

Chakras are structured in three ways. These divisions include front and back sides, left and right sides, and inner and outer wheels. Knowing this information will help you both diagnose and problem-solve energetically. For instance, if illnesses constantly appear on the left side of the body or chakras, you can examine issues of femininity. If all the back side chakras are blocked, you can analyze the unconscious or soul issues.

Front and back. The in-body chakras have a front and back side. In general, the front side governs everyday behavior and regulates our relationship with the physical world. The back side responds to our own unconscious programs and manages our relationship with the less-tangible reality.

Left and right. The left side of the chakra is feminine and regulates female-oriented issues, while the right side is masculine and governs male-oriented issues. Our feminine functions involve receptivity, attraction, relationship, intuition, and programs regarding one's own femininity or the female gender. Our male functions involve action, domination, success, rationality, and programs about one's own masculinity or the male gender.

Inner and outer. Each of the chakras also has an inner and outer wheel. Our inner wheel reflects the programming from our own higher consciousness or spirit. This programming enables actualization of our spiritual gifts, the abilities necessary to carry out our spiritual mission. The outer wheel holds our personal issues, private desires, and the heartaches and hurts that can throw a wrench into the chakra spin cycle for years on end. The job of the outer wheel is to help us adapt to the surrounding reality. Our tribal or soul issues also appear primarily in our outer wheel, which means that most subtle energy healing is aimed at shifting the outer wheel. We can, however, greatly enhance the effectiveness of healing work by expanding the spiritual energy incumbent in a chakra's inner wheel, as it is composed of our essential energy. The most direct path I know of to accomplish that is to breathe fully and with intention into a particular chakra, expanding it and opening it up to spirit. As we do this, every part of us is nourished—literally. Ideally, the inner and outer wheels should operate in concert with each other. While they might not move at the same speed, their relationship should be rhythmic and consistent. I know of few things that are as powerful as expanding the spiritual light from our inner chakra wheel into the troubled outer wheel to invite life changes.

In a healthy person, the inner wheel establishes the actual speed and direction of both wheels. Both wheels usually circle clockwise, but there are exceptions. During menstruation, a woman's wheels, especially those of the first and fourth chakras, might move counterclockwise in order to release built-up emotions. The outer wheels of all the chakras will often circulate counterclockwise when someone is in grief, shock, near death, or performing a physical cleanse.

As subtle energy healers become adept at intuitively analyzing these three chakric structures, they can use the structures to determine what is happening inside of a chakra and, therefore, a client's physical body.

CHAKRA DEVELOPMENT

While we are born with a fully intact set of chakras, each chakra unfolds to the light of life at a different time. This is so we can access the energy available to that chakra at the appropriate time, in a process that hopefully results in all of the chakras achieving maturity by age fifty-six.

For instance, when in utero and until six months of age, we are primarily focused on our first chakra, the center devoted to safety and security, as well as the development of our primary feelings. What are our initial life experiences about but survival and the encouragement of the parent-child bonding that gives us the knowledge that we are wanted and safe? Unfortunately, we don't always receive the welcome and nourishment required for this chakra to be programmed with the confidence we need to be internally secure no matter what occurs in life. This chakra will now be "wobbly," the result of which can be physical, emotional, mental, or spiritual issues that arise during our life.

The developmental ages of the seven in-body chakras follows:

Chakra	Age
One	Womb to 6 months
Two	6 months to 2 ½ years
Three	2 ½ to 4 ½ years
Four	4 ½ to 6 ½ years
Five	6 ½ to 8 ½ years
Six	8 ½ to 14 years
Seven	14 to 21 years

As implied, our first "run through" with the chakras can result in misperceptions and wounds that inhibit our ability to express our true self. Fortunately, as our life continues, we reprocess our chakras and are thus provided an opportunity for a "do-over."

While chakra seven is developing for the first time during our adolescence, between ages fourteen and twenty-one, the first six chakras undergo reprocessing. This allows us to shift the dysfunctional perspectives so we can emerge from childhood healthier. For instance, during ages fourteen to fifteen, we are activating our seventh chakra and working toward figuring out our higher purpose, but we are also revisiting the primary concerns of our first chakra, or security issues. From age fifteen to sixteen, we are simultaneously awakening our seventh chakra and reexamining our relationship with creativity. During our last year in this cycle, we are fully investing in uncovering our spiritual purpose, the key concept of the seventh chakra.

Chakra	Age	Key Concept
One	14 to 15 years	Security
Two	15 to 16 years	Creativity
Three	16 to 17 years	Personal power
Four	17 to 18 years	Loving relationships
Five	18 to 19 years	Self-expression
Six	19 to 20 years	Self-image
Seven	20 to 21 years	Spiritual purpose

After age twenty-one, our higher chakras—chakras eight through twelve—develop in seven-year spans. After age fifty-six, the development cycle begins again with chakra one. No matter our age, we revisit chakras one through seven within each new seven-year span. For instance, between the ages of twenty-one and twenty-two, we are working on karma, the subject of the eighth chakra, but also reactivating our first chakra. Between the ages of twenty-two and twenty-three, we get to re-explore our second-chakra issues against the backdrop of our karmic issues. There is always an opportunity to heal, change, and renew ourselves, no matter our age.

Chakra	Age	Key Concept
Eight	21 to 28 years	Karma
Nine	28 to 35 years	Soul purpose
Ten	35 to 42 years	Purposeful survival
Eleven	42 to 49 years	Creative success
Twelve	49 to 56 years	Powerful mastery
One	56 to 63 years	Awareness of a Greater Power
Two	63 to 70 years	Creativity with peace
Three	70 to 77 years	Success, inner and outer
Four	77 to 84 years	Relationship with All
Five	84 to 91 years	Speaking for "Above"
Six	91 to 98 years	Visions from heaven

There are many healing modalities and exercises throughout this book that can be augmented with this development information. The following examples might spark other ideas as you move forward in your exploration.

In chapter 11, "Healing the Auric Field," there are practices for assessing the auric field, and then sealing energetic leaks and tears in it. Childhood or adolescent wounds (often emotional) that continue to negatively impact adults correlate with the particular chakra under development at the time of the wounding, but also with the partnered auric field. For instance, a first chakra wound will also be reflected in the first auric field. Working with development cycles can help you pinpoint where a wound, shock, loss, or disappointment might still be undermining your health and happiness and invite healing within the chakra as well as its kin auric field.

Similarly, in chapter 13, "Modern Esoteric Healing," a process called "Uncovering Your Storyline" will help heal long-held pain, resentment, and regret. Knowing the patterns of chakra development can potentially be useful when preparing for this process, so you can go through the steps of healing past hurts with great awareness and readiness.

CASCADING LIGHT: An Exercise

MANY SUBTLE ENERGY healing practices involve clearing your chakras, freeing you of stress and balancing your energy systems, leaving you refreshed and invigorated. The easiest way to conduct this exercise is to sit in a quiet space and softly close your eyes.

1. Breathing deeply, imagine a brilliant white light entering your in-body chakra system through the top of your head. As this shimmering white light streams through you, it frees you from everything you need to let go of and fills you with inspiration and love.

2. See the light cascade downward, descending through all the chakras until it exits your feet. Even then, it continues to flow through and beyond your tenth chakra, which lies under the ground.

3. From this place under the ground, the light turns to reflow upward through the chakras and around your body, completely enveloping you in grace and protection. Continue this exercise until you feel renewed and clear.

PART II
PREPARING FOR HEALING: YOUR ENERGY MEDICINE BAG

In these pages, you will prepare for service as a subtle energy healer. You can apply these concepts in your healing practice, whether you are providing service in a professional or lay capacity. And because we are all our own healers, the ideas in part 2 are as essential for self-healing as they are for healing others.

Subtle energy medicine is "original" medicine. It is grounded in the sands of time and deeply rooted in shamanic ideology, which means any person, not just trained, licensed professionals, can stand between heaven and earth and receive the healing bounty of nature, spirit, and mind. There are rigors and safety measures we all need to take, however, when working on ourselves or on others, so that we direct the subtle energy appropriately. This is one of the reasons that the concepts and techniques in part 2 are important to all of us.

This section will also help you determine which subtle energy practitioners you might want to seek help from. By learning about the ethics, practices, and concepts that effective and honorable subtle energy specialists follow, you can better assess the professionals—or even friends—you would like working on you. After all, you don't want just anyone in your energy field!

Professional practitioners must contemplate factors that aren't as vital to the self-healer. When someone asks us for subtle energy treatment, they are entrusting us with their welfare. This awesome responsibility complicates our energy practices. Our ethics must be impeccable, as should our ability to use both our traditional and energetic skills. We must be devoted to ongoing professional development, yet be approachable and kind.

Part 2 offers concepts and tools that will bolster any practitioner's abilities in all areas of subtle energy medicine. These topics include the role of intention and the importance of ethics, as well as the influence of intuition and energetic boundaries. We'll discuss the many facets of trust and tangible ways to set goals for self-healing or healing others. You'll also be provided a worksheet you can use to establish objectives for yourself or someone else.

An entire chapter is devoted to what I call essential energy techniques. Each is a doorway into the intuitive healing realms. I've developed them through my twenty-five years as a practitioner, and most are based on cross-cultural studies. I recommend that these techniques become the foundation for all other exercises in this book, as they are designed to prepare, support, and protect subtle energy practitioners when they are engaged in healing. They can be used as stand-alone processes or combined with any other healing technique. For instance, you can use Spirit-to-Spirit, a practice described in chapter 9, to initiate any healing experience or combine it with color and sound-healing practices. All of these essential energy techniques can be safely and ethically used for any self-healing or healing work with others.

Part 2 finishes with a thorough discussion of what to expect during a subtle energy medicine session. What might you or a client experience during or after a session? How do you prepare yourself or another for the many changes that might occur?

Despite the seeming complications of subtle energy work, it's important to remember that we are all, always, performing energy healing. To smile at a crying child, to administer a bandage, to stroke the arm of an ailing parent—these and other activities are energetic healings. Ultimately, our heart will lead the way.

INTENTION AND ETHICS

> Two things fill my mind with
> ever-increasing wonder and awe:
> the starry heavens above me and
> the moral law within me.
>
> IMMANUEL KANT

All healers, from allopathic physicians to subtle energy practitioners of all stripes, enter into their sessions with a set of intentions guiding the way. The question is, are we clear about what those intentions are? Whether we are new to healing work or a seasoned pro, are we setting our intentions purposefully and consciously? This chapter will help you answer these and similar questions from the ground of integrity toward yourself and others, whatever the goal of a session.

While most of this chapter is focused on healing others, it will also be of interest to self-healers. After all, self-healing is a result of setting intentions for ourselves. We want to treat ourselves with the same level of uprightness that we guarantee others. At any given time, even the at-home healer might need to journey beyond the circle of their own skills and seek help elsewhere. This chapter will assist you in evaluating the subtle energy clinicians who could serve you. Bottom line, all parts of our lives evolve from the twin concepts of intention and ethics. We can never go wrong if we steer our lives correctly through these matched eyeglass lenses.

SUPERCHARGING INTENTIONS

Intention is a word and a concept that is frequently discussed, but what is intention, really?

At the most basic level, intentionality is the projection of awareness toward a desired outcome or object. When we set an intention, our personal field interacts with someone else's field as we transfer energetic information back and forth. Research in resonance and sound shows that when living beings operate or resonate on similar vibrations, one can affect the other. In that sense, our intentions are an important aspect of creating a healing resonance that is energetically uplifting. During a healing session, as we set clear, positive intentions, our learned skills and intuitive abilities will naturally align to help achieve those intentions.

How is an intention different than any garden-variety idea or a desire? To understand, it's useful to look at the process of creating an intention—a process often referred to as "setting an intention."

Setting an intention is the same as making a decision to which you can be committed on all levels—emotionally, mentally, physically, and spiritually. If an intention doesn't work, if the results you are getting are contrary to your stated intention, it's likely that you are not yet committed to it on all of these levels.

So what does it take to be committed on all levels? It takes becoming familiar with the *Subtle Energy Power Summit*, a visual summary of your work as a healer. Figure 5.1 shows the relationship between your subtle energy medicine work and not only your intentions, but also your values, ethics, and commitments.

Clarifying and stating your values, and making commitments based on those values, gives rise to your intentions. Therefore, the first part of this chapter is devoted to helping you to identify your values and the ethical commitments that will have everything line up for you as a healing practitioner—your thoughts, attitudes, behaviors, and actions. As you do this, you will be supercharging your intentions, because they will now be resting upon a bedrock that includes your own ethics—an extraordinarily powerful foundation.

FIGURE 5.1
THE SUBTLE ENERGY POWER SUMMIT

Intentions
Your intended purpose or outcome

Commitments
The decisions you make and the actions you take in accordance with your values and ethics

Values and Ethics
What matters to you as a healer, your moral codes of conduct, your values and ethics

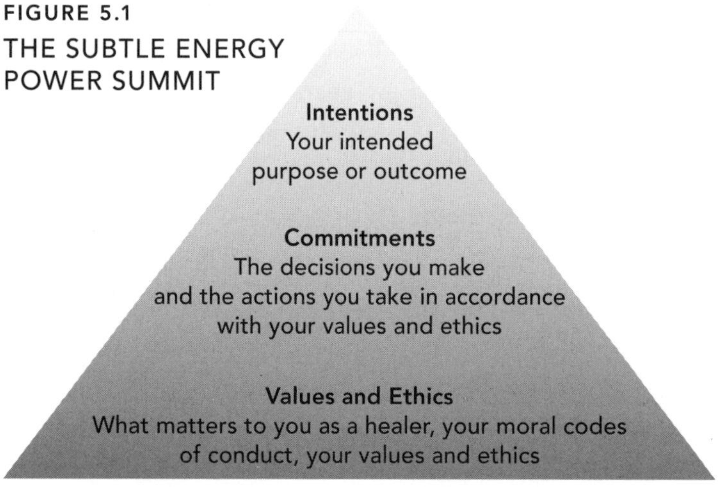

Tip: If you could use some extra assistance in clarifying and setting intentions, there is a great process for that in chapter 9, called "Six Steps to Setting a New Intention." As that exercise is one of the essential energy techniques that I frequently use and teach, I've bundled it with some of the other tools that fit into that category, so that the group of techniques will always be easy to find when you're looking for them.

YOUR ETHICAL COMMITMENTS

Being a healer involves following a code of honor that guides your decisions and choices and determines your behaviors and actions. If you are a professional subtle energy practitioner, you must decide how to operate in terms of methods, techniques, tools, values, and ethics. This is true even if you don't make a living doing healing work, and your "clients" are your friends and family and not the general public. It is also true if you are working on yourself. Are you not your own client? It would not be ethical to cause further injury to yourself in the course of trying to heal yourself.

One of the most challenging ethical issues involved in working with clients, or even on yourself, is selecting which subtle energy practices or techniques to use. You might have a strong sense of what healing approach would be beneficial, but you might not be certain. Regardless of how clear you feel, it is important to ask your client if an approach is acceptable to them before you undertake it.

For instance, you might believe that your client would benefit from hands-on healing. Before you start working on your client, explain why you think this

HOW TO EXPLAIN YOUR ETHICAL COMMITMENTS TO YOUR CLIENTS

THE MEANS BY which practitioners establish strong, healthy relationships with their clients vary greatly. Think about and create an action plan that includes what you would like to state *verbally*, what information you want to provide in *written* form, and what you might not chose to explicitly state even though it is an important part of the foundation of your work.

In the Healer's Code, there are commitments that are essential for you to make internally, but not essential for you to tell each client. For example, you may not need to tell clients that you're committed to continuing to learn and increase your knowledge and skills, but letting your clients know that you are committed to their confidentiality will give them a sense of safety and comfort.

Tip: If you have an intake form for new or returning clients, consider adding to that form a brief paragraph like the one below, a clearly stated encapsulation of the ethical commitments that you decide are most important for your clients to know:

My practice is based upon a strong foundation of ethical commitments, each of which is the result of clearly defined values, principles, and boundaries. Chief among them are complying with the laws that govern my profession, honoring and protecting the confidentiality of my clients, and referring clients to other practitioners to augment or replace my services if that is in their best interest.

CHANCES ARE THAT, at some point in your life, you will seek out the services of a professional subtle energy practitioner—or perhaps you already have. While we can easily search the Internet for a list of top surgeons, dentists, or therapists, it's more difficult to find a list of top subtle energy practitioners; after all, at some level, they are working with invisible energy, which can be hard to measure, and that makes their abilities difficult to assess.

As discussed in this chapter, one of the hallmarks of a great healer is a developed code of ethics. Some practitioners can actually provide you with a written code, and many share their philosophies on a web site or in a brochure. It's important to read through this material and decide if the stated principles match your own. For instance, if a subtle energy healer asserts that you must give up prescription medicine or stop all allopathic care to work with them, you might question the efficacy of their overall care.

If the subtle energy practitioner's ethics or work style isn't apparent, ask about it. Ask about ethics, modalities used, general principles, as well as other key factors that will help you determine if this is the subtle energy practitioner for you. Questions you can ask, either on the phone or through email, can include the following:

- What is your general healing philosophy?
- What are your codes of ethics, in terms of the use of touch, provision of care, privacy, anonymity, and more?

- Are you a licensed or unlicensed professional? (In most states, subtle energy practitioners are considered unlicensed professionals, although there are still laws pertaining to their practices.)
- What do you need or expect from a client?
- How do we set goals together?
- What is your training?
- Have you ever worked with issues similar to mine, and if so, in what way?
- What can you share about the results?
- What called you to your profession?
- How do you work with clients? (Length of session, how and when sessions are conducted, fiscal responsibilities, and more.)
- Can I talk to one of your current or former clients? (Know that this might not be possible. The sharing of client contact information negates client confidentiality.)

Ultimately you need to pay attention to your gut instinct. Many practitioners come highly recommended, but might not align with your needs or personality. Because of this, it's important to start with an initial appointment and avoid signing up for a package plan or several appointments until you have a good sense of who the healer is, how they work, and whether their style is a good fit for you and your circumstances. I also recommend that you avoid any subtle energy practitioner who insists that you can work only with them. There is no one-stop shop in the integrative world.

And again, never see someone who says you can't participate in allopathic medicine. All medicine is energy medicine, even allopathic care, which holds a vital place in the holistic field.

practice would help them and ask if it is acceptable to them. While hands-on healing may be the perfect practice for that client, they might be scared of any hands-on processes, perhaps because hands-on work triggers an abuse issue for them. Or perhaps they have a strong intuitive sense of their own about what practice will work best. Whatever the case, always honor their response and do not try to sell them on any practice they're uncomfortable with.

Apply the same standards to yourself. Perhaps you sense you would benefit from prayer, but praying reminds you of frightening experiences in church. You might need to seek a different practice to achieve the same healing outcome.

THE HEALER'S WORKSHEET

The Healer's Worksheet will help you to clarify *why* you do healing work (values), *who* you want to work with and are qualified to work with (clients), and *how* you want to work (boundaries, methods, and more). If you are working on yourself, you are simultaneously the client and the practitioner. I encourage you to actually imagine separating yourself in two and filling in this worksheet as if you were your own healing professional. The resulting objectivity might reveal new ways to look at the problem and additional means for arriving at antidotes for your "client self."

Once you complete the worksheet, you will be well prepared to take the step that follows: embracing the Healer's Code—the ethical commitments that can ensure your effectiveness and success as a practitioner of subtle energy medicine.

THE HEALER'S CODE

The Healer's Code was inspired by the great Hippocratic Oath, which has served as a beacon for physicians and healers since the fifth century BC. The cornerstones of that enduring oath have been expanded and intentionally shaped into potent commitments that will boost your confidence and courage as a subtle energy practitioner.

After you have completed the Healer's Worksheet, you are ready to review the Healer's Code and determine whether you feel alignment with the twelve commitments it asks you to make.

You might wonder if the code is significant if you are an informal practitioner or only working on friends, loved ones, or yourself. While it is unlikely that friends and family will press charges if we make a mistake, it is important to take the role as subtle energy healer seriously. By embracing our responsibilities, we can actually more effectively embrace the healing power available to us. Great things happen to those who consider themselves worthy of great energies.

As you consider the Healer's Code, know that a client isn't necessarily a paying patient. A client is anyone you work on, including yourself, whether you are performing a subtle energy service for a fee or as a gift. Anyone who receives a treatment might be considered a client.

You may want to find a peaceful place to relax and focus with care and presence. Perhaps you can light a candle and play some beautiful music that helps you to feel centered and connected to your higher guidance. Review the Healer's Code, point by point, and notice the thoughts and feelings that arise with each point. Notice where you feel clear and ready and where you may have some additional work to do in order to feel aligned.

At the end of the twelve commitments, you can include any additional commitments that may be important to you.

THE HEALER'S CODE
Ethical Commitments of the Subtle Energy Practitioner

As a practitioner of subtle energy medicine:

I am committed to helping and not harming my clients.

I am committed to respecting and knowing the tools of my trade. I understand that all energy is medicine, and I will not use the tools and techniques of subtle energy healing without full knowledge of their effects. This might include sound, music, words, light, colors, touch, fragrance, herbs, and many other tools.

I am committed to seeking out trainers, schools, and teaching programs of integrity.

I am committed to treating only those whom I am qualified to treat.

I am committed to not overstepping my professional boundaries to engage in practices that are outside of my training and knowledge base.

I am committed to not overstepping my professional boundaries to recommend that a client either engage in or abstain from other outside treatments.

I am committed to referring clients to other qualified professionals or specialists when doing so might better serve their healing process.

I am committed to contacting appropriate authorities when I know that my client is in danger or when my client could cause danger to self or others.

I am committed to honoring and respecting myself and my boundaries. My personal values, principles, and morals are important, and I will not sacrifice them for my work.

I am committed to honoring and respecting my clients and their boundaries. I will not get involved with my clients, sexually or romantically, unless they have not received treatment from me for two or more years.

I am committed to honoring and protecting the anonymity and confidentiality of my clients.

I am committed to researching, understanding, and abiding by the regional, state, and federal laws that govern my profession. And I am committed to remaining current with any changes to those laws.

I am committed to _____.

I am committed to _____.

I am committed to _____.

I am committed to _____.

Date: _____ Signed: _____

THE HEALER'S WORKSHEET

VALUES: What are my top five values as a subtle energy practitioner?* What holds the greatest meaning for me as a healer? What matters to me, and what are my priorities?

1.

2.

3.

4.

5.

BOUNDARIES with self: What are the five primary boundaries that I hold as a practitioner who values my integrity and wellbeing? Most importantly, how do I care for my physical, emotional, mental, energetic, and spiritual wellbeing in relationship to my work?

1.

2.

3.

4.

5.

BOUNDARIES with clients:** What are the five primary boundaries that I will not cross as a healing practitioner? Most importantly, what behaviors and activities will I not engage in or allow within the bounds of my healing practice?

1.

2.

3.

4.

5.

CLIENTS/PATIENTS: Who am I qualified to treat, and what types of energetic imbalances am I qualified to treat?

THE HEALER'S WORKSHEET

TRAINING/SKILLS: Do I need to engage in further research or training in order to fulfill my intentions and goals as a practitioner of subtle energy medicine? If yes, what might that look like?

RESPECTED COLLEAGUES: When I refer clients to other practitioners (either to work in conjunction with the treatment we are engaged in or in the event that we end our working relationship), who are my top recommendations and why?

LEGAL COMPLIANCE: What are the regional, state, and federal laws that govern my practice? What steps do I need to take in order to be in compliance with them?

OTHER: What else do I need to contemplate, learn, know, or do so that my healing practice is in alignment with my values and commitments?

* *Practitioner* refers to a formal or informal practitioner, whether you are collecting a fee or not, as well as the "healer within" if you are performing self-healing.

** *Client* refers to the person receiving your subtle energy work, regardless of whether you are a professional or lay practitioner, performing a healing in a formal or informal setting, or receiving a fee or not. It also refers to the "client within," if you are self-healing.

6

INTUITION AND TRUST

> Healing, Papa would tell me, is
> not a science, but the intuitive
> art of wooing nature.
>
> W. H. AUDEN

Intuition is a form of perception and internal communication. It is the inner resource that, when tapped into and utilized, differentiates a subtle energy medicine practitioner from any other practitioner. When you are relying on intuition as one of your primary healing tools, you need to embrace your strongest intuitive faculties and wisely use them when healing yourself or others. One of the ways to do this is to figure out which of the four main ways of being intuitive is most accurate and available to you.

FOUR TYPES OF INTUITION

Clarifying your strongest intuitive abilities is really quite easy. There are actually twelve different types of intuitive gifts, each available through a different one of your twelve chakras, as I share in my book *The Intuition Guidebook*. These gifts can be divided into the four main categories outlined below.[1] Read the following descriptions and see which type resonates most strongly for you—the one that elicits a response like, "That happens to me *all of the time!*"

Physically kinesthetic: *feeling gifts.* Your body tells you what is happening within others. You are especially aware of what is happening physically and emotionally inside of them. If they have an ache, you have an ache; if they are exhausted and running on empty, you can momentarily feel drained of energy; if they are fearful or anxious, you can feel that fear too. For those who are physically kinesthetic, it is especially important to have vibrant, strong energetic boundaries in order not to absorb others' physical and emotional energies (see chapter 9).

Spiritually kinesthetic: *spiritual gifts.* You sense or simply know the basic nature of a person, a place, or a situation. You also know what is true in a particular moment, such as when someone you're communicating with is being honest, is in denial, or is outright lying. You just sense it. You are aware of and sense "good" or "bad" energies in a room or around a person.

Verbal: *hearing gifts.* You can hear messages in your head. What you hear might sound like tones, music, noises, or spoken words. You might be meditating on a question, then turn on the radio or television and hear a spot-on response. You could read a meaningful phrase in a book, discover you've written a powerful message to yourself, or recognize the hidden meaning in something that someone said seemingly out of the blue.

Visual: *seeing gifts.* Visual intuition involves inner and outer sight. You see pictures in your head, or you see things outside yourself, with your eyes,

INTERPRETING VISUAL INTUITIVE INFORMATION

IF YOUR STRONGEST intuitive gift is visual intuition, answers to subtle energy questions often come in the form of pictures or images, which you then need to interpret. One way to help ensure you're interpreting meaning of the vision correctly is to discern what type of vision it is.

There are five types of visions: *hindsight, current sight, foresight, full sight,* and *half sight.* The following questions can help you to "type" a vision:

- Is this vision about the past? If so, it is *hindsight.*
- Is it about something occurring right now? If so, it is *current sight.* And the next question is, is there something you are supposed to do with this knowledge?
- Is this vision about the potential or probable future? If so, it is *foresight.*

- What is the truest form of the source of this vision? To ask this question is to seek *full sight.*
- Are you getting all the information as accurately or as completely as possible? If you are receiving all of the messages at once, you're receiving *full sight.* If you are only receiving a part of the message, it is *half sight.*
- If you have not received all the information accurately or completely, is there more that can be revealed so you can fully understand the message? When you ask this question, your first image might be enhanced or made larger in scope, or you will receive new images until you are in full sight. If no more information is forthcoming, you are supposed to remain in half sight and the mystery of not fully understanding the message.

that others might not perceive. You might receive images of colors or shapes in response to a question or while examining an issue. Higher guidance often comes as a vision (a visual revelation), messages in nighttime dreams, or sometimes through daydreams.

INTUITIVE INFORMATION AND THE CHAKRAS

In order for intuitive information to really qualify as helpful, it must lead to a life-enhancing awareness that brings greater freedom, whether it be on the emotional, mental, spiritual, and/or physical level. This new awareness will have a balancing effect on one or more of the in-body chakras and should produce at least one of the following results.

Chakra Balanced	Result
First	Improves your physical wellbeing
Second	Frees you from imprisoning feelings and emotions and moves you toward joy
Third	Releases you from negative beliefs and moves you toward higher self-esteem
Fourth	Unbinds you from harmful relationships or patterns and encourages more loving ones
Fifth	Allows you to share yourself powerfully and communicate lovingly by removing old tapes and increasing your ability to set respectful boundaries
Sixth	Can rid you of false impressions about yourself and allow you to see yourself and your potential more realistically
Seventh	Helps spiritually by enabling you to better understand God's love and accept divine assistance and support
Eighth	Helps you work through the experiences of the past that are holding you back and claim the gifts you have yet to use
Ninth	Removes the blocks to living your purpose
Tenth	Leads you to take practical, concrete steps toward a life of contribution and fulfillment
Eleventh	Encourages the ethical applications of your personal and positional power, and leads you to generously use your abilities and gifts to uplift others

TRUSTING OUR INTUITIVE GIFTS

As important as it is to identify our intuitive gifts, it's also important to expand our intuitive gifts and develop the skills that will allow us to *trust* the psychic information we're picking up. No matter what healing modalities we choose to work with, when we merge thorough training and practice with our innate intuitive capacities, we become more effective practitioners.

When we make a commitment to continuously grow, learn, and refine our skills as practitioners, we increase our ability to correctly interpret the psychic information we receive, to trust our interpretations. As you practice, you become increasingly familiar with your gifts, strengths, and talents. This creates a solid ground of trust within yourself—and one that can be felt by your clients.

However, in order to trust your intuitive faculties, it is essential that you both develop your intuitive skills *and* have strong energetic boundaries and filters. Energetic boundaries are the subject of the next chapter.

THE POWER OF ACQUIRED KNOWLEDGE

What I have observed in my years of teaching individuals in the fields of intuition and subtle energy healing is that many people believe that being intuitive is enough. They believe that with strong enough psychic abilities, they can simply hang their proverbial shingle and be open for business. However, as important as intuition is, there is so much more to being a well-rounded and effective practitioner.

In my own case, I'm constantly reading, studying, and refining my knowledge and skills. Why? *Because intuition can go only as far as your mind can stretch.* You can't tell someone to take an herb if you don't know what that herb *is* or does. You can't recommend acupuncture if you have no understanding of that system. I could list hundreds of other examples, but I know you get the point. Having intuitive abilities is not an excuse to ignore or abandon the pursuit of knowledge, because our intuition often has to work *with* the knowledge that is already stored within us. Whether you are a chiropractor, massage therapist, naturopathic doctor, Reiki practitioner, intuitive coach, or another kind of practitioner dealing with the subtle realms, you must have a wide, deep body of knowledge to draw from.

In your own practice, think about the kinds of recommendations you make to your clients. What types of foods, natural remedies, physical exercises, inner-reflection activities, or other methods do you tend to suggest? What specialty disciplines have you delved into, even if informally rather than scholastically? Are you ready to expand your knowledge of these information areas? Are there additional lines of interest that might further benefit your practice or your self-healing?

After concentrating on these questions, I recommend that you prepare a training program for yourself, deciding which areas of interest you might want to further through educational programs or through your own research. Whether you've been in practice for one month or thirty years, there is always something new to learn that can benefit you and any clients. As you expand your inner intuitive capabilities and your externally derived knowledge base, your entire skill base expands.

HUMILITY

A healthy dose of humility is necessary for becoming masterful in the art of subtle energy medicine. As profound as intuition is, it should not and cannot operate alone. As a practitioner and teacher, I have found that, at best, most of us are 80 percent accurate, and we have to assume a 20 percent margin of error. On any given day, we might be energetically off, or our client might be off.

If committed to self-healing, we also need to apply the 80/20 percent yardstick to ourselves. We are simultaneously our own healer and our own client. The "healer" part of our self might receive intuitive information in a way that is different than the way our "client" self can understand. Maybe neither self likes what we're intuitively sensing, and so both of our selves distort the input. One of the ways I deal with this fact, when working on myself, is to apply yet another rule, which I call the "three-clue rule." If I receive intuitive counsel for myself or someone else, and I have any doubt about it, I ask for three signs to confirm the recommendations. Perhaps someone besides myself suggests the same path. Maybe I read the equivalent guidance in a book. Maybe I have a dream that shares the same instruction. I might also seek the counsel of other subtle energy professionals or intuitive friends to triple-check my information.

You can also apply this three-clue rule to client work. If offering intuitive advice that could be questionable or could really affect a client, I advise them to check out the data with at least two other sources and tune into their own inner wisdom. They could work with a couple other subtle energy practitioners, but I always ask clients to back up the information about therapeutic or medical issues especially with standardized measurements like medical tests or psychological evaluations. I'd like to say that intuition can always spot a tumor or a critical condition, but it can't. And I believe in some situations, it's not supposed to. In certain situations, clients need to be directed toward allopathic care, and doing so will be keeping the ethical commitments you made in the previous chapter.

With certain clients, the synergy of subtle energy work with standardized testing creates a kind of healing safety net.

Most important is to share intuitive information in a straightforward but humble way. We might be receiving accurate information, but are unable to clearly convey it, or our client might not want to hear it. The future changes every time we walk forward, making intuitive predictions highly questionable. And we can't control others' actions. Sure, we might get a sense that a particular doctor would be helpful for a client, or for ourselves, but that doctor might refuse or not be able to accept us as a patient. I constantly remind clients and myself that intuitive practices are arts, not sciences. As with a piece of art, the colors and movement of intuitive data shift and change, unlike the information of science, which likes to remain in place. Even though I share these reservations with clients, I find that they often tend to cling to intuitive insight as if it's God's words, which means that we intuitive practitioners, professional or informal, have to be truly committed to relaying intuitive guidance with great humility and with a caveat that explains its limitations.

COMMUNICATION IS KEY

The main difference between using intuition to help ourselves versus helping others is that we're not just receiving information; we're also *communicating* the information to someone else in a way that is useful, helpful, and appropriate for that person. We need not only to learn to trust our intuition and the information it sends us, but also to communicate that information in such a way that it is meaningful to those we're helping. As we communicate clearly, confidently, and appropriately with our clients, we develop the trust with them (and with ourselves) that significantly increases the effectiveness of our work.

If you are a layperson delivering subtle energy work, your informal clients might not understand exactly what you are doing because they might lack a clear description of your service. So it's important to explain the reason subtle energy works, what you are doing, and what they might do with the information or healing you are providing. If you're a layperson, you might also feel a bit squeamish or inadequate about your work. "I'm not a professional," you might say to yourself. "Who am I to be saying what I'm saying?" By explaining your practice and interactions to your client, whether the client is paying for the work or not, you are actually boosting your own self-trust and confidence in your own abilities.

TIPS FOR UNLOCKING THE ENERGY OF TRUST

As we have explored in this and the previous chapter, trust in the healing process is intimately intertwined with intention, commitment, intuition, and integrity.

More than a behavior (e.g., trusting the process, trusting the technique, trusting yourself), trust is an attitude and an interactive *energy*. Perhaps trust is also the bridge that we build by owning our gifts, practicing our skills wisely and safely, and conducting ourselves from a foundation of clearly defined values and ethics.

The following are eight things you can do to keep both trust and intuition alive and well in your practice, whether you are working with others or just working to heal yourself.

- Identify your intuitive gifts (verbal, visual, physically kinesthetic, spiritually kinesthetic).
- Determine whether you need to further develop your intuitive gifts through self-study, formal/structured training, or apprenticeship.
- Know the potentials and the limitations of your intuitive gifts.
- Know how to use your intuitive gifts in a healing context—with yourself or others. In addition to training, this requires ethical practice. Learning to use your gifts for healing or helping others often involves trial and error, but your ethics will ensure that nothing in that trial-and-error process is unsafe or costly to other people.
- Realize that while it's essential to do the work of getting trained, studying, and practicing, there always comes the point where you must let go and open to receiving intuitive information.
- Analyze the information you receive intuitively and make an assessment about how to best apply this information. Should you be offering advice about physical or emotional health? Should you share the information with a formal or informal client or simply keep it to yourself?
- Be willing to have the information you receive backed up with tests or evaluations by someone else.
- Finally, trust your inner capacities. Even the best allopathic practitioners rely on their gut instincts in certain moments. I have yet to meet someone who has said, "I should *not* have trusted my intuition!" Intuition is there because it will point us in the direction that we need to go.

7

ENERGETIC BOUNDARIES

> Healing may not be so much about
> getting better, as about letting go
> of everything that isn't you—all of
> the expectations, all of the beliefs—
> and becoming who you are.
>
> RACHEL NAOMI REMEN, MD

The subject of energetic boundaries—what they are, what they do, and how frequently you will see subtle energy issues pertaining to them—is one of the most important of this book. As you will discover, the clarity, strength, and health of our energetic boundaries directly impacts every system of the physical and subtle bodies and every level of consciousness.

Energetic boundaries are imperative for every subtle energy practitioner, professionals, informal healers, and self-healers alike. Both the lay practitioner and professional are equally susceptible to picking up others' "stuff," the main downside of poor energetic boundaries. In fact, we are all vulnerable to absorbing others' energy—physically, emotionally, mentally, or spiritually—all the time, not only when energetically working on others. We can even take on the energy of a practitioner when we are clients. Because everything is energy, it's vital that we understand these energetic parameters and learn how to establish boundaries that keep out harmful energy and attract what we need.

WHAT ARE ENERGETIC BOUNDARIES AND HOW DO THEY FUNCTION?

Our energetic boundaries act as invisible gates, keeping harmful things out of our lives and inviting helpful things into our lives. Though imperceptible to the naked eye, they mean the difference between experiencing an enjoyable, prosperous, and loving life or suffering through a sad, limited, and unhappy existence. They separate what we need from what we don't, selectively letting into our lives only those energies, people, guidance, thoughts, situations, opportunities, and healing that bring our spiritual essence further into our real lives. Our energetic boundaries also go a step further and separate us from those receiving our subtle energy treatments, enabling a healthy flow of information and energy to both of us, without entanglement. If we're doing self-healing, they insert a space between our wounded selves and our whole, healer selves, inviting clarity and objectivity.

I often describe our energetic boundaries as roadblocks staffed by conscious border patrol agents. These discerning and good-natured guards are our internal

WHEN YOU ARE THE CLIENT: An Energy Protocol

SOMETIMES THE BEST of subtle energy practitioners get mixed up. They might read intuitive information or provide subtle energy input that fits themselves, not you. They might interpret information or answers to your problems through their own experience or training and at least partially miss the mark. Perhaps they don't have well-established energetic boundaries themselves, and their own energetic issues leak out of their energy field or they pull energy from others' fields without knowing it.

We are especially vulnerable to our own energetic codependent patterns when in the position of being a client. Most of us lower our boundaries to receive the desired inspiration, assistance, and energy, or to release the energies we no longer need. We might also unconsciously start to take on practitioners' problems or send them energy in an attempt to help them.

As much as we'd like to depend on the practitioner to monitor these occurrences, we are ultimately responsible for our own boundaries. So it's good practice to establish a healthy "being the client" protocol, which can be used in other areas of life as well.

Start by being really clear about your goals. (See the "Taking AIM" worksheet in chapter 8 for more on establishing your healing goals.) Then take a few deep breaths before you enter the practitioner's office and do the following:

Visualize yourself having achieved your goal(s). Sense how different you feel physically, but also emotionally.

Ask your inner spirit to infuse your four energetic boundaries with the various colors, communiqués, and vibrations needed to allow in only the energy that will help you accomplish your goal(s). Also request that your boundaries be shifted so that they will release the blocked energies safely, causing no harm to yourself or others.

programs. They aren't supposed to keep *everything* out. They're designed to let in that which is good for us and our clients. The multilevel boundaries can, therefore, serve three basic functions:

Protection. They keep out the energies that fail to support our emotional wellbeing and spiritual essence.

Filtering. They let in the energies that enhance our spiritual essence, keep in the energy we need, and emanate the messages to the world that will only enhance our lives.

Magnetizing. Our energetic boundaries can draw what we need to us, including healing, information, guidance, people, events, jobs, money, healthy relationships, and life lessons.

Ask also that your inner spirit provide you with clarity regarding any information or healing energy offered by the practitioner.

During your session, pay attention to your intuitive senses, especially those that are body based. Information or energy that doesn't fit will feel, sound, smell, or just seem off. Quite simply, it won't connect with you. You might also experience a sensation of dread or fright, both indications that what is happening doesn't suit you. If these situations arise, you can do any or all of the following:

- Ask the practitioner for further insight or explanation.
- Tell the practitioner that you'll have to think about the information or healing solution more to see what fits for you and what doesn't.

- Suggest that the information or energy doesn't fit and ask the practitioner what he or she thinks might be going on. (Once in a while our systems resist truth because it's hard to face. This step provides the practitioner space to double-check his or her boundaries or insights, but also go a step deeper into your issues, if need be.)
- Mentally compartmentalize this information or energy so you can energetically reexamine it or dispose of it now or later. Picture yourself putting the energy into a box. Imagine an angel, guardian, the Divine, or some other helper assisting you with carrying out the box so it can be assessed later, or ask this spiritual assistant to safely dispose of it in the moment.
- If you are truly uncomfortable—and you are sure that you aren't simply "triggering" your own issues in order to avoid stress or emotions—you can always leave the room, either for a break or to end the session.

ENERGETIC BOUNDARIES AND THE AURIC FIELD

There are many types of energetic boundaries around our body, but the primary one is the auric field (see chapter 2 for a review of the auric field). This auric field contains several layers, each corresponding to one of the twelve main chakras. As we grow and evolve, our spirit activates the appropriate auric layer or energetic boundary, infusing it with the spiritual truths or programs explicitly and elegantly suited to our unique self. However, our spirit isn't the only influence on these boundaries. Our parents, relatives, ancestors, schools, religious institutions, friends, enemies, co-workers, bosses, news sources, and the culture at large also have their say—for our good or ill. Challenging life events, from the chronically negative to one-time traumas, can also keep our boundaries from fully developing or operating in harmony with our true spiritual essence.

It is useful for subtle energy practitioners to know that our clients' energetic boundaries are great transmitters of information and receivers of healing vibrations. In other words, energetic boundaries are interactive; they both take in and emit energy. That is why you can sense someone when they walk into your space, often getting a read on them before a session even begins and sensing the energy of their personality, fears, and traumas, as well as that of their needs, desires, and hopes.

FOUR TYPES OF ENERGETIC BOUNDARIES

Based on my studies, professional practice, and personal life, I have grouped the twelve auric layers or energetic boundaries into four types, based on their jobs or functions. Each type is associated with a particular color:

- Physical (red) boundaries
- Emotional (orange) boundaries
- Relational (green) boundaries
- Spiritual (white) boundaries

Within each of these boundaries are subsets of other colorations. For instance, gold and silver are members of the white family, while yellow belongs to the emotional. For an in-depth exploration of energetic boundaries and their subsets, you may want to reference my book *Energetic Boundaries: How to Stay Protected and Connected in Work, Love, and Life*.

As you learn more about energetic boundaries in the following pages, you can begin to practice noticing how these four colors (and variations of them) may appear in certain clients.

WHAT HAPPENS WHEN OUR ENERGETIC BOUNDARIES ARE VIOLATED?

As you work with clients, you are likely to find that their personal issues or health challenges are related, in part, to boundaries that have been violated in some way. When our boundaries are violated, there are three basic repercussions energetically:

Our boundaries become rigid or immobilized. Think of an icy wall. Getting near it makes us and others feel cold and shut down. Rigid energy boundaries have the same affect on others and us. People stay away, perceiving us as unavailable or disinterested in them. Our boundaries also repel potentially positive events or opportunities: promotions or new jobs, financial opportunities, referrals to the right healthcare professionals, healing energies, or friendships that might warm our hearts.

Our boundaries become permeable. A permeable boundary is loose, flimsy, and downright weak. In fact, it's almost like having no boundary at all. People with permeable boundaries are easily swept aside, ignored, used, taken advantage of, or unrewarded. These people are often the proverbial people-pleasers or doormats.

Our boundaries are sliced, diced, and cut full of holes. Gaps in our energy boundaries leave gaps in our lives, doorways through which anything and anyone can walk. We easily absorb others' energies, from diseases to poverty issues and, in so doing, lose our own life force. The more disturbing the issues in our lives, the greater the possibility that we have holes in our energy fields. In people who often find themselves in the role of victim, we will usually find energetic boundaries in this state.

Do you believe you enter client- or self-healing sessions with some of these problems in your own boundaries? If you are a practitioner, you are already aware that many clients have boundary issues. Many of the exercises in this book will assist you in healing and developing your energetic boundaries. The most important techniques for setting boundaries for self and other healing are found in chapter 9, "The Essential Energy Techniques." But you can use the steps in the next section right away to set up positive client interactions.

UPLEVELING YOUR ENERGETIC BOUNDARIES

The single most frequent question I hear from practitioners and caregivers is, "How can I keep my boundaries?" The following ten steps are practical ways to establish energetic boundaries for your work with clients. As you practice each of these ten steps, notice how it affects your energy level at the end of your work-day. You may very well find that not only are you not depleted, but your energy reserves also may actually *increase*.

Step 1: Preparation. Before work, move your body in some way (with an activity such as walking or yoga) and set a clear intention for the day. Also, let your intuition select your wardrobe, and pay extra attention to the colors you are drawn to. For example, if you find yourself reaching for red, it may be that red will help you to be forceful and to do your work with a dramatic flair. If you're going for a dark outfit, you might be dealing with a needy or angry client, and a shade of black or gray might help you to hide your personal reactions (or your entire self) so you can better assist the client.

Step 2: Setting. One of the strongest ways to set up your client room or office so that it supports your energetic boundaries is to include objects that

WORKING ON A LOVED ONE

IT CAN BE especially challenging to perform healing work on a loved one, whether you are a professional, layperson, or a student of subtle energy medicine. We always want to make someone feel better, and this motivation is exponentially increased the closer someone is to us. It's easy to overlook obvious or intuitively provided signs of a critical issue because we don't want to believe the signs are true. Conversely, we might be oversensitive to an insight because we feel compelled to perform perfectly to "save" our loved one.

I usually recommend that subtle energy practitioners of all levels refer relatives, friends, children, or others who are close to them to other practitioners. When you are unable to do this, I suggest the following:

Explain what your subtle energy process is capable and not capable of accomplishing. I use the same statements I use with new clients, including:

- "Energy is information that moves. I am working with energy that moves so fast that it is considered subtle or spiritual."
- "My intuitive and energy work is not meant to replace anything you are doing professionally or with licensed caregivers. It is a supplemental way to look at your issues and life."
- "Intuition is an art, not a science. At best, it is 80 percent accurate."
- "It is important to pay attention to what fits you or not. Just because I offer advice, that doesn't mean it is completely accurate or that you will be able to use it."
- "Ultimately my work is meant to broaden your horizons and help you examine what is occurring at a deeper level."
- "Please interrupt and ask questions whenever you need to."

hold deep meaning for you. Choose photos, art, sacred objects, gifts from nature, healing tools, and other items that resonate at a high vibrational frequency and always reflect back to you your highest ideals, your professional commitments, and your true essence. Also, at the most basic level, you will want a workspace set-up that establishes a boundary between you and your client. (Refer to the section, "Setting Up Your Workspace," for ideas on ensuring that your workspace is set up to support the best experiences and outcomes for you and your clients.)

Step 3: Protocol. If you don't already do so, consider starting your sessions with a short statement that verbally creates boundaries. For example, I tell clients my intention, which is to invite healing and to assist them. I also tell them that I ask the Divine to form parameters and boundaries, so at least I cause no harm and at best I can assist. Then I make sure they understand that I can't guarantee my work or information and that it is

Maintain a professional pose and, if possible, work in your office space. I often tell my loved one that I might seem cold and distant, but that this is because I am maintaining a professional composure in order to be as objective as possible.

Give yourself emotional support. You might intuitively receive information that is hard for you to embrace. If you discover that it is too difficult for you to manage what arises for you when working with a loved one, know that you can gently end a session or refer the loved one elsewhere for further support.

I once helped a friend who went to the emergency room with severe heart contractions. She called me, desperate. I immediately went into professional mode but struggled inside because I didn't want to "get it wrong." I was also very concerned about my friend.

I did receive intuitive insight, but made sure to say that everything I provided was simply intuitive and my friend should do only what the physicians recommended.

In this case, I was able to suggest that she run tests for a bacterial or viral infection in her heart and described two areas that might be weakened by microbes. Her physicians discovered that she did indeed have a viral infection in her heart, which had originally been weakened by strep, a bacterial infection. There were two valves that were weak.

As accurate as my assessment was, the truth is, I could have easily misinterpreted the data—or conversely, not shared any of it, because I was stuck in my own fears. Remain humble and help, but keep your common sense about you.

their job to decide what information is helpful and what is not. I also answer any questions they might have about what we're doing. Clear communications is necessary for establishing and maintaining strong energetic boundaries!

Step 4: Physical boundaries. As noted in step 2, your workspace should be set up to establish boundaries between you and your client. For example, you might have a table or desk between you and your clients (depending on the type of work you do). In my work, I pick up a lot of information from and for my clients through my physical energetic boundaries and, therefore, need a physical barrier for filtering purposes. I only do hands-on healing if I feel like I'm safe and strong that day. Sometimes I recommend that hands-on practitioners employ a cloth, gloves, or special jewelry programmed to deflect negativity and boost the healing energies. You can also take a quick break between clients to wash your hands, visualizing your client's energy being lovingly washed away so that you are refreshed and ready for the next client or activity.

Step 5: Emotional boundaries. Your imagination can support strong boundaries. Imagine a clear screen of energy between you and your clients, one that filters their emotions, so you can always discern your emotions from theirs. You can also adapt this screen according to your particular needs. For example, because my work relies on my ability to sense others' feelings and thoughts, I program my energetic screen to allow me to subtly sense their emotions, to allow those emotions to register with me, but to prevent me from taking in the energy of their emotions.

Step 6: Relational boundaries. Sometimes it can be difficult to keep from getting overinvolved in a client's problems. For example, when a child is being abused, a spouse has been abandoned, or a hard-working person has lost their job and income source, our heart can't help but go out to the other person. This is when I make sure I've disengaged my relational boundary, or heart field, at the end of a session. I do this by sensing the outer edges of this field before the client leaves the room. Try this for yourself. If you sense that your relational field (or any other layer) is not back around you, and attached only to you, conduct a few deep-breathing exercises until it is completely intact.

Step 7: Spiritual boundaries. Calling on higher guidance or the Divine to link your clients with any needed healing is a powerful way to begin and end a session. You can also request the same for yourself, so that both you and your client are energetically supported by the clearest and highest frequencies. Two techniques that you will learn about in chapter 9 have become a seamless part of my professional protocol, Spirit-to-Spirit and Healing Streams of Grace. Employing these simple practices can transform your boundaries from good to great.

Step 8: Dealing with your own issues. Ask your higher guidance to alert you when your issues are triggered during client work and to hold these issues in safekeeping for you. What I do, energetically speaking, is set the issues in a white box that I keep inside of my heart. At the end of the day, I spend a few minutes reviewing the contents of this box. Committed to doing my own work, I will say that some of these issues have then made their way to my own therapist's office!

Step 9: Coworkers. If you have business partners or employees, ask your higher guidance to hold space for your higher efforts. In addition to business partners, I sometimes have co-teachers. During meetings, workshops, or classes, I like to envision a white bubble of healing grace surrounding all concerned. This energy protects each of us, teachers and students alike, from each other, keeps our issues from blurring, and enables a safe and loving connection.

Step 10: Being done. At the end of the workday, ask your higher guidance to assist you in coming to completion for that day—to recognize, acknowledge, and release all that has occurred. I like to call upon the Divine to release me from my daily work. Very seldom do I obsess about my workday, which leaves me free to be present for the other aspects of my life.

SETTING UP YOUR WORKSPACE: THE OUTER REFLECTION OF YOUR INNER COMMITMENTS

Whether your focus is self-healing or working with others, creating an environment that is conducive to the healing process is essential. Once you have done the phenomenal work of clarifying your intentions, values, and commitments, it's the perfect time to ensure that your physical healing space is a match for them. Does your office or healing room outwardly reflect your inner intentions and ethics? The following questions can serve as your guidelines for setting up a new healing space or revamping an old one.

IS THE SPACE PRIVATE?

It doesn't matter if your healing space is situated in the corner of your house, under a lush tree in your back yard, or in a commercial office building, it needs to be a *contained* space. This is one of the ways that your internal boundaries are reflected externally. Work with the container of your space (the visible boundaries of it) so that only positive subtle energies can be at work and play. As *Star Trek*'s Captain Kirk would say, you don't want "The Trouble with Tribbles"—you don't want to allow annoying or destructive little energies to infiltrate and diminish the high-vibration environment you wish to provide. Buoyed by your clear intentions and boundaries, subtle energies can be exponentially strengthened rather than disbanded or disintegrated. Like creates like, so the more uplifting healing energy you intentionally generate and invite, the more you have available to you.

IS THE SPACE UNCLUTTERED?

Environments and objects hold and emit subtle energy. Methods such as the Chinese system of feng shui (see chapter 24) show that we are continuously affected by what surrounds us. One of the foundational theories of feng shui is that chi, or universal energy, is encouraged or limited, depending on many different factors. To create a healing space that supports the free flow of chi and welcomes transformation for your clients and yourself, ensure that it is free of clutter.

DOES THE SPACE CONTAIN BEAUTY?

One of the most potent ways to shift the energy of any room or space is to intentionally infuse it with beauty. In addition to the beauty that can be crafted by your selection of furniture, carpet, curtains, and other basic components, include objects that have meaning for you, such as art, sacred objects, or amulets that hold the resonance you wish to support. Of course, you can also choose to include beautiful objects that possess perceptible, natural healing properties, such as plants, flowers, crystals, gemstones, water fountains, and even the tools of your trade.

DO YOU HAVE THE TOOLS OF YOUR TRADE?

Speaking of tools, be sure to regularly take inventory and make sure that you are well-stocked with any of the items that allow you to do your work and function with ease, elegance, and confidence. Depending on your methods, you might have some of the following: tissues, essential oils, flower essences, massage oils, clean sheets for your bodywork table, acupuncture needles, and drinking water.

If you discover mid-session that you don't have a particular tool or material that you need, or if you know that you're running low on something, it can cause a bit of free-floating anxiety that can detract from the energetic experience you want to provide. Being well stocked is an important way to take care of yourself and your clients.

IS THE SPACE PHYSICALLY AND ENERGETICALLY CLEAN?

In addition to keeping your space clutter-free, as noted in question 2, it's also essential to keep it physically and energetically *clean*. Beyond removing piles of paper or stacks of dusty books, set an intention to clean your space on a consistent basis. Open the windows to air it out. Let the sunlight stream in, if you can. Because my healing space doesn't have a window, I use a full-spectrum light bulb during the long winter months. In addition to vacuuming, sweeping, and dusting, make a practice of continually releasing emotions and other energies. I do it mentally, through my intention for a clean, clear space. You can also cleanse through prayer, meditative techniques, burning sage or lemongrass, lighting a candle, or even posting a guardian angel or other spirit guide at the door. In any case, all cleansing and clearing techniques come back to intention. So choose the ones that you enjoy and that work for you.

SAYING NO

SOMETIMES THE BEST boundary a subtle energy practitioner can set is a practical one: we can decline to use our skills if we are not in a safe position—physically, energetically, mentally, and emotionally—to do so.

Like doctors and nurses who are often asked to give medical advice outside the office, subtle energy practitioners are asked to give intuitive insights or perform energy work in informal settings. When people know you're an intuitive or a subtle energy practitioner, they will often believe everything you say is authentic, accurate information, even if you haven't taken the time to really focus, protect yourself, and warn them not to overempower the intuitive input, as described in chapter 6.

This is one of the reasons I hardly ever use my intuitive gifts in an informal setting. Yes, sometimes people get mad. One of my best friends once asked me to check in on a situation for one of her friends when we were out to dinner. I said no, and my friend was upset. But I knew it was better to upset someone than to incompletely administer advice and potentially compromise my safety, my ethical standards, and the recipient's wellbeing.

WHAT IS THE RESONANCE OF YOUR HEALING SPACE?

As you tend to each of the points above, you are shaping the energy, resonance, and reverberation of your healing space. One of the most effective ways to change or up-level the resonance of your space is to play music that is carefully chosen to help set the emotional and energetic tone. In addition to the tangible items and action steps we have covered, there are also the immeasurables—feeling states such as hope, peace, optimism, and love that you can intentionally infuse into your healing space. What other immeasurables are important to you and in alignment with your intentions and commitments?

PREPARING TO HEAL SELF OR OTHERS
SETTING GOALS

[I]f I can ease one life the aching,
Or cool one pain,
Or help one fainting robin
Unto his nest again,
I shall not live in vain.

EMILY DICKINSON

When preparing to heal yourself or another, all of the philosophical questions *about* healing turn into a quest *for* healing. The quest is one of activating and bringing to the surface that underlying wholeness. So what is the key to this activation?

What I have usually found is that the real shifts—whether they are physical, emotional, relational, or another type—begin once the client is able to accept some level of self-responsibility. If we're engaged in self-healing, the shifts usually begin to happen when we ourselves accept some level of self-responsibility. In either case, we must understand that self-responsibility is not about self-blaming. We must avoid the trap of "I caused a problem." The root cause of the problem might be genetic, or stemming from a childhood trauma, or spurred on by an accident. Even if our wounds were self-inflicted, what I have seen in working with many thousands of individuals is that we usually didn't know better at the time.

One of the most empowering perceptions we can hold is the assumption of wholeness rather than guilt. If we are a practitioner, this attitude sets the resonance for healing to take place. If we are a client, it is the precursor to deciding not to wait for someone else to do the healing for us. When we stop blaming ourselves, a healing shift in consciousness can get underway.

FROM SELF TO OTHER: DEEPENING EMPATHY

For practitioners, understanding the significance of self-responsibility marks the beginning of true empathy. In working with others, it is important to understand that pain is sometimes the doorway for change. Even if the urge to swoop in and "save" someone bubbles up, we must instead acknowledge that the other will not change (in the way their soul may intend) unless they, not us, take responsibility for owning the healing process, while remembering that ownership has nothing to do with self-recrimination. If we are our own client, we must simultaneously assume responsibility for our own issues and be kind to ourselves.

We can't fix another's dilemmas, nor can we assume responsibility for their outcomes. What we can assume responsibility for is *how* we work with them. We can assume responsibility for our integrity, attitude, knowledge base, and commitment to do our best.

COMMITTING TO THE HEALING PROCESS: OPENING TO THE MIRACLES

Paradoxically, showing up strong, clear, and competent as practitioners is what allows us to get out of the way and allow the healing current to flow. In truth, the healing is done by something bigger than us. Whether we relate to that power as a force beyond us or simply as the greater part of ourselves, the impact of subtle energy is anything but subtle. In some way, all healing is a miracle—a big or small miracle.

When we're in the role of client or patient working with a practitioner, or when we're acting as our own self-healer, doing our part and welcoming self-responsibility eventually comes down to specific and tangible behaviors. For example, if I have some weight to lose, Spirit will come in to help me, but I have to do my part and not eat the cake. If I'm working on myself, I have to differentiate between fantasy and reality. There might be a miracle available, but I'm only setting myself up for disappointment if I expect overnight success.

As subtle-energy healers, one of the key ways we commit to the healing process is to set reasonable goals, both for ourselves and with our clients. This always starts with being aware of what is actually within our own control. Our job is to take care of the following:

- Training and practice
- Knowledge and understanding
- Perception and attitude
- Intention and commitment
- Self-care and encouraging self-care in others

Beyond that, energy will do what energy is going to do. In my own practice, I have been reminded again and again that subtle energy is extraordinarily powerful. Our goals must be set based on what we can define and move toward. And as we open the doorway to the potency of subtle energy, *more* may actually happen than what we, or our clients, anticipate. In that regard, we always have the wonderful opportunity to be open to the miracle at the heart of all healing, while keeping our feet grounded in the world of the utterly practical.

MANAGING EXPECTATIONS

Early in my career, I thought that I had failed if a client dealing with a life-threatening illness wasn't miraculously and instantly healed. (No pressure there, right?) I remember working with a woman who had stage-four cancer. One of our first sessions together was so powerful that both of us left the room thinking that the cancer would be gone by the next day. And yet it wasn't. There was improvement with her cancer right away, but I distinctly remember the feeling of wanting it to be entirely cured overnight. It turned out to be an eye-opening moment in my career. Although I'm happy to report that this client did eventually heal completely, it was the gradual improvements she made along the way—and the unpredictable timing of the healing process—that were some of my greatest teachers.

Working with subtle energy, we don't know what is going to improve or when. I once worked with a woman who had lung cancer. Although her cancer didn't disappear overnight either, she discovered that she had actually grown taller after our first few sessions together! Her spine had actually straightened out. She also found herself experiencing moments of inexplicable joy, even in the midst of dealing with cancer. These disparate and unpredictable signs of healing perhaps pointed to a rebalancing that was taking place on different levels, as her cancer eventually went into complete remission.

What makes working with subtle energy so uncanny is that you don't really know *what* is going to shift or what is going to *cause* the shift. For instance, I have found that sometimes subtle energy medicine enabled clients' healing by making their allopathic treatments more effective. This is an example of why managing our expectations as subtle energy practitioners is inestimably important. The energy work may not be the method that heals a client, but it may enable them to be receptive to a conventional treatment protocol—and markedly more peaceful while going through it.

As subtle energy practitioners, we concentrate on what we *can do*—what we *can work with*. But we can't make promises. Energy has a life of its own. Again, working with the subtle body may allow surgery to go more smoothly, or it may facilitate an openness that helps someone to embrace their emotions. It might also connect a client to their inner wisdom, allowing them to approach their situation with greater equanimity, confidence, or clarity.

BEYOND DIAGNOSING: THE POWER OF A HEALING PLAN

As subtle energy practitioners, we cannot legally diagnose an illness or condition; that must be left to licensed healthcare professionals. Even licensed practitioners who integrate subtle energy work into their practices can't *precisely* diagnose when working within the realm of the subtle body. For example, a doctor of Oriental medicine (an OMD) might assess that your Liver meridian is stagnant, but they can't say, "You have liver cancer, and here is the protocol that will get rid of it." Also, they cannot say that they can cure cancer. The OMD must accept the limitations of working with subtle energies.

As subtle energy practitioners, we just can't make promises to our clients, but we have something even better, and stronger, than promises: we have commitments. So rather than making promises, we can start by making a commitment to managing ourselves—managing our own internal process (which might include processing our beliefs, agendas, and projections, as well as tending to our energetic boundaries, for starters), and managing the practices and protocols we use with our clients. There is no guarantee what the outcomes will be and what our tools and techniques will do for others. The results may be less than what we, or our clients, are hoping for, or *the results may be more.* In any case, by understanding and acknowledging the nature of subtle energy medicine, we are better able to get out of the way and let the healing take its course in whatever way the energy chooses.

Rather than diagnose, subtle energy healers utilize their training and skills to accomplish the following:

- Accurately analyzing what is occurring in the subtle realms
- Remaining flexible about *how* to work with the subtle energies—about which tools and techniques to draw upon
- Working in collaboration with clients to set reasonable goals

SETTING REASONABLE GOALS AND MARKING PROGRESS: TAKING AIM

If you, as a subtle energy practitioner, are (1) grounded in the importance of self-responsibility (yours and your client's), (2) focused on the imbalance or challenge that has presented itself, and (3) clear about the tools and techniques you are going to proceed with, it is time to set goals with your client.

Whether you are working on your own self-healing or with a client, it is important to set *reasonable* goals. Rather than setting yourself up to fail by creating potentially grandiose goals (where the progress isn't good enough or big enough), set yourself up to win. In determining your goals, I recommend "taking AIM"— in other words, basing each of your goals on the following criteria:

- Is this goal achievable?
- Is this goal important?
- Is this goal measurable?

Taking AIM is a practical and effective way to approach goals for healing on every level, be it physical, emotional, spiritual, relational, psychological, or mental. For example, on the relational level, you might be working with your client to set goals for their intimate relationship with their spouse or how they conduct themselves socially. Mentally, goals might be focused on their belief system, their thinking process, or how to express what they have learned. Or, on the psychological level, goals could be focused on inner-child work or the deep issues involved with becoming a healthier and more integrated human being, such as identifying the interpretations and perceptions that are having the greatest impact on their health and life.

I believe that progress is being made when we see some measurable success in any of these core areas. In other words, if your client is experiencing progress in any part of their life, you are being effective.

However, you also don't want to see a slip in any of those areas, which is one of the reasons that goal-setting is so valuable. Setting achievable, important, and measurable goals will prove to be one of the best tools in your subtle energy medicine bag, which we will continue to add to chapter by chapter.

The worksheet on pages 100 and 101 can be used when you are beginning to work with a new client or when you reach a new healing phase with an existing client. If you are performing self-healing, you can change the pronouns and use the worksheet to evaluate and set healing goals for yourself. Obtaining a more objective viewpoint will only benefit you.

On page 102 is a separate worksheet that you can use to remind clients of key steps they've agreed to take outside of your session work with them.

TAKING AIM: CLIENT GOAL-SETTING WORKSHEET

Step 1: Clarifying the presenting problem
Write down your initial understanding of your client's presenting problem.

Step 2: Assessing the bigger picture
Interview your client to discover their level of satisfaction, fulfillment, or happiness within each of the primary areas of life, with 0 being no satisfaction and 5 being high satisfaction.

Body/health	0	1	2	3	4	5
Business/career	0	1	2	3	4	5
Money and financial wellbeing	0	1	2	3	4	5
Friendship/community	0	1	2	3	4	5
Family life	0	1	2	3	4	5
Home/physical environment	0	1	2	3	4	5
Love/romance/partnership	0	1	2	3	4	5
Fun/recreation	0	1	2	3	4	5
Spirituality/personal growth	0	1	2	3	4	5
Purpose/meaning/contribution	0	1	2	3	4	5

Step 3: Identifying top priorities and objectives
Based on the information gathered in Step 1 and Step 2, what are your client's top one to three priorities in their healing work with you? What matters most to them right now and in the future? List these priorities in order of the importance your client has expressed:

1.

2.

3.

TAKING AIM: CLIENT GOAL-SETTING WORKSHEET

Step 4: Taking AIM—setting achievable, important, and measurable goals

Goal #1:

Timeframe:

In-session plan (techniques, tools, processes):

At-home plan (specific action steps, regular activities, processes):

Goal #2:

Timeframe:

In-session plan (techniques, tools, processes):

At-home plan (specific action steps, regular activities, processes):

Goal #3:

Timeframe:

In-session plan (techniques, tools, processes):

At-home plan (specific action steps, regular activities, processes):

Step 5: Marking your progress

Based on the number of sessions you and your client agree to do together, assess and track their progress with each stated goal during each session. Here is a basic template for marking and staying mindful of their progress.

Goal #1/Session #2

Measurable change:

Client action(s) taken:

Client's level of satisfaction on the 0 to 5 scale: 0   1   2   3   4   5

TAKING AIM: CLIENT GOAL-SETTING WORKSHEET

Goal #1/Session #3

Measurable change:

Client action(s) taken:

Client's level of satisfaction on the 0 to 5 scale: 0 1 2 3 4 5

Goal #1/Session #4

Measurable change:

Client action(s) taken:

Client's level of satisfaction on the 0 to 5 scale: 0 1 2 3 4 5

Practitioner Notes
Client's at-home assignments for health and wellbeing

Date assigned:	Date assigned:	Date assigned:
Activity or action step:	Activity or action step:	Activity or action step:

TAKING AIM: CLIENT REMINDERS

This is what I (the client) am agreeing to do:

Date assigned:

Activity or action step:

Next session date and time:

Date assigned:

Activity or action step:

Next session date and time:

Date assigned:

Activity or action step:

Next session date and time:

9

THE ESSENTIAL ENERGY TECHNIQUES

The winds of grace blow all the time.
All we need to do is set our sails.

RAMAKRISHNA

One of the things I enjoy about subtle energy medicine and intuitive healing work is that I never do it alone! Grounding myself in the natural world, rooting myself to the earth, and calling on the invisible forces of clarity, compassion, and divine guidance are truly essential to my practice. The energy techniques contained within this chapter are *elemental* for me now, like breathing in air. Having taught them to my apprenticeship students over the years, I see the difference they make for many practitioners in the effectiveness of their treatments, as well as in their overall enjoyment and satisfaction in their work.

These techniques are elegantly simple and can be applied across the wide spectrum of modalities outlined throughout this book. Although I won't explicitly tell you each time you might find these tools (from the Light Wand to Healing Streams of Grace to the Five Steps to Grounding) most useful, know that you can dig into this treasure chest any time you want to complement any exercise in this book.

As you will see, these energy techniques will help you to keep your energy clear and flowing, assist you in being receptive to intuitive guidance, strengthen your energetic boundaries, and protect you from energies that could be draining (whether those energies are emotional, psychic, or electromagnetic in nature). They will also support you in experiencing more of the wonder of healing work, the beauty of collaborating with higher consciousness (be it your own or that of a spirit guide), and the joy of interacting with others on our journey back to wholeness.

SPIRIT-TO-SPIRIT: THE THREE-STEP TECHNIQUE FOR HIGH-VIBRATION HEALING

I developed this exercise to use during sessions with clients, but have gone on to employ it in every area of my life. At workshops, I teach it to professional healers, doctors, nurses, therapists, and intuitives, and afterward, most of them say, "This is the only technique I really need—for *anything!*"

Spirit-to-Spirit is a three-step process for establishing the spiritual borders needed to engage in any activity with another person or a group. They ensure clean and pure boundaries, leaving us able to receive highly accurate and clear information, guidance, directives, or healing for ourselves or to offer to another person.

I also suggest you use this exercise whenever you are engaged with a client or group that is sending you into an energetic tailspin, causing you to lose your personal or professional sense of self. It will immediately shift your energetic boundaries, disengage unhealthy connections, support loving bonds, and call in the assistance of a greater presence.

The three steps of Spirit-to-Spirit:

1. Affirm that you are a full, powerful, and loving spiritual being. Breathe into your heart while making this affirmation, and feel the resulting shifts in your energetic fields.

2. Affirm that the other person is also a fully developed and loving spiritual being. Sense the presence of his or her personal spirit and engage with this aspect of the other. Feel how the unhealthy connections release and only love remains. (This step can also be done between you and an entire group of people, such as your family or business community, or even between you and an animal.)

3. Call upon the presence of the Great or Holy Spirit, which immediately shifts the situation into whatever it is supposed to be, providing any necessary insight, protection, healing, or act of grace.

Can you still use this process outside of the professional setting, such as when you're by yourself? Absolutely. When I'm alone, I do the following for step 2: I affirm the presence of a spiritual guide, angel, or master who is there to love and assist me. Personally, I use Christ. Several of my clients call upon the Virgin

Mother Mary; others affirm a quality of the Divine, and still others connect with the Buddha, the goddess Kwan Yin, or a guardian angel. If in doubt, ask for the Divine to attend you in step 2 as well as in step 3.

HEALING STREAMS OF GRACE: THE UNSTOPPABLE FLOW OF EMPOWERED LOVE

The technique that I call Healing Streams of Grace is one of my most treasured allies in my counseling work. In fact, it is far more than a technique for me; it's become more like a state of being that permeates how I work and how I interact

THE FIVE STEPS FOR GROUNDING

THE EXERCISES AND techniques in this chapter and throughout the book will help you gain access to many different sources of information and healing—such as intuitive, energetic, emotional, mental, or other invisible frequencies coming from your clients, your higher guidance, or your innermost self. For each of us, the subtle nature of this information is sometimes difficult to see, feel, and interpret.

The following five steps for grounding can serve as your access point to uncovering the invisible. You can utilize them at the start and conclusion of any process, exercise, or work session. Incorporating these steps into your work on a consistent basis will help you to maintain your energetic boundaries, access your intuition, and remain clear and receptive throughout your work day.

Step 1: Grounding. Grounding is the process of bringing yourself fully into your body and linking with the natural world. When grounded, you will be able to feel all parts of your physical body, from your toes to your head. You will also be able to feel the full extension of your energy system, including parts of you above and below your feet and head.

Step 2: Centering. Centering is the process of bringing yourself to your center, or middle. To be centered is to be fully connected to the part of your body that serves as the meeting ground for all your energies. This meeting ground is usually found within the abdomen, solar plexus, or heart.

Step 3: Protecting. Protecting is the process of clearing, repairing, and erecting energetic boundaries in order to keep yourself safe. The safer you feel regarding visible and invisible elements or beings, the more heightened your intuitive abilities will be.

Step 4: Opening. Opening is the process of opening your energy centers. Once you have opened to these centers, you can accomplish what you set out to accomplish. You may remain open after an exercise (if you are appropriately protected) or choose to close back down when finished.

Step 5: Closing. Closing is the reverse of opening. It includes appropriately closing (or partially closing) energy centers, reprotecting, centering, and grounding.

with clients throughout each day, whether I'm working with them in person or over the phone.

For me, the healing streams are incredibly practical, while deeply moving and inspiring too. Grace, as a force of the Divine, is empowered love. It is love in motion, continually available to us in every moment and ready to be used for our greatest benefit. We could say that the overflow of this empowered love is the divine tributary that we can access in any situation, for any reason. And allowing that love to do its job is the greatest type of subtle energy medicine in the universe.

As I invoke this energy in my work, I perceive it as infinite streams of grace or healing waves. Not simply "energetics," the streams are conscious aspects of the Divine; they are living. My job, whether I'm healing myself or another, is to open to the needed streams of grace. This is why I don't decide which streams are needed and what they need to do. I let Spirit decide. Spirit might assign one stream to my cause, and spirit might assign many streams. When I ask for streams to be put in place, I trust that they will do whatever is needed. Because they flow from the infinite, I figure they are smarter than me. But that doesn't mean that there is no skill involved in working with the streams. As with all techniques described in this book, the human element is an important part of the equation.

Although there are no limits to how you can use the healing streams with your clients, here are a few of the ways that I frequently employ this technique.

Illness. If you are working with an illness, or with a manifestation of an illness, such as a tumor, you can ask that the organisms of the illness be replaced with healing streams of grace.

Medications. If you are working with someone who is on medications (whether allopathic or natural), you can infuse the medicine with grace so that the medicine is most optimally useful.

Emotional and mental blocks. If you are working with a client who is struggling with an emotional or mental block, you can ask that the block be dissipated by or replaced with a healing stream or wave.

Energy clearing. If your work involves energetic clearing, such as cord-release work, you can ask the Divine to substitute a stream of grace for that particular interference.

Addiction at the psycho-spiritual level. If you're working with someone who is struggling with an addiction, you can ask that the aspect of the person that holds the emotional or spiritual wound be bathed in healing streams of grace.

Addiction at the physiological level. When working with an addiction, you can envision the healing streams of grace serving as an antidote or medicine that responds to the physiological compulsion taking place in the brain. You can ask that the streams soothe the neurological response.

Protection. If a client is in need of protection (or if you don't feel safe at some level while working on someone), ask to be surrounded with a bubble, sheath, or wave of protection made of the healing streams—the strongest protection available.

As you can see from these examples, there is no need to label the stream that is needed. Calling on the healing streams of grace is a way to step into that place of compassion, actively holding an intention for the best outcome for each client, and let Spirit do the rest.

THE GATEKEEPER: PREVENTING INTERFERENCE, ASSURING LOVE

A gatekeeper is a being sent from and appointed by the Divine to protect and guide you. A gatekeeper might be the Divine or any other divinely sanctioned being that guards your boundaries and psyche and invites in only that which is good for you. A gatekeeper undertakes many tasks. These include:

- Regulating the flow of psychic information inside and outside of you.
- Helping you pay attention to necessary messages or energies from both psychic and sensory sources.
- Attracting and summoning help and energies that are supportive.
- Protecting you from harmful energies, information, and sources; deciding which sources might communicate with us.
- Selecting which personal prayers and questions should be directed to which external sources (a client, a loved one, oneself).
- Overriding you if you might harm yourself or someone else.
- Building your self-esteem and capabilities.
- Helping you learn your lessons in a gentle way.
- Encouraging you to heal your own issues.
- Strengthening your connection with the Divine.

In qualifying a gatekeeper or other psychic contact, sometimes we search for intuitive inspiration; other times, it simply comes to us. How can you tell what is worth paying attention to or not? Even more importantly, what is dangerous versus helpful psychic information—or for that matter, harmful versus healing energy? The key is to qualify the source. You can determine the validity of a potential gatekeeper or any psychic source by first analyzing it completely. This will tell us if it is compatible with you.

Use the following steps to find and qualify a gatekeeper or other psychic source.

Step 1: The request. Seclude yourself in a quiet place, and make sure you won't be disturbed for the duration of this exercise. Now breathe deeply, ground, and center. Establish your psychic boundaries, set the intention to meet a gatekeeper, and fully open your chakras. Bring your concentration to your fifth chakra (throat chakra), and ask the Divine to connect you with a gatekeeper, or spiritual guide, who can serve as your celestial filter and psychic information interpreter. You can make this request through your thoughts, aloud, or through your chosen form of prayer.

Step 2: The introduction. Now ask the Divine to introduce you to this appointed gatekeeper, helping you to intuitively see, hear, and sense it.

Step 3: The connection and agreement. If you are absolutely confident in this being's ability to represent the Divine, as well as your own needs and interests, continue this communication with questions of your own. Decide if you would like to employ this being as a gatekeeper in everyday life. If so, discuss the various ways you can further this spiritual relationship and then close the line of communication when you feel complete. If you have any concerns, however, conduct step 2 again to qualify the gatekeeper before cementing the agreement.

SIX STEPS TO SETTING A NEW INTENTION

For the subtle energy practitioner, an intention is a conscious decision made for healing the self or another. It is one of the most vital tools in your medicine bag and can be used in nearly every setting to establish goals for your healing. The following six steps can be used at any point before, during, or after a session, in connection with your healing objectives.

1. Focus on your perceived need.

2. Take a slow, deep breath, centering your attention in your heart.

3. Now ask your higher guidance to completely cleanse you (and your client, if applicable) of any old intentions, agendas, beliefs, or energies that

might be in the way of a bright, new intention that can better serve you at this time.

4. Allow a new intention to arise within you, seeing the impact you would like your work with subtle energy to have. Sense, feel, embrace, visualize, or otherwise fully experience this new intention.

5. Create a ball of light in your mind's eye and visualize within it your intention, along with the full sensation of it. See this ball of light within your heart. Allow yourself to see or feel how this newly established intention flows from your heart, expressing your highest values and commitments through your words, actions, and healing resonance.

6. Release this intention to your higher guidance and commit to paying attention to any information, guidance, or signs you receive that will support positive activity on your part.

Special step: Create an intention journal that is dedicated solely to writing about your intentions—intentions for your work, body, health, love and relationship, life purpose, money, creative expression, or any other area of your life. Your intention journal can help you to expand your awareness of how you are focusing your thoughts and what kind of outcomes you're experiencing in relationship to your awareness.

USING INTENTION TO BLESS AN OBJECT

The following is an adaptation of the six intention steps you just learned, but this time used for blessing an object that is a part of your healing toolkit while simultaneously clearing your energetic boundaries.

1. Hold or think about the object you are going to use (e.g., a stone, crystal, pendulum).

2. Clear your mind of everything you've been thinking about.

3. Center in your heart.

4. Sense any feelings, thoughts, experiences, people, resentments, or obstacles that might be compromising your energetic boundaries, especially in relationship to your healing work.

5. Release these factors, allowing your own spirit or the Divine to flush them out of your system and your energetic boundaries.

6. Now ask the Divine to completely cleanse you and this object of all intentions, decisions, or energies that might interfere with the process of healing.

7. Reflect on the new intention you would like to set. Sense, feel, embrace, visualize, or otherwise fully experience this new intention.

8. Create a ball of light in your mind's eye and visualize this intention, along with the full sensation of it, being inserted into this object. You can feel this new intention flow from your heart down through your arms and hands and into the object.

9. Acknowledge that this object now carries the energy of your intention and that holding, carrying, or thinking about the object will reenergize your new intention.

10. Believe that the Divine is accessible through this object, flowing through it for the healing benefit of all concerned.

THE LIGHT WAND

From an energetic perspective, everything is made of sound (sonic waves) or light (electromagnetic radiation). Based on this simple yet powerful knowledge, one of my favorite tools for distant healing work is the light wand—an energetic wand. Students in my apprenticeship training program learn to use the light wand to bring the energy of the shaman into their practices, as it is a modern shaman's tool for conducting universal healing energy. (Practitioners can also use a sound wand for healing. For more information on the healing properties of sound and light, see chapters 21 and 22, respectively.)

Whether you are working with a client in person or at a distance, the light wand is a brilliantly simple way to focus and direct healing energies and intention. You can also choose to incorporate the light wand into your practice in the way that best suits your goals and the flow of your work. For instance, you might choose to use the light wand at the beginning of a session, at the end of a session, or as a stand-alone healing practice. However you choose to use it, here are the basic steps for doing so:

Step 1: Grounding and centering. Using the power of your breath, take a moment to ground and center yourself. Then attune to the person you are working with, whether they are in your office or on another continent.

Step 2: Choosing your sending and receiving hands. Now imagine that you are holding a wand in each hand; one is for sending healing energy, and the other is for receiving or collecting energy. (You can choose which hand is responsible for the sending and which for the receiving.)

Step 3: Opening to universal healing energy. Imagine that the wand in your sending hand is a wand of light that is a conduit of universal energy. This pure energy is received through your heart chakra, where it travels down your arm, through your wand, and into the person you are treating.

Step 4: Sending light energy. Envision the light passing through the wand and directly into or toward your client's area of distress or their issue. (Although the light wand is often used for specific physical ailments or wound healing, it can also be used to transform emotional, mental, or situational blockages.)

Step 5: Collecting old energies. Imagine that whatever energy needs to be released by your client is collected by the wand that is in your receiving hand. See that old energy collected into a ball of energy that will be released after that session. It is crucial to know that the receiving wand doesn't allow this old energy to enter into your energy field or physical body, but instead holds this energy for later release.

Step 6: Releasing and clearing energy. Once your session is complete, it is time to release the collected energy into the universe, where it can be recycled. Every practitioner is partial to his or her own methods of releasing energy. Those who are very tactile can select a rock, crystal, or gemstone to deposit the energy into. Others prefer to symbolically place their receiving wand in a bowl of water with baking soda or in a sunny spot outdoors. Each of these is a way to merge the subtle energies with the physical domain. My preferred method of releasing and clearing energy is through decision-making, which is deeper than intentionality and a fast way to transform energy.

FREEDOM FROM INHIBITING ENERGETIC CONTRACTS

As we are exploring throughout this book, and as you likely observe with your clients, there are many types of energetic influences that result in lost energy, physical and emotional imbalances, the acceptance of others' toxic energy, and the ability to tolerate all sorts of harmful connections. Here is a list of some of the most common energetic restrictions and what they look like psychically.

Cords are energetic contracts or connections that intuitively appear like garden hoses. The older and more limiting the cord, the thicker the tubing. Energy flows through the middle of these cords. If you psychically read this energy, you can interpret the nature of the contract. Yellow energy, for instance, means exchange of beliefs; orange might indicate that feelings are being swapped. You know you have an energy cord if you can't detach from a certain person, group, or system no matter how hard you try. Certain cords or codependent contracts are held in place or vibrate in circular form. If the energy is spiraling clockwise, it is bringing energy (most likely undesirable energy) into you. If counterclockwise, it is costing you energy.

Life-energy cords look a lot like regular energetic cords, but are psychically red or orange in color because the energy flowing through is basic life energy. These cords can exist between parts of the self, such as current life and a past-life self, or between a person and any other individual or group. Life-energy cords work like wires running off a mainframe to deliver electricity to different end users, thus splitting your basic life energy into several streams going to several outlets. Energy depletion, chronic or severe illnesses, chronic fatigue, and adrenal problems usually stem from life-energy cords.

Codependent contracts or bargains are unique cords usually formed between a parent and child to engender a two-way flow of energy. We create these in order to ensure our survival while in the womb or during our infancy. They basically assert that we will take on another's energy in exchange for giving away our own.

Curses look like tubules of thick, dark filaments bound together. They, too, can run between a person and any other individual or group. Curses are not empty at the center; the energy is bound in the tubes themselves. Curses hold many diseases or sexual and monetary disorders in place.

Bindings are elastic-like bands that connect at least two beings. A binding keeps the beings stuck together, usually lifetime after lifetime. Unlike cords, they might not involve an exchange of energy, merely a gluing together of two or more souls.

Energy markers look like clumps of counterclockwise, swirling charges forming a symbol, most often an X. This symbol will instruct others how to treat the marked. For instance, if you're always treated disrespectfully, no matter your behavior, you might have an energy marker. An energy marker on one field will affect all other fields. See chapter 23 for more on the helpful and unhelpful effects of different symbols on the subtle energy system.

Miasms are energetic fields that program a group of souls or family members; miasms often create disease patterns within family systems. To check for a miasm, look for brown areas in the red physical boundaries. These areas will have a cross-stitch pattern and a cord that travels backward in time to an ancestor or an event that occurred a long time ago.

Filaments are energy strands that connect pathways or layers of realities. Many healers move filaments and, by doing so, open an entryway to the energy or forces of a previously unexposed pathway.

Implants are energetic devices that are usually carried over from a past life. While an energetic marker looks like an X, an implant will appear like a mechanical device of nearly any size or shape. This is because it most likely started as a mechanical device inserted in a victim's physical body in a previous incarnation; it will have been programmed by authority figures in order to either control or use the victim's gifts or prevent them from using their powers. Even though, in the current lifetime, the implants are no longer physically present, they often continue to function according to their original design and can block the flow of physical energy, leading to soreness, tumors, tension, and restricted access to the spiritual gifts. They can also allow others to tap into the victim's spiritual and life energies and use those energies for themselves.

RELEASING ENERGY CONTRACTS

This exercise can be used to release energy contracts of all kinds, from cords to filaments. It centers on determining the *payoff*, or the reason we are holding onto our end of the contract, as well as the healing streams of grace.

Conduct this exercise for yourself or another while in a meditative state. Ask first to psychically perceive the intrusive contract. Now ask these questions of yourself or the client, changing pronouns as necessary:

- Am I one of the original creators of this contract, or is something or someone else?
- If I did not create it, how did I come to receive it?
- If I did enter this agreement, when did I do so? For what reason?
- What is the nature of the contractual agreement? What am I giving? What am I receiving?
- How is this contract affecting me? How is it affecting others around me or in the contract?
- What do I need to know to release myself from, to change, or to better use this contract? What feelings must I understand or express? What beliefs must I accept? What energy must I release or accept? What power or gift must I be willing to accept or use?
- What forgiveness or grace must I allow myself or the other(s) involved?
- Am I now ready for this healing? If not, why or when will I be?

- Am I ready to accept full protection so I can safely live my purpose in this world?

If you work through these questions and find yourself willing to release the contract, I suggest using the following exercise for accepting a healing stream of grace:

1. When you are absolutely willing to release the contract, ask the Divine to substitute a healing stream of grace for it.

2. Accept the gift of this stream of grace, acknowledging it as perfect for you.

3. Ask the Divine to cleanse you of any remnants or effects of the contract.

4. Ask the Divine to provide a healing stream of grace for all others concerned in this contract.

5. Ask the Divine to now heal you internally and to restore your energetic boundaries so you can now live freely and in harmony with divine will.

6. Feel the gratitude that accompanies this life change.

For additional exercises on releasing cords and shifting energetic fields, see chapter 13, "Modern Esoteric Healing," specifically the sections "Uncovering Your Storyline" and "The Vivaxis: Your Earth-Energy Body."

10

WHAT TO EXPECT FROM A SESSION

> It's supposed to be a professional
> secret, but I'll tell you anyway.
> We doctors do nothing . . .
> We are at best when we give the
> doctor who resides within each
> patient a chance to go to work.
>
> ALBERT SCHWEITZER, MD

This is a special chapter for those of you offering subtle energy work to others and anyone receiving subtle energy work. The purpose is to clue you in to the many experiences that can occur during and after a subtle energy session.

One of your critical jobs as a practitioner is to understand what is occurring energetically in your client, yourself, and the environment. This three-way task can be arduous, but it is simplified when you know how to set up a session and what to look for during and after one. In essence, this chapter outlines a formula for a subtle energy session, and you can adapt this formula to suit your practice and personality. It will guide you, step by step, through a session protocol, beginning with the intake process and ending with ways to debrief a client post-session.

If you are a client, you might be fascinated (and educated) by the possible reactions to energy work. When receiving energy work, I often like to remind myself about what might occur so I can track changes and adjust my expectations.

CLIENT INTAKE

It can be helpful to ask certain questions of your client to ascertain if you are the correct practitioner for the work ahead. An intake questionnaire can also determine the nature of your interactions and the direction you might take with your energy work. Finally, it can pinpoint challenges that might deter you from working with the client.

Suggested intake questions include the following:

- What do you expect from this session?
- What are the issues you would like to address?
- What outcome do you desire overall?
- Have you done this kind of work before? If so, what have been your results?
- Do you have a professional diagnosis for the issues you are facing?
- Are you under the care of a licensed professional?
- Are you taking any prescribed medication?
- Do you have authorization from your licensed professional to conduct this work?
- Do you understand that you need to continue working with your licensed professional and taking your medications while working with or receiving services from me?

BLOCKS AND STRONGHOLDS

BLOCKS ARE POINTS of resistance to our wellbeing that keep us from living as our authentic self. A block is any physical condition, belief, feeling, or spiritual misunderstanding that prevents us from living our purpose. A block can be caused by

- a physical problem,
- a false mental belief,
- an unresolved feeling, or
- a spiritual misperception.

A block is a problem because it inhibits the free flow of our natural energy and spiritual self. There are many types of blocks; the majority of them operate as strongholds, or stuck beliefs or feelings. A stronghold is a mental or emotional program that keeps us stuck in a pattern that isn't good for us. There are three basic types of strongholds.

A *mental stronghold* is made of two or more beliefs that join together but never come apart. An *emotional stronghold* is formed from at least one thought and one feeling. There are also *spiritual strongholds,* which are composed of beliefs or feelings that bond together and relate specifically to spiritual issues. Examples involve ideas relating to deserving divine love or accepting universal abundance.

A stronghold becomes a block when it fails to release when we're through with it. Strongholds are ultimately programmed into our energetic system, primarily into the external wheel of a related chakra. When we work with a client, it can be important to zoom in on the chakras related to the blocks or strongholds and focus the healing work there.

- (If applicable.) Do you understand that the care you are receiving from me is unlicensed and that you need to check with your overseeing professional before following any of my advice?

It's important that you always tell clients to check with their primary care physician, or whatever other licensed professionals they are working with, regarding the use of subtle energy medicine and its impact on their health. If you are working with a client who is under the care of a licensed mental healthcare provider, always require that they obtain permission before using any form of subtle energy medicine.

SOURCING ENERGETIC INFORMATION DURING A SESSION

Subtle body practitioners often use intuition to obtain insight and healing energy during a session. It is helpful to have available a list of questions you can ask of your own inner or higher guidance in order to obtain initial information, seek additional data, and construct a healing plan for your client.

After beginning your session with Spirit-to-Spirit, connect with a gatekeeper and request healing streams of grace. (See chapter 9 for details on each of these practices.) Now use the following questions to call forth the information and guidance needed.

INFORMATION-ORIENTED QUESTIONS
- What am I supposed to see, sense, hear, or know?
- If you are receiving an image, ask if it is a *vision* or a *fantasy*. (Visions cannot be altered; fantasies can.)
- Who or what is sharing information with me?
- Who should be sharing information with me?
- Is this information about the present? The past? The future?
- Is it a guarantee? A possibility? A probability? A have-to-do?
- Is this about an action to take? Not take? Something to avoid?
- Is this data for the client? For someone else?
- Should I be the one sharing this information or not? If so, what is the best way to communicate it?
- If this data is about the future, is it a must-happen? Can it be altered? Is it a red flag? Can it be shifted? Should it be? If so, how or by whom?
- Can I be provided more information to help me interpret or clarify the given data?
- Can I be given this information in other ways for validation or clarification (e.g., images, words, senses, smells, impressions)?

- What additional questions should I ask of the intuitive source(s) or ask of the client?
- Can you reveal what hidden information I am supposed to share?
- What's the best way for the client to respond to these insights?
- What client actions will bring the most healthy responses or responses supporting wholeness?

HEALING-ORIENTED QUESTIONS

- What needs to be healed?
- What issues are underlying the presenting problems?
- What energies, guides, activities, or other professionals can provide healing?
- What's the best way to achieve a healed or higher state?
- How much of this situation is affected by others' energies?
- How much of this situation is affected by entities or negative influences?
- How can I best clear others' energies? Or how can I best clear the entities or negative influences?
- Are there cords, attachments, or other types of energetic contracts involved?
- Should I do releasing work on any external influences?
- How should I direct the healing streams of grace?
- What am I missing?
- If a thousand angels were attending my client, what would he or she now be experiencing?

ENERGETIC EXPERIENCES DURING A SESSION

During a healing session, it's very common for you and your client to experience many energetic, emotional, and physical reactions. In fact, each of you might have very different experiences. So it is important to keep track of what is occurring in your own body and to see if it holds meaning for your client, and it is important to continually ask your client to share their experiences. The following is a detailed accounting of the different types of experiences either of you might have during an energy session and what these experiences might mean. Based on these observations, you will make decisions about how to interact with your client or what healing steps to recommend.

In general, your client will have more physical and emotional reactions when working on issues that are deeply entrenched in the psyche and when dealing with issues stemming from the distant past. Often, the older the issue, the bigger the reaction in the physical body.

The following are common reactions, shifts, and changes your clients may experience during a session. Note that you might pick up on their experiences and register them in your own body. Sometimes a practitioner also feels what the client might or should be feeling, as a way to gauge hidden issues.

TEMPERATURE CHANGES

Temperature changes are common during healing sessions. Your client may experience what seems like extreme fluctuations in body temperature—from really hot to really cold, and sometimes both at once, such as hands and feet feeling very cold and face and chest feeling very hot.

In general, heat indicates that new healing energy is coming in or old energy is being burned out. If someone has an infection, the heat could be jump-starting the immune system. The element of fire might be burning away shame. In general, cold has to do with the release of energy. Cold too can signify the release of microbes, old beliefs, or even an entity leaving the body.

As a practitioner, you too might feel various temperature-related sensations. For example, you might be feeling the movement of subtle energy within yourself or within your client. You might be feeling cold because you're inviting the release from the client. Or your sensing of temperature changes might be mirroring what your client is experiencing.

You and your client may experience temperature sensations and changes on different ends of the spectrum. For example, sometimes when I have my hands on a client, my hands feel cold to me, but my client experiences them as emitting heat. In situations like this, I might be helping them to *release* energy. So while I feel the cool temperatures of release, they might be one step ahead to receiving the warmth of the new healing energies.

I frequently experience what my client is going to experience about thirty seconds before they do. This is called *registering*. With strong energetic boundaries in place, registering allows you, the practitioner, to sense or receive information about your client without taking it on. You might say, "I'm feeling a lot of heat. What are you feeling?" Communicating with them in this interactive way helps them to feel companionable with you. They feel safe within an environment of empathy.

OTHER PHYSICAL SENSATIONS

You and your client may experience any number of physical sensations. For example, one or both of you might feel a distinct tingling or a slight internal trembling. I find that this often happens when there is a shift in perception in the client's psyche. The nervous system responds to the moment of realization or awareness, and the psycho-spiritual shift becomes a physical shift. This is often an "aha!" moment for a client.

If a client experiences numbness, it's often due to blockage. When a client goes numb, they are usually reliving a shock that could be the cause underlying the condition or situation that has brought them to your door. People can also get numb in a specific area of their body where they are *holding* a past shock or trauma.

In either case, the healing for shock is grieving. You can get a sense of the event by asking your client a few gentle questions and also by accessing your intuitive guidance, then creating a safe space for them to feel the feelings that they weren't able to feel at an earlier time. If that type of therapeutic process is outside of the scope of your work, it's important to refer your client to someone who is trained in helping people through the steps of the grief process. If a client comes to this threshold in your session, you can assure your client that it's a good sign. Now they are in the *aftershock* of the original experience and much closer to healing than before.

THE MOVEMENT OF EMOTIONS

When people are undergoing healing, it's common that they will feel a wide range of emotions. Very often these emotions are old feelings that have been repressed. Although there are many nuanced emotional states and types of feelings, there are five core feelings: anger, sadness, fear, disgust, and happiness. As a healer, you can help your client figure out what they are feeling and, just as important, what their feelings mean. They might also need to address a block or a stronghold, as described in the sidebar "Blocks and Strongholds."

We can best support a client by "holding space," a phrase commonly used in the subtle energy community. To hold space means to create an atmosphere of sacredness that inspires healing. It's an energetic space that's filled with optimism, care, compassion, and connection to Spirit as we understand Spirit.

If your client is experiencing repetitive emotional states and having trouble moving through and beyond them, we need to ask if all the emotions they're experiencing are *their own* emotions. With persistent worry, anxiety, fear, or anger, I ask my client to ask themselves what percentage of what they are feeling is their own energy versus belonging to someone else. People often tune into this percentage quite easily. "It's thirty percent mine!" they might say.

We can only process our own emotions. If seventy percent of the anger is your dad's, you can hand it over to *his* higher self. If the remaining feelings belong to your client, help them determine the meaning of the feelings. The following are the deeper perspectives posed by the five main feelings:

Sadness asks us to perceive the love under a loss.

Fear asks us to move forward, backward, or out of the way.

Anger asks us to set boundaries.

Disgust tells us that something or someone isn't good for us.

Happiness tells us that we want more of the same.

It's vital to keep the process moving and not get derailed. There is an important balance between knowing when to continue an emotional exploration and when to move on. Because I'm very kinesthetic, I often feel the emotions of my clients. But I have learned the importance of providing and managing the structure of the healing process and to keep it moving. Acknowledging what they're experiencing and offering an optimistic light is often the key. "I know that you're in pain, and I know it's hard, but let's keep going to see what we can do about it."

EMERGING MEMORIES

HEALING WORK OFTEN triggers memories for clients. We all have a story, and it relates to many times, places, and people. A client's memories can be the product of any of the following:

- Past lives
- In-between lives
- Childhood
- Adulthood
- Ancestral memories
- Memories that are not their own, perhaps assumed from family members, the culture, or entities

Overt memories are what actually happened. For example, we may have a memory comprised of what our five-year-old self experienced with his or her five senses—what he or she saw, heard, touched, smelled, and possibly tasted. *Covert memories* come from someone else's feelings. Resentment is often related to a covert memory. Maybe Mom fed us, but was silently resentful about having to do so. Or maybe Dad tucked us in at night, but we felt icky about it; if sexual boundaries weren't overtly crossed, there might have been something off with the energetic boundaries. That old discomfort is the covert memory.

Sometimes clients experience the opposite of past memories, receiving future possibilities, such as warnings, foreshadowing, foretelling.

When working with any memories, it's important to first figure out if they are overt, covert, or futuristic; if they belong to the client or not; the circumstances under which they originated; and how they are affecting the client today. You can use exercises such as Uncovering Your Storyline, in chapter 13, to help a client find the silver lining in the memory.

UNUSUAL CIRCUMSTANCES AND PRACTITIONER CHALLENGES

Being a subtle energy practitioner sometimes invites unusual circumstances. When a client is triggered by the past or strong emotions, they can sometimes get angry or violent. They might also become nauseous, ill, or spacey. I have witnessed clients undergoing panic attacks and full-blown paranoid episodes. Your job as a practitioner, first and foremost, is to keep yourself and the client safe. Calm and soothing talk usually pulls the client through the shift. Ask your client to connect to their breath and remind them that they are letting go of an issue that has been stored inside and that they will soon feel better. In an extreme situation, know that you can always end a session or call for help. Never try to manage a situation that is spiraling out of control.

Quite frequently, subtle energy practitioners and their clients report the presence of otherworldly beings. Many of these beings are helpful and might include ancestors, deceased loved ones, guides, angels, and other forms of assistance. Entities—also commonly called interference, dark forces, evil, or fallen angels—might also attempt to negatively influence the outcome of a session. (See chapter 16, "The Subtle Spirit," for more on entities.) In my own practice, I've experienced lights flickering on and off, phone lines dying, doors banging, and shadows emanating from the corners. I often employ the healing streams of grace to sweep out the space so my client and I can continue working. When a client gets scared, I usually tell them that the dark presence is a good sign—it indicates that we are closing in on a real issue.

One of the most vital challenges is dealing with our own and our client's fear, if it arises. Sometimes we're afraid that there won't be a healing or change. But sometimes a client is actually afraid that there *will* be change.

For instance, I worked for about six months with a woman who had multiple sclerosis. I'd go to her house because she was in critical shape. Through our work, she started to improve and was starting to lead a near-normal life. I asked her if she was ready to go all the way with healing. She said no! She wanted to torture her husband because he wasn't in love with her. Within two weeks of making this statement, the client returned to her former state of being wheelchair bound.

Sometimes it seems like absolutely nothing happens during a session. When this occurs, our client might be experiencing a block or interference. Perhaps the healing energy is still held in their energy field and hasn't landed. Maybe the client will feel the session later, after arriving home or even weeks later. Know that healing energy is never lost. Ask your client to pay attention to shifts or changes that occur over the next few days or to ask for signs or dreams telling them what else they need to know or do.

CONCLUDING A SESSION

At the end of a session, I ask a client if they are willing to let the healing energy continue working within them. I suggest that they pay attention to their dreams, emotions, and needs, even their food cravings, so as to continue the healing. You might also share what they might expect upon arriving home, such as the following:

Healing crises. Many people become physically ill or dissolve into a torrent of emotions after a session. Energetic healing often occurs first in the spiritual or mental arenas and then lands in the physical body, setting off physical or emotional detoxification and chemical adjustments. For instance, someone might purge a long-held virus or repressed anger. The most common symptom I find with clients is that they get a cold or flu symptoms, in addition to undergoing a grieving process.

Changes in behavior. Clients often find that long-held behaviors or habits start to change. They might suddenly stop eating sugar or want to wear new clothes. This indicates that the subtle energy shifts are locking into the body's neurological software.

Reactions from others. Sometimes other people or the external world will act differently. Someone who has been nasty might now be supportive. Others will want us to be who we were before. Clients need to be supported in retaining their newfound equilibrium when meeting adversity, to the point of working with a therapist or a coach.

Nothing happens. Sometimes you are not the right practitioner for this client, and the session produces no changes. The client might also be unconsciously resisting change or could be under the influence of interference. In these cases, it is best to suggest that the client work with a different practitioner.

More difficulties. Sometimes a session creates a watershed moment. Life becomes more challenging, not less, after the session. This often occurs when we are asked to make a breakthrough via our breakdown. Forces might be gathering to stop the movement forward, in which case it's all the more important for the client to continue their personal growth process.

THE BLESSINGS OF THIS WORK

One thing that is assured: serving people in the capacity of a subtle energy practitioner is equivalent to walking what the Navajo call the Beauty Path, the way of wisdom and truth. If you show up in service, know that only blessings will flow through you.

PART III
THE UNIVERSAL PATHWAYS AND PRACTICES

As you might have surmised from its title, part 3 is a compilation of tools and practices from many subsets of the expansive field of subtle energy medicine. I call them *universal pathways* because they are derived from energy healing practices from many cultures around the world. The practices in this section are sacred technologies—*sacred* in the sense that they address our human needs with care, kindness, and reverence for our right to pursue healing with dignity and freedom, and *technologies* because they are processes and methods that marry science and soul. Many can be blended for optimal uses, not only with other practices in part 3, but also with the essential energy techniques presented in chapter 9.

With clear and simple instructions, you will learn how to use the tools with your clients and loved ones, as well as for your own healing purposes. (As in earlier chapters, know that when the text says "clients" and "your clients," it refers to anyone that might be using the practices, including yourself.) You will discover also helpful (and often fascinating) ways to use these tools—from hands-on healing to shamanic journeying to using color, sound, and the elements of nature—across a wide spectrum of healing needs. Each of the applications outlined in part 3 is fundamentally connected to the first four chapters of the book; they each tie back to the interconnectivity between the fields, meridians, and chakras that make up the subtle body.

Having explored the essential topics of intentions, ethics, intuition, trust, and energetic boundaries in the previous section, you are well prepared to now have a splendorous walk through the universal pathways—an adventure into territory old and new.

11

HEALING THE AURIC FIELD

Though outwardly a gloomy shroud,
The inner half of every cloud
Is bright and shining:
I therefore turn my clouds about
And always wear them inside out
To show the lining.

ELLEN THORNEYCROFT FOWLER
"The Wisdom of Folly"

Working with the auric field—to assess, clear, mend, or recharge it—could become the technique that you come to value the most as a subtle energy practitioner. As a stand-alone practice, it can provide the energetic support your client may need to heal in body, mind, or spirit. Also, in a relatively short amount of time, tending to the field can prepare your client for any other type of healing modality you choose to use.

Working with the aura, you can obtain information and guidance on many levels, from intuitive information to visual information to the data that your client directly conveys. Therefore, it's useful to remember that you will be accessing and integrating information from the rational mind and the intuitive mind. (In chapter 15, we will deepen the adventure into even more subtle distinctions of the mind.) Additionally, there are many notable practitioners who specialize in working with the auric field, such as Stephen Barrett, the founder of Chios Energy Healing.[1] Several of the assessment and healing exercises in this chapter have been inspired by the thoroughness and clarity of Stephen's work.

GATHERING INFORMATION

Before working with your client (or yourself) to address any energy leaks and to clear and recharge the auric field, you will begin by assessing your client's condition. In addition to the information they tell you (such as how they are feeling physically and emotionally, what challenges they may be dealing with, and what caused them to seek your support), your assessment will involve three main perceptual tools:

- The intuitive information and guidance you receive regarding the condition of your client's auric field and chakras.
- Your observations of their aura and chakras based on what you see with your eyes.
- Subtle energy sensations in your hands, especially as you practice the passing-of-hands over your client's energy field.

The information you receive from these means will be combined and used together. You will use these perceptual tools to look for energetic leaks, tears, impurities—anything that may be depleting or disturbing the energy of the client's auric field. You will also assess whether specific chakras are blocked.

TWO STEPS FOR INTUITIVELY ASSESSING THE AURIC FIELD

The most fundamental way to assess the auric field is to do so in your mind or through your intuition. This hands-off process can be used if a client is present, but unable to be touched for some reason, if the client is not present, or if you are working on yourself. It requires only concentration, receptivity, and a willingness to access your intuitive gifts.

Step 1: Concentrate and receive information. Stand over or sit next to your client with your eyes softly closed, fully focusing on your client with your intuitive gifts activated. If your client is not present (or you are assessing your own field), imagine the shape of the body in your mind's eye. Focus your awareness on the outline of the body, allowing all other thoughts and emotions to drift away. While you are doing this, hold the intention that you will be receiving information about the auric field of your client. Releasing all effort, open yourself up to receiving the information, which will just come.

Step 2: Focus your intuition. Focus on the information that pulls you the strongest emotionally or intuitively. The information you receive may include some of the following:
- Colors
- Fuzzy areas
- Patterns on the body

- A discoloration or blotch over a chakra location, possibly indicating a blocked chakra
- A muddiness around the head or other specific parts of the body that you sense as auric impurities
- Tears and damaged areas in the field that are leaking vital energy
- An energy depletion or weakness in various layers of the field
- An overall disturbance of energy flow in the entire field

This exercise may only take a few minutes and can be repeated for a second or third time, if you feel it would be beneficial. Whether you take one pass with this technique or more, allow all the information coming to begin to integrate and to reveal an overall understanding of the condition of your client. Again, trust the intuitive information you are receiving; your intuitive mind is as valid a tool as your rational mind.

In addition to assessing the condition of the overall auric field, you can also locate and identify issues in its specific layers, which will tell you the exact nature of the presenting problems. (See figure 11.1, "Energetic Issues in the Auric Field," to better picture the energetic anomalies you might discover when assessing the auric field.)

Note: It is possible that while you are assessing the auric field, you might simultaneously receive information regarding potential healing solutions for these areas.

GETTING TO KNOW THE AURIC LAYERS: CHARACTERISTICS, COLORS, AND SHAPES

Where exactly are the layers of the auric field and what do they look like intuitively? The following list explains the location of each of the main auric layers in relation to the physical body.

First Layer. The first layer of the aura is often visible as a reddish color, although some practitioners envision it as light blue, grayish, or colorless. It surrounds the surface of the body at a distance of **one or two inches** and interpenetrates the skin. (Some practitioners call it the *physical body* and others the *etheric body* or the *gross body*.) The color may deepen in hue as you become better able to perceive this field. This layer of the subtle body also includes the energy pattern on the surface of and within the physical body; thus, it is an energetic mirror of the structure of the physical body.

Second Layer. The second layer, also called the *emotional body*, is composed of clouds or areas of color that are often indefinable shapes of various sizes.

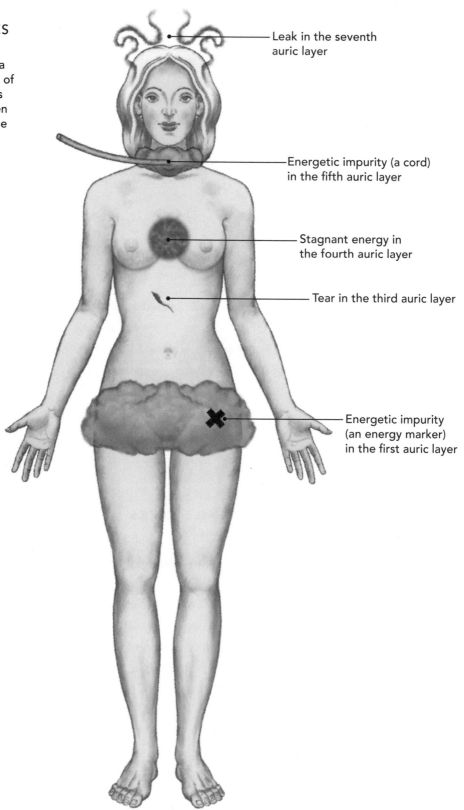

FIGURE 11.1

ENERGETIC ISSUES IN AURIC FIELD

This figure shows just a few of the many types of energetic disturbances that can be found when intuitively assessing the auric field.

Leak in the seventh auric layer

Energetic impurity (a cord) in the fifth auric layer

Stagnant energy in the fourth auric layer

Tear in the third auric layer

Energetic impurity (an energy marker) in the first auric layer

These multicolored clouds extend **four or five inches** above the surface of the body and are usually in a condition of constant flow, change, and movement. These moving colors typically correspond to the psychological state of the client and the current circumstances of their life. Healthy colors will appear vibrant and radiant. Unhealthy or potentially harmful auric phenomena might have a muddied, smeared, or streaked appearance, and the colors might be muted or have a basically unhealthy look and feel.

Third Layer. The third layer, the *mental body*, primarily appears yellow in color. In actuality, it is not composed of yellow light, but has a radiance that makes it appear light yellow or golden. This layer does not have clouds of color, like the second layer, but has a shell-like shape, similar to the shape of the physical body yet less defined. It exists about **eight to ten inches** from the body surface.

Fourth Layer. The fourth layer, the *astral body*, is similar to the second layer in that it is composed of multicolored clouds. The colors in this layer are finer, paler, and lighter than those of the previous layers; however, they can also be less vivid and harder to see. The cloud colors often include green, pink, or gold. These multicolored clouds, like those of the second layer, are always in motion and are similarly connected to the life experience and current state of psychological wellbeing of your client. This layer exists in the area approximately **one foot to a foot and a half** above the surface of the body.

Fifth Layer. The fifth layer, the *etheric template body*, primarily appears to the eye as a deep blue radiance, although its radiance is not as bright as that of the third layer. Its overall shape is that of an egg (although it is not as large or wide as the seventh layer, which is also egg shaped). It exists approximately **two feet above** the body surface. Like the first and third layers, this layer appears as a pattern that mirrors the surface and inner structure of the physical body. This layer is a vibrational mirror for the layers above and below it.

Sixth Layer. The sixth layer, also known as the *cosmic* or *celestial body*, appears as multicolored, softly flowing streams or streaks of light that emanate from the center of the body in all directions. This layer has no clouds of color and no particular shape; it consists only of these streams and gentle streaks alone. It often encompasses tones of purple or other violet energies.

Seventh Layer. The seventh layer, sometimes called the *ketheric body* or the *causal body*, appears as a fine, transparent eggshell with a soft, glowing light that may appear bright, white, or golden to your psychic sight and your physical eyes, but is actually composed of a light that contains all colors. This layer is approximately **three feet** from the body surface.

Additional layers. There are several other layers to the auric field, and they are labeled with different names according to the system you are using. My twelve-chakra system incorporates five more bands of auric layers as well as a final energy egg or protective mechanism that encloses all the layers. The auric layers in this twelve-chakra system are described in chapter 2 (see figure 2.1 specifically). The twelve auric layers are located atop each other, with the exception of the tenth auric layer, which is found between the first and second auric layers and contains the codes to our natural self and our link with nature. (Refer to *The Subtle Body* encyclopedia for a more detailed accounting of the twelve-layer auric field.)

As you become increasingly skillful at distinguishing the auric field in general, you will likely move from detecting one or two predominant colors to seeing many colors interspersed.

SEEING THE LAYERS OF THE AURIC FIELD

With time and practice, you can learn to discern the different layers of the auric field, one by one, working your way up from the first layer and then learning to bring all the layers into view simultaneously. Here is a handy process for doing just that.

Before you begin, make sure that the lighting in your work environment is neither too bright nor too dim. You also want to have a neutral-colored background your client can stand or sit in front of.

When your client is in position, set the intention of perceiving their first auric layer. Briefly glance at their body and then look away, averting your eyes (which are still open) to an empty area or space off to the side of their body. Allow yourself to become aware of what your mind's eye perceives.

Quickly glance again at their body and look away. You might want to repeat the quick glance several times over, each time opening to whatever your mind's eye may perceive in regard to the first auric layer.

After you have gained a good impression of your client's physical auric field, or their first layer, located in and just outside of the skin, it is time to try to view the next layer up. Each layer will extend approximately four to five inches above the maximum extent of the previous one. As you move to higher layers, you will need to use a more soft-focused gaze, and you will also have to stand farther back from your client's body—up to six feet or more for the higher layers.

Don't rely on distance alone to recognize which layer you're perceiving. The auric layers interpenetrate; one layer can blur into another. It isn't physical distance from the body alone that defines the layers; rather, it is the differences in each layer's energetic characteristics. As well, these layers fluctuate in breadth and distance from the body on a daily or even moment-to-moment basis. When we're really emotional, for instance, the second emotional layer might enlarge and extend out three or four feet. When we are at peace, it will condense and might be found only three inches away from the body.

The location, depth, and breadth of each auric layer can provide clues as to what is occurring in your client. As in the example above, an expanded second auric layer might indicate a high degree of emotional turmoil. If your client seems open to discussing the matter, you might ask your client about events that have caused or are causing them emotional strain. Perhaps the first auric layer is distended and a scarlet red, perhaps indicating an enflaming security issue or even an overwhelming sexual passion. Allow your intuitive senses (and common sense) to direct the conversation so you can invite observations from your client.

SEALING ENERGETIC LEAKS AND TEARS

After assessing the overall condition of your client's auric field, the first thing you may choose to do is repair any leaks or tears you have discovered. Sealing leaks and tears restores the integrity of the field and prevents further energy loss. By making these subtle energy repairs, vital energy becomes available for healing and for enjoying life.

Sealing of leaks and tears is generally performed with the hands. Using only one hand at a time, you move your hand over the area where you've identified a leak or tear. Although you may choose to use your dominant hand at first, with even a little practice, both hands can become equally effective in this technique.

SIMPLE TIPS FOR IMPROVING YOUR AURA VISION

- Relax your eyes and use a soft, slightly unfocused gaze. Don't try to see an aura by staring or making an effort.

- Maintain a higher focus by gently concentrating on the third eye (sixth chakra) area.

- Don't force yourself or over-concentrate.

- It helps if your client wears white. The color white contains all the colors equally and therefore doesn't create an afterimage, or a halo effect. Other colors will taint the image of the aura.

- Look for subtle color impressions rather than solid or vivid colors.

- As the aura is impacted by one's state of relaxation, help your client relax—suggest that they use their breath to do so—and observe the difference in their aura before and after they relax.

- While regular practice will increase your skill, don't deplete yourself by trying too hard or for too long.

Thanks go to Reiki masters Leslie and Elmarie Swartz for inspiring these tips.[2]

Tip: When choosing whether to use your right or left hand, know that everyone has an energy-generating hand, which sends energy, and a receptive hand, which receives or takes in energy. Most people send energy with their right hands and receive it with their left. You can return to the "Palm-to-Palm" exercise in chapter 1 to assess your hands. You can also skip ahead to chapter 12 and the section titled "The Five Elements in Your Hands," which shows you how to activate the power of the five elements that are reflected in each of your fingers and incorporate that information into various subtle energy endeavors—from working with the auric layers in this chapter to several other modes of hands-on and distant healing described elsewhere in the book.

As you move through the following steps for sealing leaks and tears, you will want to keep your eyes open. While some techniques require practitioners to remain in a more passive, receptive state (to emphasize sensing and assessing energy), for this technique you will take a more active role.

Step 1: **Position your hand.** Hold one of your hands over the first leak or tear you wish to seal. The hand should be palm down and inside the auric layer that you are repairing. The fingers are gently held together; the palm is open and held flat (instead of relaxed).

Step 2: **Move your hand.** Slowly move your hand in a gentle back-and-forth (or circular) motion. Your kinesthetic intuition will often guide you in how to move your hand. To be most effective, move your hand at a speed of approximately two inches per second. If you move it much slower or much faster, the technique will not be as effective.

Step 3: **Visualize the repair.** As you move your hands, visualize the leak or tear being repaired. Sense that the area in which the leak is occurring is being sealed shut. The energy in your hand, in conjunction with the inner-eye visualization, works to fully repair the damaged or compromised area. It may also help to see yourself smoothing over the damage and melding the field. Again, visualize the repairs as you go. You are sealing the fissures closed with your conscious awareness so that the energy can no longer escape.

Making these subtle repairs generally takes only a moment or two.

LEAKS AND TEARS IN MULTIPLE LAYERS

Tears can be found in any or all of the auric layers. Many begin in the first layer but then extend to the second, third, or even higher layers. In a case like this, you will need to seal the tear in each layer.

Use the three previous steps to seal the tear or leak in the first layer (figure 11.2). Then progressively move your hands farther out from the client's body, onto each layer where the tear continues, and seal that layer using the technique given above.

For example, after sealing the first layer with the palm about two inches above the body, you may need to move the hand an additional four to five inches upwards and seal the next level. Then, you may need to proceed another four to five inches up to the third level or higher. Using your intuition and felt sense, you will know when such tears are present and how high you need to go to seal them.

Tip: Small tears sometimes occur over a chakra. It is not usually the chakra that is torn (a torn chakra is a rare occurrence), but the auric layer or layers above the chakra. This damage is often the result of emotional or mental traumas. When you encounter a tear over a chakra, simply seal the tears as instructed above. See the sidebar "From the Auric Layers to the Chakras" for more on caring for the chakra connected with a damaged auric layer.

AURA CLEARING

For the health of your client, it is essential that the flow of energy in the auric field be free from stagnation or energy impurities.

Stagnation is blocked energy. It can be comprised of emotions, beliefs, psychic toxins, or even others' energies. At one point, this energy might have served, but no longer does. The resulting congestion is preventing healthy energy from flowing.

Energy impurities can include stagnated energy, but also undesirable energies, including energetic contracts, such as cords and curses (covered in chapter 9 in the section "Freedom from Inhibiting Energetic Contracts"). Sometimes

FROM THE AURIC LAYERS TO THE CHAKRAS

BECAUSE EACH AURIC layer also relates to a specific chakra (for example, the first auric layer relates to the first chakra), you can decide to work in the corresponding chakra(s) as well as in the auric layers. Knowing the affected chakras enables you to work in their related physical organs and address the emotional and mental states that might be interrelated. Quite often, the chakra issues being explored in the present have their roots in the distant past—in infancy, childhood, or adolescence. Not only were our teeth, bones, and brains developing then, but so were our chakras! The chakra-development information on page 58 in chapter 4 can be enormously helpful for connecting the dots with your client and assessing how to proceed with a healing plan.

FIGURE 11.2

SEALING THE FIRST AURIC LAYER

Seal a leak or tear in the first auric field by holding your hand about one to two inches away from the body. Then proceed about four inches higher to assess and seal the next auric layer. Repeat in each of the subsequent layers as necessary.

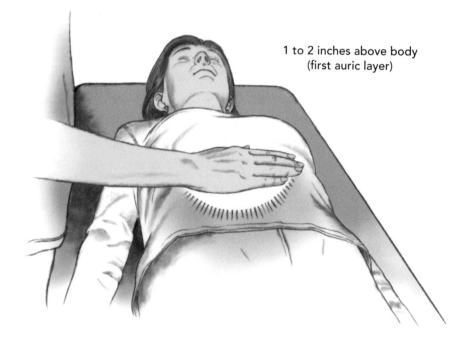

1 to 2 inches above body (first auric layer)

FIGURE 11.3

AURIC CLEANSING: THE FIRST AURIC LAYER

To cleanse the first auric layer, first hold your cupped hand in it, the fingers falling downward like spider's legs. Then lift your hand upward about 15 inches, extending your fingers to point to the sky, and lightly fling or release the energetic impurities into the universe for disposal. You can clear any of the auric fields in the same way, starting in the pertinent field and flicking off the impure energy 14 or 15 inches up from there.

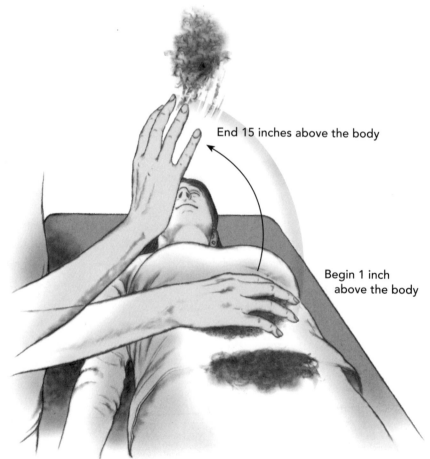

End 15 inches above the body

Begin 1 inch above the body

energy impurities, especially those linked to an entity or intrusive being, such as a ghost or ancestral spirit, can completely lock down the corresponding auric layer, or even several layers.

If you detect either energy stagnation or impurities in your client's aura, they may be cleared using a procedure aptly known as *aura clearing*.

Like the technique for sealing leaks and tears, this technique is performed over the various areas of the body where energy impurities commonly occur, as well as over chakras when indicated. It is also done using only one hand at a time and with the eyes open. In this case, the hands, especially the fingers, are used to remove undesirable energies from the layers of the energy field. Your hand and its outspread fingers have their own auric field, which acts as an attraction device—*an auric net*. It catches and detaches the harmful or stagnant energies from the client's field. Those energies stick to your hand (primarily the underside of the palm and fingers) and are released from the client's field by your hand motion. Now separated from the body, these impure energies lose their charge and their ability to cling to the client's field. The impurities simply dissolve and have no further effect on your client.

Also like the technique for sealing leaks and tears, this technique utilizes your ability to visualize. While you perform the hand motion, you see the removal of unwanted energies with your inner vision and/or your physical eyes.

Clear away auric energy impurities or blockages that you have detected in your client's field with the following steps.

Step 1: Position your hand. Place your hand, palm down, over the first area to be cleared, with fingers spread a moderate amount—wider apart than during the sealing technique. Your hand and fingers should be slightly cupped, with the fingertips facing downward, just like the legs of a spider. If you're clearing the first auric layer, your hand should be about one inch above the body surface.

Step 2: Draw out the energy. Draw your hand upward until it is about fifteen inches above your client's body. As you do this, also raise your fingertips upward toward the sky. Imagine that you are "flinging" the impurities out of the auric field. (See figure 11.3.) This entire motion should take approximately five seconds. While performing this motion, visualize, intend, and sense that the auric impurities are being removed. Feel and see the part of your own auric field around your fingers attracting, pulling, and clearing away the undesirable energies as you draw your hand upwards.

Step 3: Shake out your hand. Some practitioners like to shake the impurities off their hand after it is fully drawn out and away from their client's body, before they return the hand to its starting position and begin the next drawing-out motion.

Step 4: Repeat. Repeat this technique as many times as necessary to clear the auric impurities away from each area or layer in which they occur. You might methodically assess each auric layer, continuing the process at four-inch intervals, or allow your hands to intuitively move wherever they need to. In each case, draw your hand about fourteen inches above the starting point. Typically, it will take two to ten motions—between one and three minutes—to remove an impurity or block in a given area.

FOR CHALLENGING SITUATIONS

Certain blocks or energetic impurities, especially energetic contracts, can be difficult to remove. I recommend using one or both of the following techniques, which were covered in chapter 9.

The Light Wand. When the stagnant energy refuses to budge, imagine that you are holding a wand in each hand. One hand is for sending, the other for receiving. Open to universal healing energy, which will pass like a light through the sending wand and into the stuck energy. The blocked energy, which is now diffused, will be collected by the receiving wand and recycled through intention by the universe.

Healing Streams of Grace. Use intention or ask Spirit (using the Spirit-to-Spirit technique, also described in chapter 9) to swap the stagnant or undesirable energies or contracts with streams of grace. Know that Spirit can select the appropriate streams for you.

Note: You may find that aura clearing will be required over specific chakras. The second, fourth, and sixth chakras are particularly susceptible to these sorts of impure energies or energy blocks, as they are very receptive chakras. When performing aura clearing over chakras, be aware that you may also be smoothing or attuning the energy flow in the chakra. In keeping with the whirling motion of the chakra, draw your hand up above the chakra as if you were cleansing and smoothing the flow in a funnel of energy.

AURA CHARGING

Energy depletion can be an insidious problem for people, sapping their vital life-force energy and making them more susceptible to diseases and

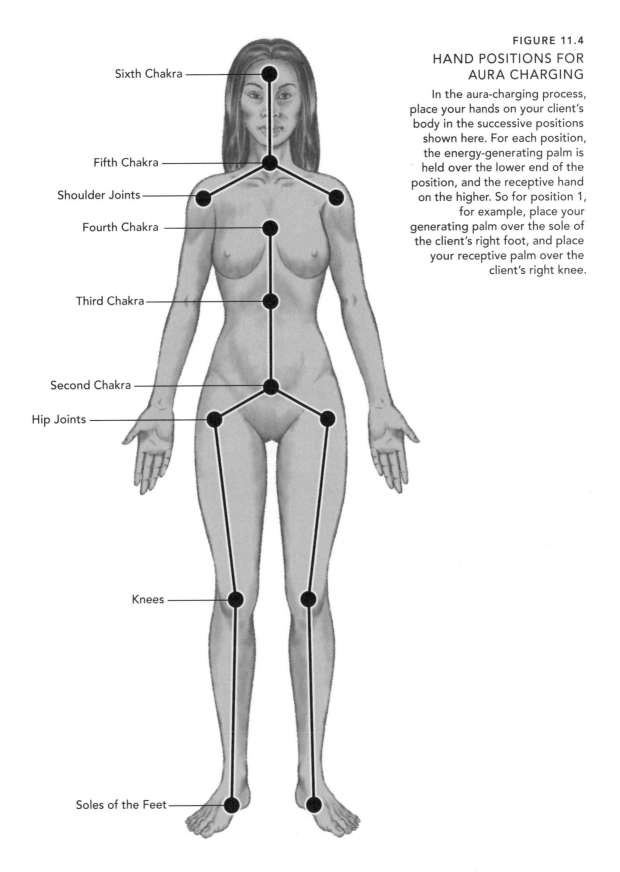

FIGURE 11.4

HAND POSITIONS FOR AURA CHARGING

In the aura-charging process, place your hands on your client's body in the successive positions shown here. For each position, the energy-generating palm is held over the lower end of the position, and the receptive hand on the higher. So for position 1, for example, place your generating palm over the sole of the client's right foot, and place your receptive palm over the client's right knee.

Sixth Chakra

Fifth Chakra

Shoulder Joints

Fourth Chakra

Third Chakra

Second Chakra

Hip Joints

Knees

Soles of the Feet

imbalances. It can also inhibit the effectiveness of any other healing work that is being performed.

The aura is like a porous seal emanating from the body. Energy from our physical body, as well as our mind and soul, continually renews it, as does energy we attract from outside of our auric field. External energy sources include other people, companion animals, as well as all of nature and the various putative and verifiable fields described in chapter 2. While we can lose energy through leaks and tears, as described earlier in this chapter, and because of blocks and energetic impurities, we might also simply lose too much energy during the day because of our codependent nature. Or our body might be recovering from an acute illness or struggling with a chronic pain, disease, or problem, and it is therefore using much of its natural electrical energy for survival or recovery, in which case we also generate a lower magnetic field.

HEALING YOUR OWN AURIC FIELD

SOMETIMES WE NEED to work on our own auric field. We can accomplish the same goals as a practitioner—assessing, repairing, clearing, or charging the field—by employing the following techniques.

It's very hard to assess our own aura visually or move our hands over all parts of our body or field. The good news is that we don't have to if we ask the Greater Spirit, accessed through the Spirit-to-Spirit exercise (see chapter 9), to do the work for us. Acknowledge your own inner spirit and the invisible spirits in attendance. Now ask the Divine to help you sense what is adversely affecting your auric field. You can also request that Spirit cleanse and repair your field, as well as charge it.

Ask also that the appropriate healing streams of grace be inserted wherever they are needed in your auric layers. These streams of grace can do everything from sew rips to release entities. (See chapter 9 for more on healing streams of grace.)

When working on my own auric field, I usually put one of my hands on the center of my heart chakra. The physical heart, which is the endocrine center of the heart chakra, generates 5,000 times more magnetic energy than does our brain. It generates the most intense magnetic field produced by our body. The very center of the heart chakra is metaphysically known as the center of the energy system, as well as the location of the "inner child," the self who holds our wounds but also our sweet strength. By putting your hand on your heart chakra, you are tapping into your field's energetic powers, sweeping the healing through all layers of your physical body and energetic fields, and gently providing healing for the self who needs it most of all.

If you sense that every layer of the auric field is depleted, you'll want to use aura charging. This process will enable you to strengthen the entire auric field, not only deal with blocks or rips. It also enables a more secure attachment between the body and the field so that they can work together better. Sometimes when we supercharge the entire field, other auric issues are naturally healed. They might also become more apparent, in which case you can seal the rips or clear the specific fields that require cleansing.

In this aura-charging process, you will place your hands on your client's body in the successive positions shown in figure 11.4, beginning with the feet. In each position, the energy-generating palm is held over the lower end of the position, and the receptive hand on the higher. For example, for position 1, place your generating palm over the sole of the client's right foot, and place your receptive palm over the top of the client's right knee.

Step 1: Transfer energy. Beginning with your hands in the first position, conduct energy into your client, radiating the energy into the client's body and their auric field *to create a bond between the body and the field.* Radiate the energy from both of your hands equally as you are doing this.

Step 2: Visualize the bond. Visualize the bond between the client's body and auric field in the area where you are working, seeing the field filling and expanding with energy. Continue visualizing and transferring the energy into the client for one to two minutes, or until you get a sense of completeness, such as a diminishment of the energy flow or the intuitive sense that their auric field is starting to brim with energy.

Step 3: Continue with the next hand position. Place your generating palm on the sole of the client's left foot and your receptive palm on the client's left knee. Again transmit the energy, seeking to create a bond between the client and their energy field while visualizing the field filling and expanding. Continue treating this second position until you gain a sense of completeness. This time, also make sure that you sense a balance between this side of the client's field and the side that you previously treated.

Step 4: Work successively through the other hand positions. Continue working through the other positions in numerical order, as shown in figure 11.4. Transmit the energy in the same way for each position, ending when you feel that that position is complete. Some positions have several points within them; you can visit each point or slide your hand between them. Each position will probably require between one and two minutes of treatment (although certain positions may require a little longer, depending on your client's particular needs). Remember, as you move upward, proceeding from one side to the other, treat until you feel you have achieved balance between the two sides.

As you proceed up the client's body, you will sense their aura charging, and you may feel the energy radiating outward as it fills. Observe their aura filling with vibrant energy, brightening and expanding.

Note: Occasionally you might find that only certain regions of the body will exhibit energy depletion. For example, you might work with a client who has been overworking at a computer and experiencing energy depletion in their lower arms and hands. This depletion, caused at least in part by repetitive motion, can be alleviated with aura charging in that region only.

For energy depletion in the lower arms, charge each arm from the hand to the elbow joint by placing your right hand palm-to-palm with the client's hand and placing the other palm on the inside of the elbow joint. The arm to the shoulder may be charged on each arm also, if needed. For energy depletion in the lower legs, charge from the foot to the knee (as in positions 1 and 2 in the full procedure above), as well as from the knee to the hip joint, if you sense it is necessary.

12

HANDS-ON HEALING

The wound is the place where
the Light enters you.

RUMI

As subtle energy healers demonstrate on a regular basis, the keys to our health are literally in our hands. Simply by rubbing our hands together, we can experience the heat and energy that is easily generated. When we add the power of intention—transmitting energies such as love, care, hope, and optimism—the results can be remarkable.

In this chapter, we will explore a rich variety of hands-on healing techniques that you can use to support the health and wellbeing of your clients, and also to tune up and amplify your own healing powers. Some of these techniques use our hands to transmit energy or move energy within the subtle body. For others, we use our hands to press, tap, massage, or otherwise manipulate the acupoints and meridians in order to promote a healthy, balanced flow of energy through these channels.

THERAPEUTIC HEALING TOUCH

In her exceptional book *Healing Touch: Essential Energy Medicine for Yourself and Others,* my colleague Dorothea Hover-Kramer, EdD, RN, DCEP, provides clear and inspiring instruction in the practice of Healing Touch (HT), an energy therapy in which practitioners consciously use their hands in a heart-centered and intentional way to support healing. Similar to practices outlined in the previous chapter, HT affects the auric field, the chakras, and other aspects of the energetic biofield. As Dorothea says in her book, "Healing Touch is literally as close as the presence of a caring person."[1]

The first technique that Healing Touch students learn is called *Magnetic Passes*. As a practitioner, you visualize your hands as small magnets that draw out congestion and energetic stagnation and restore balance to a client's field. Magnetic Passes work well for releasing headaches and other types of bodily pain. Although HT is used for many purposes, relief from pain is probably the most appreciated outcome that people report.

MAGNETIC PASSES FOR HEADACHES

There are two parts to Magnetic Passes, and their names describe what your hands do in relation to your client's field: *Hands in Motion* and *Hands Still*. When your hands are in motion, you will be moving them in a circular fashion, either clockwise or counterclockwise. Clockwise often brings energy in, while counterclockwise often ushers energy out. When your hands are still, you're simply holding them motionless and allowing them to sense and receive energy.

You can position your hands directly on the body, with your client's permission, or over the body in the auric field. If your hands are on the body, apply a light pressure, just enough that the client is aware of your presence. If your hands are in the auric field, you can intuitively gauge how far away from the body to hold them, or return to chapter 11's descriptions of the auric layers and select a specific layer to work in. Most practitioners assess intuitively, and they will move from a hands-on to a hands-off position during a session. Many also work with a twelve-chakra system, and five of these chakras (and corresponding auric layers) are found outside of the body (see chapter 4). Wherever you place your hands, you are using them as gentle but potent healing magnets.

The following step-by-step process for headaches can be easily adapted to eliminate pain in other parts of the body as well.

1. Prepare inwardly by centering, grounding, and creating an atmosphere of calm and safety. (See chapter 9 for suggested techniques.)

2. Obtain consent from your client to proceed.

3. Attune to your client and intuitively assess the area of discomfort around their head. (Refer to "Intuition and Trust" in chapter 6 for tips about how to apply your intuitive faculties to perceiving energy.)

4. Using *Hands in Motion*, move your hands lightly over the painful area. If the area is large, start at one end and work your way to the other,

continually moving your hands in a circular motion. Your hands can be on the client's head or just over it, unless you sense that some of the causes of the headache lie in one of the outer energy fields, in which case you will want to shift to this auric layer and work there for a while as well.

5. Follow with *Hands Still* to further calm the disturbed area. You will know when to stop because you will feel a shift in your client's body.

6. Once you complete the Magnetic Passes, use your hands or your intention to ground your client.
   - If using your hands, place them over or under their feet; you can either touch their feet or let your hands hover a few inches away. It doesn't matter if they are wearing socks or shoes; the healing energy gets through.
   - If using intention, intuitively link your client's feet with the deep earth or any of the elements of the earth. (See chapter 20 for more on the elements.)

7. Complete the treatment by asking your client for feedback about how they are feeling.

In the case of migraine symptoms, your hand movements may need to be done several feet away from your client's head. Find a distance where your client feels no discomfort from the presence of your hands. Use *Hands in Motion* to clear out congestion, continuing with it until you can move both hands closer to your client's head. Then change to the *Hands Still* position, holding your hands directly above your client's head and continuing until a sensation of symmetry and balance is established.

HEALING THE REIKI WAY

Reiki is a holistic spiritual healing practice developed in 1922 by Japanese Buddhist Mikao Usui, and it has since been adapted and changed by different teachers. Drawing from ancient traditions, Reiki employs both hands-on and hands-off healing.

Reiki uses life-force energy to heal and balance the subtle body, and the practitioner is the conduit for this universal energy. Reiki also uses mystical symbols that channel the energy toward a directed end. For decades, these symbols were kept secret, which is why different traditions explain them differently, but they are now available over the Internet and in many publications. Many people believe that the symbols are merely focus points for the practitioner and do not have power unto themselves.

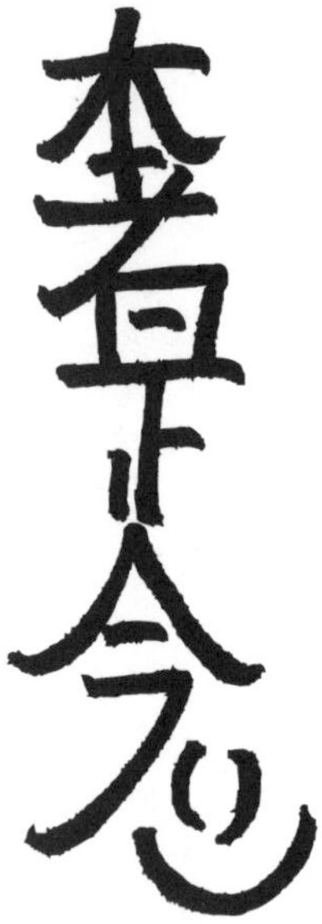

**FIGURE 12.1
THE REIKI
SYMBOL
CHO KU REI**

Cho Ku Rei
(pronounced
choh-koo-ray)
can be drawn
clockwise to bring
in or generate
energy, or
counterclockwise
to cleanse and
discharge energy.

One of the Reiki symbols you can use when practicing Reiki on yourself or someone else is Cho Ku Rei, which acts like a light switch to invite manifestation, increased power, and accelerated healing. The symbol consists of a horizontal line, which represents the Reiki source; a vertical line, which represents energy flow; and a spiral that touches the middle line seven times, representing the seven chakras (see figure 12.1). Cho Ku Rei is very versatile. You can draw it with your finger or your hand or visualize it in your mind. You can draw it on each of your palms before you do hands-on healing. You can draw it on a chakra, in an auric layer, or on a meridian acupoint. It can be sketched directly over an impaired or wounded area or traced on an object, on an image or picture, or into food or water. This symbol is often used in the beginning or the end of a healing session.

Here is a simple exercise you can use to catalyze healing and manifest a new reality using this power symbol.

Step 1: Decide which version of the symbol to use. When traced clockwise, the Cho Ku Rei symbol moves energy from spirit into matter, empowering, enabling manifestation, and promoting healing. When drawn counterclockwise, or in reverse, the symbol shifts energy from matter into spirit, discharging and releasing negative energy and cleansing.

Step 2: Set your intention. Select what you will activate and why. The most important part of the work is coming up with an intention (where to draw the symbol and why) and deciding if you should sketch the symbol clockwise or counterclockwise.

Step 3: Activate the symbol with intention. While tracing the symbol, focus on your intention. Imagine that the symbol works like a light switch, turning on the flow of life-force energy.

A few simple ideas for using Cho Ku Rei:

- Use it with other symbols or healing techniques. The Cho Ku Rei symbol can be used to bolster any other healing intention or process. For instance, you can add the clockwise symbol to the aura-charging technique explained in chapter 11 in order to energize the process, or you can use the counterclockwise symbol when releasing energetic impurities when cleansing your aura, as also explained in chapter 11.
- Use it to open or seal a healing. You can open a healing session for yourself or someone else with this symbol. Use the clockwise version if you or the

client need to bolster energy at the beginning or the end of a session, and use the counterclockwise if you need to release negativity or impurities.

- Draw the symbol directly over a wounded area to promote pain relief.
- Sketch it over an image of something you want to encourage the object in question to manifest.
- Draw in front of you (in the air) with an intention of protection.
- Draw the symbol over your home's windows or doorways with an intention of protection.
- Sketch it on or over a chakra or into an auric field layer to promote healing for that area of the subtle anatomy.
- Sketch it on your hand or your client's hand with a desire, such as empowering your writing or opening to healing energy.
- Bless your food and water by drawing the symbol above them. You can use a clockwise motion to add vitality or a counterclockwise motion if you are using the food or water to cleanse your body.
- Draw the symbol on and focus an intention into a crystal or a piece of jewelry for healing or magnetizing a wish.

You can also incorporate the Cho Ku Rei symbol into the essential energy techniques described in chapter 9.

For example, when using the Spirit-to-Spirit technique, after affirming your own spirit and that of another, ask the Greater Spirit to work through the Cho Ku Rei symbol to perform healing or manifesting.

You can also bolster the symbol with a healing stream of grace. As covered in chapter 9, healing streams of grace are powerful energies for change. When calling in a healing stream of grace to replace a block or impurity in a client's energy field, intuitively perceive the unhelpful energy being released and stream of grace attaching to the field, filling the void left by the unhelpful energy. Then perceive the connection point being sealed with the Cho Ku Rei symbol.

THE FIVE ELEMENTS IN YOUR HANDS

In the five-phase theory of traditional Chinese medicine, the human body is a reflection of the universe and the primary five elements—earth, metal, water, wood, and fire. These same five elements are reflected in and directed through each of our fingers. In the system developed by the Taoist master Mantak Chia, whose tradition is thousands of years old, each finger corresponds with the following elements:

- Thumb: earth
- Index finger: metal

- Middle finger: fire
- Ring finger: wood
- Little finger: water

In traditional Tibetan healing, the five elements are seen as space, wind, fire, water and earth. Each is similarly reflected in each finger, as is the color associated with that element:

- Thumb: space/white
- Index: wind air/green
- Middle finger: fire/red
- Ring finger: water/blue
- Little finger: earth/yellow

Whether your focus is acupressure, massage, Healing Touch, or another hands-on healing modality, being aware of these two systems and invoking the healing energies of the elements can increase the effectiveness of your healing practice.

FINGERS AS DIAGNOSTIC HEALING TOOLS

In deciding which finger or set of fingers to use for a subtle energy practice, consider the following questions as they relate to your client (or yourself, if you're engaged in self-healing):

Traditional Chinese medicine theory (Taoist):

- Is this issue about worry or the stomach? If so, use your thumb to bring in the earth element.
- Is this issue about sadness, grief, or depression, or the lungs and/or large intestine? If so, use your index finger to bring in the metal element.
- Is this issue about impatience or hastiness or the heart, small intestine, or circulatory and/or respiratory systems? If so, use your middle finger to bring in the fire element.
- Is this issue about anger or the liver, gallbladder, or nervous system? If so, use your ring finger to bring in the wood element.
- Is this issue about fear or the kidney(s)? If so, use your pinky finger to bring in the water element.

Traditional Tibetan system:

- Is this issue about higher ideals or principles? If so, use your thumb to bring in the element of space.

- Is this issue about ideas, thoughts, or beliefs? If so, use your index finger to bring in the element of wind/air.
- Is this issue about inflammatory conditions, passions, or the need to manifest? If so, use your middle finger to bring in the element of fire.
- Is this issue about emotions, creativity, or intuitive flow? If so, use your ring finger to bring in the element of water.
- Is this issue about practical concerns, physical healing, ancestors, or a need for groundedness? If so, use your pinky finger to bring in the element of earth.

You can also use your fingers themselves as diagnostic tools, employing each finger, one at a time, as you explore the following questions:

- As you begin to work on your client, are you drawn to use any of your fingers?
- Does a particular finger evoke a sense of strong feelings?
- Do certain fingers call forth images, words, or other intuitive messages?
- Do you feel compelled to use certain fingers more than once or use two or more fingers in any particular sequence?

The fingers that "talk" the loudest might be the ones that carry the most healing potential for you or your client.

SIMPLE FINGER HEALING

Using either the Traditional Chinese (Taoist) understanding of your fingers or the Tibetan understanding (or any other system you are comfortable with), you can bring instant relief to an issue by simply wrapping the fingers of your right hand around the left-hand finger related to the present issue and squeezing three to six times. You can then do the same on the opposite hand.

If you are employing the Chinese system, for instance, and you're dealing with anger, you can use your right hand to hold the ring finger of your left and squeeze it. In the Tibetan system, you'd hold your left index finger. If you feel overwhelmed and cannot figure out the problem, squeeze each finger, one by one, three to six times, and then reverse hands. Want to increase the effectiveness? Do deep abdominal breathing simultaneously.

ACUPRESSURE FOR EVERYONE

Acupressure is an ancient healing art in which the fingers press and hold key acu-points in order to stimulate the body's natural self-healing abilities. Sometimes referred to as acupoint massage, the acupressure that we will focus on in this chapter is derived from traditional Chinese medicine. As we explored in chapter 3, chi circulates throughout the body through energy channels called meridians. Each meridian corresponds to a different internal organ. Pressure points lie along the meridians, and these points are the focus of both acupuncture and acupressure. While acupuncture employs needles, acupressure uses gentle to firm finger pressure. When these acupoints are stimulated, they release muscular tension; promote circulation of chi, blood, and lymph fluid; and enhance the body's overall balance of life-force energy to aid healing.

Acupressure accomplishes two primary goals.

- When you **massage a point** in a small, circular motion, you release any blocked chi along the meridian and release tension in the related organ.
- When you **press and hold the point,** you draw chi more abundantly into the meridian, invigorating the organ system.

THE TEN GOLDEN ACUPOINTS

Out of the nearly 500 acupoints that exist within the human body, ten points are considered to be *the* points—the ten golden points that are most important for preventing and treating illnesses and imbalances of all kinds. At the center of acupuncture, acupressure, shiatsu, and other meridian-based therapies are the following acupoints:

Stomach 36 (ST 36): Revered by ancient physicians for its ability to treat all disease states, ST 36 restores and builds digestive energy in the stomach and the spleen. It is known to alleviate digestive disturbances, including constipation, gas, bloating, nausea, diarrhea, and abdominal pain and distention. It is also used to treat arthritis and weakness associated with aging.

Large Intestine 11 (LI 11): This is one of strongest points for boosting immunity to heal persistent infections. It expels excess heat, such as the heat associated with high fevers, hot flashes, and burning diarrhea. It alleviates damp-heat skin eruptions, such as acne, hives, and herpes zoster. It is useful for blood-circulation issues, such as anemia. Finally, it can be used to treat tremors and tennis elbow.

Large Intestine 4 (LI 4): This is one of the best analgesic points for any type of pain, including headaches and pain in the shoulder and arm. It is one of the most well-known points and is often referred to by the name *Hoku.* It is very helpful for clearing the excess heat in the body that can cause nosebleeds and fevers. It strengthens the body's defensive chi and is used for alleviating allergies, sinus congestion, colds, sneezing, runny nose, sore throat, sore eyes, and toothaches. *Use of this point is contraindicated during pregnancy.*

Bladder 40 (BL 40): This point is very useful in easing back pain (including acute low-back pain), muscle spasms, sprains, knee stiffness, and leg pain. It is also used to treat arthritis, skin-related issues (itching, inflammation), and heat conditions such as heat exhaustion and heatstroke.

Liver 3 (LR 3): This is a primary point for the liberation of chi, for releasing pent-up energy that can contribute to irritability, aggression, anxiety, depression, tension headaches, and premenstrual syndrome (PMS, including painful breasts). It nourishes tendons and ligaments by alleviating overall tightness and tension. Liver 3 is also known as a potent point for alleviating hypertension, insomnia, and even diabetes.

Gallbladder 34 (GB 34): This point controls the wind rising up to the head that causes insomnia, migraines, and anxiety. It is also used to treat indigestion, nausea, vomiting, and bitter tastes in mouth, and to prevent gallstones. It is useful for treating cramping, pain, spasms, sciatica, and other issues with the low back, hips, knees, and leg muscles.

Lung 7 (LU 7): This is a very good point for relief from asthma and breathlessness. It is also a key point for any conditions involving the head and posterior neck, including migraine headaches. It addresses the internal wind that can cause spasms, twitching, and Bell's palsy. And it is also effective for treating exterior wind issues such as alternating chills and fever, runny nose, scratchy and sore throat, sneezing, and body aches.

Heart 7 (HE 7 also known as HT 7): This point calms the mind and invites relaxation when overactive thinking has induced anxiety. It relieves insomnia due to overexcitement. It also reduces heart palpitations and regulates the heart by harmonizing its function, balancing emotions, and strengthening the spirit (or *shen*).

Spleen 6 (SP 6): Nourishing the spleen and building the blood, this point is important for addressing all gynecological, sexual, urinary, digestive, and emotional imbalances. It is often used to treat anxiety, insomnia, headaches, and menstrual cramps. And it's valued for relieving the feeling of heaviness and tiredness. *Use of this point is contraindicated during pregnancy.*

Kidney 1 (KI 1): This is a powerful point for grounding and connecting with earth energy. In this way, it is useful for calming and soothing someone who is highly anxious or has experienced a shock. It is used to treat headaches, hypertension, diarrhea, and insomnia. And it is also a vital point for nourishing the inner fire, especially in the elderly.

Thanks to the team of NaturalNews Network for inspiring this adapted roundup of acupoints. Identifying the top ten points from the vast number that exist is an invaluable distillation for the subtle energy healer.[2]

LOCATING YOUR TEN GOLDEN ACUPOINTS

Here are brief descriptions of the locations of your golden points, which are pictured in figure 12.2. A *cun* is the width of your thumb. Acupoints are found in depressive or slightly indented areas, often near the bones. You'll often feel tenderness in the spots that are blocked. (Note: Several of these points should not be used when pregnant or low on energy. Discuss these matters with a professional meridian specialist if you are concerned.)

Stomach 36 (ST 36): Three cun below your kneecap, one fingerbreadth toward the anterior crest of your tibia.

Large Intestine 11 (LI 11): Found at end of crease line on the outer side of your bent elbow.

Large Intestine 4 (LI 4): Press together your thumb and first finger to form an elevation. The point is at the highest point of the mound.

Bladder 40 (BL 40): Behind the knee, at the center of the crease.

Liver 3 (LR 3): On the top of your foot between your first (largest) and second toe bones, about three cuns in from large toe.

Gallbladder 34 (GB 34): On the outside of the leg just below your knee, in the tender depression about one cun below the head of the fibula.

Lung 7 (LU 7): Extend your thumb with the nail up, away from the palm of your hand. Find the depressed area at the base of your thumb, near your wrist. About another thumb-length (not a cun, which is the width) down this left side, you'll find another bone that sticks out. LU 7 is in between those two tendons.

Heart 7 (HE 7 also known as HT 7): At the wrist joint on the inner side, palm up, at the side of the pisiform bone. (About one cun from pinky side of wrist.)

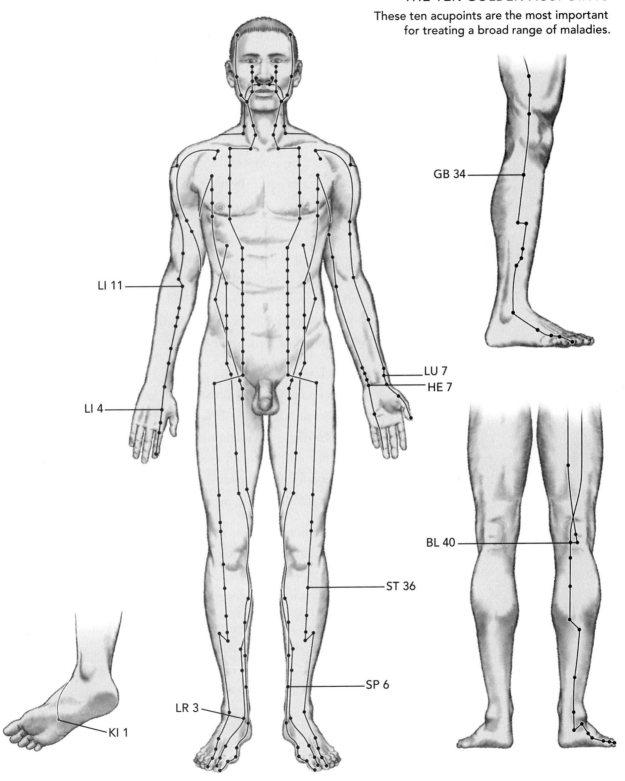

FIGURE 12.2
THE TEN GOLDEN ACUPOINTS
These ten acupoints are the most important
for treating a broad range of maladies.

GB 34

LI 11

LU 7
HE 7

LI 4

ST 36

BL 40

SP 6

LR 3

KI 1

Spleen 6 (SP 6): On the inside of the lower leg, one hand width above the tip of the anklebone and on the back of the shin bone.

Kidney 1 (KI 1): On the sole of your foot between the second and third toes, about one-third of the distance between the base of the second toe and the heel—in the depression that appears when your foot is extended or bent downward.

SIMPLE GUIDELINES FOR APPLYING ACUPRESSURE

The following guidelines for using acupressure are inspired by Michael Reed Gach, PhD, founder of the Acupressure Institute in Berkeley, California, and author of several books, including *Acupressure's Potent Points*.[2]

Tools of the trade. The middle finger is typically the longest and strongest of your fingers and is well suited for self-acupressure and applying acupressure with your clients. You can also use your knuckles, fist, or other tools, such as a tennis ball or a pencil eraser. Additionally, refer to the information on the five elements and the fingers (earlier in this chapter) to potentially increase the power of your application.

Finger pressure and holding acupoints. Use gradual, steady, and penetrating pressure directly on an acupoint for approximately two to three minutes. (You can increase the amount of time as you wish, but spend no longer than ten minutes on a single point.) While you might want to gently massage the point before applying direct pressure, avoid massaging the entire area around a point. When your finger or fingers are comfortably positioned on the spot, gradually lean your weight into the point, without straining.

Sensitivity and pain. Each point will feel somewhat different when you press it. You will likely encounter a few points that feel tender or sensitive when touched. If you feel extreme (or increasing) sensitivity, gradually decrease the pressure until you find a balance between pain and pleasure.

Mindfulness when applying and releasing pressure. Applying and releasing pressure gradually allows the tissues time to respond, which promotes healing. Moving your fingers into and out of the point with awareness will increase the effectiveness of your acupressure treatment.

Signs of chi. Hold a point for a few minutes until you feel a regular pulse (the pulsation of energy) or until the soreness at the point decreases. Then gradually release the pressure, finishing with a soothing touch.

Timing. Avoid working on a single area of the body, such as the face, head, or abdominal area for longer that fifteen minutes at a time. The effects of acupressure can be quite strong, and too much energy being released in one area can cause complications, such as a headache. And limit your self-acupressure sessions to one hour at the most.

Frequency. Practicing acupressure routines daily offers the best results. However, using acupressure two or three times a week is also highly beneficial.

Environment. Find a comfortable, private environment that is conducive to deep relaxation.

Body position. Choose whatever position you find most comfortable and convenient, either sitting or lying down.

Clothing. Loose, comfortable clothing is ideal.

Food and beverages. Avoid practicing acupressure on a full stomach or right before eating a large meal. Avoid iced drinks, as the extreme cold can counteract the benefits of acupressure. After a session, a cup of hot herbal tea is very good, along with a period of deep relaxation.

QUICK RELIEF WITH ACUPRESSURE: SEVEN ACU-EXERCISES FOR FAST RESULTS

The following seven acu-exercises are for self-care. They will help you do everything from easing anxiety to eliminating headaches to getting rid of neck pain. Given the accessibility and simplicity of each exercise, you can also use them with clients, including teaching them to clients, whenever that is appropriate. They include some acupoints beyond the top ten points featured above. For these, you will find a clear explanation of the location and benefits of each point.

Metabolism Boost

Good digestion involves much more than the stomach alone. A powerful way to fire up your metabolism is to liberate your liver chi (eliminating what is known as *liver chi stagnation*). The two acupoints you want to locate are Liver 3 (LR 3), also known as the "Great Surge," and Liver 2 (LR 2), known as "Moving Between." (See *The Subtle Body*, figure 4.15, page 198, for the location of LR 2.) Just find the depression on the top of each foot between the big toe and second toe. Press down gently but firmly, and either hold the spot or massage it for a few minutes. Using three fingers, you will be sure to contact both points simultaneously.

Note: Both LR 2 and LR 3 points will also help to relieve irritability, headaches, and poor circulation to the hands and feet (all signs that liver chi is blocked).

Anger and Tension Release

When irritation, tension, and anger build up, it is common to experience body aches and stiffness, along with the emotional upset. One of the best acupoints for releasing and melting this angst away is Conception Vessel 17 (CV 17), also know, aptly, as "Sea of Tranquility." At the center of your chest, above the sternum (level with the nipples, for many people), you will find CV 17 (see *The Subtle Body*, figure 4.16, page 199). One especially peaceful way to hold this point is to place your palms together in a prayer position, and then press the knuckles of your thumbs into the point. Remember to use your breath as your ally, breathing in deeply, and exhaling fully. Hold the point until it's no longer tender or until you feel some relief.

Neck Pain Relief (Plus)

In truth, this simple acupressure exercise will not only help to relieve neck pain, but it can also relieve neck stiffness, headaches, mental stress, nervous tension, irritability, eye strain, hypertension, tinnitus (ringing in the ears), and insomnia. By holding the pair of points known as Gallbladder 20 (GB 20), also called "Gates of Consciousness," you are helping to regulate chi circulation for the brain, relaxation, and the release of endorphins. They are very easy to find, and most of us intuitively rub these points from time to time. Just below the base of your skull, you will feel the two indentations or large hollows that are between the two vertical neck muscles. Using your fingers or knuckles (whichever is comfortable), press firmly but gently into those two hollows underneath the base of your skull. Your fingers will be approximately four finger widths (or three inches) apart. Close your eyes, tilt your head back very slowly, and take slow, deep breaths for two minutes or so. Repeat as necessary.

Stress Relief

Not surprisingly, one of the most effective stress-relief acupoints is found along the Heart meridian. Heart 7 (HE 7 or HT 7), also called "Spirit Gate," helps to relieve stress and anxiety at the level of the emotions. Whether you're experiencing a mild wave of worry or fear, or even outright panic, you can hold this point, which is easily found on the inside of your wrist.

Turn one of your hands so that your palm is facing upward. Now trace your little finger (pinky) down to the bottom of your hand, to the crease where your palm meets your arm—and just inside your wrist bone. With one to three of your fingertips, gently hold this point for a few minutes, remembering to breathe in deeply and exhale fully. When you are ready, switch to Heart 7 on your opposite wrist, holding and breathing for a few more peaceful minutes.

Anxiety Relief

Although there are several acupoints that are very useful for alleviating anxiety, there is one that is exceptional in its overall balancing and uplifting abilities—Kidney 1 (KI 1), also called "Gushing Spring." Nourishing to the whole being, Kidney 1 roots the body, refreshes the brain, and calms mind and spirit *(shen)*. This point is easily found on the sole of your foot. Place your finger between your second and third toes and trace over the ball of your foot until you come to the natural indentation about one-third of the way along the sole of your foot. Holding the point with one to three fingertips, breathe deeply for a few minutes and then switch to your other foot and repeat.

HEADACHE RELIEF

An elegantly simple approach to relieving headaches is readily available with this special acupressure point. Located in the center of your forehead, between your eyebrows, is the point that is associated with the third eye—the outer source point of one's inner vision. In traditional Chinese medicine, this point is known as Yin Tang (or "Hall of Impression"). It is interesting to note that although the point is located along the course of the Governor Vessel, it doesn't officially belong to that meridian. Instead, it belongs to a category of points known as the *extraordinary points*. Gently applying pressure to this point, and breathing consciously, you can allow headaches to dissipate, along with any anxiety or worry that may be the root of the tension.

Backache Relief

An easy and effective way to find relief from low-back pain, whether chronic or acute, is to apply acupressure to the Bladder 40 (BL 40) acupoints. Also known by the name "Bended Middle," these points are located at the back of each knee, in the center, at the middle point of the depression when your knees are bent.

Find a comfortable place to either lie down on your back with your knees bent or to sit in chair—whichever way will give you easiest access to the BL 40 points behind each knee while feeling as relaxed as possible. Hold the points for two to five minutes, using your breath to breathe in a color or image that symbolizes ease and openness for you. Let your out-breath release any tension in your back, legs, and any other part of your body where you may have pain.

Livestrong.com, the online resource cofounded by Lance Armstrong, is devoted to helping people to create their own health and wellness success stories. The acupressure exercises above were inspired by their compendium of resources and adapted to best support the subtle body.[4]

EMOTIONAL FREEDOM TECHNIQUES: PSYCHOLOGICAL ACUPRESSURE FOR TOTAL WELLBEING

Although there are many methods for addressing past wounds and present-day symptoms, Emotional Freedom Techniques (EFT) offers an elegant and often permanent solution. EFT comprises a series of tapping techniques that help individuals release stressful feelings. Created by Stanford University engineer Gary

SHIATSU MADE EASY

SHIATSU IS A Japanese word that means "finger pressure." However, a shiatsu treatment typically involves the use of thumbs, palms, knees, forearms, elbows, and feet, in addition to finger pressure. The goal is to apply pressure to the meridians and acupoints of the body, promoting vibrant health by stimulating chi—or *ki*, as the energy flow is known in Japanese healing.

A shiatsu session is typically done on a floor mat, allowing freedom of movement for the therapist. As a tool for self-healing and self-development, shiatsu can be done almost anywhere and at any time. The following simple exercises are accessible methods for practitioners and their clients to give themselves an energy tune-up when needed.

Head-to-toe energy flow. Unleash your ki energy by separating your toes with one hand, then squeezing each toe between your thumb and index finger. This allows energy to flow from your feet all the way to your chest.

Relieve neck and back stiffness. Free yourself from the stiffness that is caused by sitting at a desk too long. Stand up and place your hands on your waist. With thumbs pointing upwards on your back, steadily apply pressure in an up-and-down motion on either side of your spine. Feel the inherent strength of your back as energy is allowed to move again.

Escape anxiety, restore courage. To reduce anxiety and revitalize the energy of courage, use your knuckles to mildly tap across the top of your head. You'll be awakening the energy of several acupoints as you do this. While keeping a steady rhythm, remember to be gentle.

Craig, EFT dissolves the pain attached to grief, sadness, anger, or fear. Based on acupuncture and acupressure principles, it involves tapping meridian points on the head, chest, and underarms to free blockages from the meridian system while you think about a specific issue and voice a key phrase, often a reminder phrase about the cause of a negative reaction. Some practitioners follow this reminder phrase, which emphasizes your desire to change, with a positive affirmation. This combination clears emotional blocks from your subtle energy field and restores the energetic balance needed for health and wellbeing.

For this section, I called on the expertise of colleague Valerie Lis, an EFT Universe certified expert and trainer.[5] Valerie and other EFT practitioners have found that this approach is highly effective regardless of the intensity of the problem and often works in minutes. In addition to releasing stress, EFT is known to dissolve emotional pain (including phobias and trauma), abolish cravings, reduce chronic physical pain, resolve headaches and acid indigestion, provide freedom from food and chemical sensitivities, and improve physical performance (such as in sports and other athletic endeavors).

To try EFT right now, just follow these steps.

1. Focus on a specific bothersome memory. Notice how much stress you feel and where you feel that stress in your body. You want to experience the emotional distress of the issue while tapping in step 3; the more intense your reaction, the better and faster EFT will work. You can even create a phrase to encapsulate the issue, such as "anger at my mom" or "hurt at being ignored."

2. Prepare to tap. You can tap on both sides of your face at the same time, but this is not necessary, and according to Valerie, most people don't. Instead, tap on one side of your face or the other. It is okay to cross over, and you can use either hand.

3. While continuing to focus on the memory, gently tap with your fingertips four to seven times on each of the following locations. Following is a suggested order, although Valerie says the order is less important than your intention:
   - Top of the head
   - Inside of the eyebrow
   - Outside of the eye
   - Under the eye
   - Under the nose

- On the chin
- On the collarbone—at the beginning where your breastbone, collarbone, and first rib meet
- Under the arm, on the side of the body, at a point even with the nipple for men or in the middle of the bra strap for women, about four inches below the armpit

See figure 12.3 for a diagram of the first seven points.

4. Continue to focus on the memory and repeat the tapping procedure, tapping on each point in succession.

5. When you notice a shift, adjust your focus and start over. For example, if you still feel stressed but at a reduced level, focus on the feelings and thoughts that remain in your awareness (what is left of the problem). If the emotion has changed from stress to fear, focus on the fear and begin again. If the energy has moved from your stomach to your neck, adjust your focus and tap again.

This simplified process may be all you need to permanently eliminate your reaction to this memory. Although there are extended versions of EFT that may be more effective for deeply rooted memories, this quick-relief process provides the opportunity for anyone to experience its stress-relieving benefits.

In the following exercise, we will explore what happens when we add a specific phrase to the process of tapping.

RETURN TO JOY: AN EFT EXERCISE FOR HEALING EMOTIONAL HURT AND CLEARING DEPRESSION

Using EFT, we can face difficult memories and related limiting beliefs head-on by adding a statement to the tapping. This statement should be a positive one, such as "I am so happy," that brings up a negative reaction, such as causing you to feel unhappy. The tapping is used to clear the negative charges preventing you from accepting the positive belief or statement.

To clear resistance to joy, use the basic tapping points and technique outlined above while repeating aloud the statement, "I am so happy!" Say the statement out loud and with great enthusiasm; repeat it at every tapping point. After a few rounds, change it to, "I am *such* a happy person." Tapping with one or both of these statements usually begins the recovery process and resolves the underlying hurt, sadness, and other emotions that can crowd out peace and happiness.

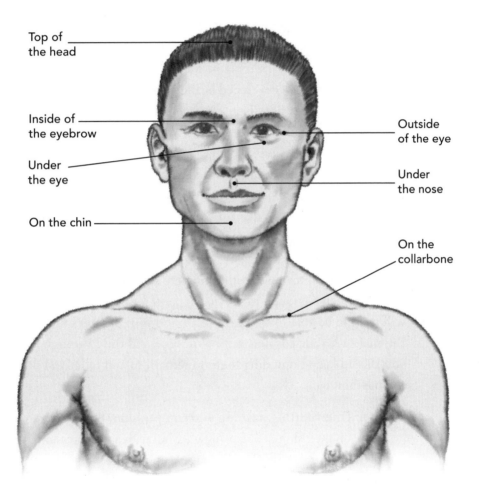

FIGURE 12.3

TAPPING POINTS OF EFT

Shown are the first seven points; the eighth point is underneath the arm, on the side of the body, at a point even with the nipple for men or in the middle of the bra strap for women, about four inches below the armpit.

Top of the head

Inside of the eyebrow

Under the eye

On the chin

Outside of the eye

Under the nose

On the collarbone

Using phrases such as these is the beginning point for some people; to clear depression that may be felt more strongly, more tapping should be done, for up to ten more minutes.

THAI MASSAGE: A MARRIAGE OF YOGA AND MASSAGE

Thai massage is a dynamic type of bodywork that brings together elements of yoga, stretching, and compression practices, a form of exercise therapy that combines pressure and massage, to elongate the muscles, increase blood flow throughout the body, and to allow chi to move freely and vibrantly.

Thai massage has its roots in Indian Ayurvedic healing techniques and is believed to have been developed by the physician to the Buddha more than 2,500 years ago. For centuries, Thai massage was performed by monks as a primary component of Thai medicine. Today, Thai massage is normally conducted by licensed massage therapists who have received this specialized training. If you are not specifically trained in this method, you can still try the following simple Thai massage techniques at home with a partner.

Before you begin, make sure you're dressed comfortably. Since Thai massage is a very active practice, you and your partner should dress in loose clothing that does not restrict movement. Also choose a location on the floor that gives you ample room to move, either on very soft carpet or a comfortable exercise mat that is large enough to provide support for both of you. If using a mat, you will need to be able to freely move around your partner's body without leaving the mat. Ask your partner to remain loose and fluid throughout this exercise; you should keep reminding them to remain so and to let you do the work during the massage.

> **Step One: Starting position and compression.** Begin with your partner lying on their stomach, face down. Start with a compression, which is one of the key strokes in Thai massage. Using the heel of your hand, press down on your partner's back, arms, and legs. Work with your partner to determine a comfortable level of pressure. According to the Associated Bodywork and Massage Professionals, this touch increases circulation, promotes the drainage of lymph fluid, and relaxes tense or overused muscles.

> **Step Two: Range of motion—arms and hands.** This exercise can be done with your partner either face down or face up. Actively move your partner's limbs. Start by moving each arm through its range of motion. Bring the arm over their head and gently pull it away from their body to provide a stretch. Also rotate the hands and feet through their ranges of motion.

Step Three: Simple bent knee stretch. With your partner face up on the mat, sit near their feet, your legs around their legs. Raise one of their legs so that their knee is facing up toward the ceiling. Tuck their foot under their hamstring near the buttock. Fold your hands together and place them on the far side of your partner's knee, wrapped around so that your partner can see them. Now gently lean back, pulling upward and toward you so as to stretch your partner's leg near the knee. You can then shift your hands a few inches further up your partner's thigh and lean back, pulling softly for a quick stretch. Raise your hands another few inches and repeat this motion. Each of the stretches lasts no more than a couple of seconds. Once you have reached mid-thigh, reverse a few inches and repeat this stretch until you return to the knee. Repeat this stretch with the other leg. Talk and work with your partner to determine other areas that can be comfortably stretched. Remember to go slow and easy.

Step Four: The torso life stretch. A common movement in Thai massage is called the torso life. With your partner lying face down, on their stomach, you kneel on the ground between their legs, enabling you to hold their arms and gently pull them up and back. Lifting their torso, head, and neck off the ground and pulling them backwards provides a lovely stretch for the back, shoulders, and abdominal muscles.

Be sure to communicate with your partner, always finding out what feels like the right amount of pressure and stretching for them. Thai massage should never be painful. If stretches are taken too far, they can cause injury. Encourage your partner to speak up if they feel uncomfortable, and keep reminding them to relax. And both of you should remember to make use of the cleansing, healing power of the breath throughout the practice.

13

MODERN ESOTERIC HEALING

> The possibility of stepping into
> a higher plane is quite real for
> everyone. It requires no force
> or effort or sacrifice. It involves
> little more than changing our
> ideas about what is normal.
>
> DEEPAK CHOPRA, MD

The nature of subtle energy healing is quite *esoteric*—mysterious, enigmatic, and perhaps even mystical. It often involves visiting other places, times, dimensions, and spaces. This chapter provides access to these esoteric places and a few techniques that can safely take you to them. After describing each place you can visit, I will share a healing process that will help you clear and resolve issues in that space. Included also is a section on performing distant healing, which involves remaining in place and sending healing energy elsewhere.

HEALING ISSUES AT THEIR ORIGIN: THE WHITE ZONE

Before embarking on a particular lifetime, our soul enters the *white zone*. Within this space, we engineer a *soul contract*, an agreement between us and our spirit guides or the Divine that covers what we want to learn and accomplish in an upcoming lifetime. The main soul contract incorporates contracts with other souls, such as our future mother, father, siblings, friends, and significant romantic partners. These individual soul-to-soul contracts outline the nature of these relationships, including when we will meet and what type of relationship we will form. These soul connections often form the basis of energetic bindings or cords; the commitment can solidify into an energetic bargain that can, unfortunately, create a locked-in issue rather than a free-flowing bond.

Also within the white zone, we establish our destiny points, the "must happens" that will occur when we're inhabiting a physical body. We might select our schools and career moves. We might also choose to experience challenging or even life-threatening events, if we believe that they are necessary for our soul learning.

In your work as a practitioner of subtle energy medicine, you may have clients come to you who desire change or healing pertaining to their soul contract, whether they are consciously aware of the contract or not. You might want to change your own soul contract. In these cases, it is appropriate to revisit the white zone to uncover the original soul plan and change it, if appropriate. The following is the basic method for accessing this dimension:

1. Always start at the eighth chakra, which is just above the head, as the portal for exploration, or your fourth chakra, your heart, through which you can also access other time periods. The eighth chakra also links to the physical body through the thymus, which is just above the center of your chest, which means you can also access it through this "high heart" area.

2. From the middle of the eighth or fourth chakra, envision the filaments that emanate from its center and surround it. Ask your higher guidance to show you which thread will lead to the white zone.

3. Journey along the designated filament to reach the white zone.

4. Once there, ask to see or reexperience the agreement that has caused an issue that is adversely affecting you.

5. If it seems that you are best served rewriting the agreement, ask for divine or spiritual help to do so.

If serving as the healer for another person, you can verbally guide your client through these steps, asking them to relay their findings so you can follow along.

If the client is unable to obtain this information, you can undertake these steps on their behalf, as shamans in many cultures have done through the ages. For the purpose of energetic safety, journey in your own inner being and energetic anatomy, asking to register the client's information within yourself. This way you remain within your own personal boundaries and are still able to read a client's energies.

THE ENERGETIC RECORDS: THE LIBRARIES OF YOUR SOUL

There are three main energetic records you can access or visit to enable healing: the Akashic Records, the Shadow Records, and the Book of Life.

The *Akashic Records* contain all knowledge of human experience. This metaphysical library or compendium of knowledge resides in a nonphysical plane of existence. These are records of the factual history of both our individual lives and the cosmos itself. One of the extraordinary aspects of the Akashic Records is that they contain the knowledge of everything ever done, said, or thought in what we experience as past, present, *and* future.

The most elegant way to access the Akashic Records is through the eighth chakra, meditatively attuning to the portal of the eighth chakra to open to and receive the information you seek. The Akashic Records are often utilized to do past-life work, inner-child work, or when engaged in a significant decision-making process.

The *Shadow Records* contain our "unfinished business"— regrets, disappointments, heartaches, and even shame—that can cause an incalculable amount of emotional, mental, and physical pain. This unfinished business is often comprised of things not done, not said, not thought, and not felt. We could simply describe this human phenomenon as "that which hasn't been and still lingers" across time and space. Another way to understand it is as the things that we believe *could have* or *should have* happened, but didn't.

The *Book of Life* contains the knowledge of the gifts of the paths you have taken. Having gone to the Akashic Records and the Shadow Records to gather pieces of the miraculous puzzle of our lives, we can then enter the Book of Life and find a transformational viewpoint, a new perspective that will allow us to deeply know and understand what is important in what did happen, what didn't, what could have, and/or what will. This way, we may come to a far deeper understanding that enables us to sincerely say, "Okay, I now see the gifts of the path I have taken."

The following exercise, "Uncovering Your Storyline" can be used to access any and all of these records.

UNCOVERING YOUR STORYLINE

A storyline is the sequence of events that led to a life challenge. Some of these events are concrete, but most of them—the most important—are invisible, consisting of our inner reactions and unconscious decisions.

This particular exercise is designed for you to use for your own process of healing and evolution and to be used for similarly assisting your clients. It will assist you with finding the cause of a current dilemma. It can be used to access past-life memories, childhood events, or more contemporary experiences. As well, you can use this process to deliberately access information about the past through your Akashic Records, uncover regrets through the Shadow Records, or find hidden gifts through the Book of Life.

There are five elements involved in uncovering your storyline or the series of events that led to your current problems. They are:

Your imprisoned self. If a trauma was really big or hurtful, the energy of it locks us into the age we were when we experienced it. That part of us never gets to grow up, to stretch, grow, and fly. She or he is incarcerated in the energetic fibers created by the people or situation that injured us. We must rescue this hidden, trapped self in order to release the negative energies sentencing him or her to prison.

The safety violation. This refers to the nature of the event, attitude, person, or chronic situation that threatened our survival.

Your security decision. In order to survive the threatening situation, you had to think quickly—maybe so quickly that you weren't even thinking when you (unconsciously) decided how to energetically protect yourself. What did you decide that you had to do in order to survive?

The syndrome. Inevitably, your survival-based decision locked up your development and impacted other areas of your life. How did it affect you short and long term? How is it still affecting you today?

The need. What was supposed to happen? How should you have been treated, if you had been loved, protected, and valued? Here is your work; herein lie the answers to the question of how to heal yourself from the past.

Are you ready to discover a pertinent storyline? The easiest way to perform this exercise on your own is to take out a pen and paper and lead yourself through questions and answers in a state of open awareness. If you are guiding a client through this internal process, have paper and pen ready to capture the information they share out loud, and adapt the following script accordingly.

The active meditation I have designed involves asking your spirit questions about the storyline. We each are a spirit, and this spirit is also our wise self. In this process, I will be asking you to see, experience, hear, or sense your wise self as a being separate from you. This is so you can obtain the necessary answers and healing that is buried within your subconscious. At the end of the process, you will reintegrate this wise self so your healing can continue.

1. Secure yourself in a quiet place and make sure you won't be disturbed for a while. As calmly as possible, settle into a comfortable position and breathe deeply, guiding yourself into your heart.

2. Ask that your own inner spirit, or wise self, appear on your mind's inner screen. Take a moment and engage with this wise self. What does he or she look like? How is your wise self dressed or clothed? Does he or she hold any objects of power or talismans?

3. Ask this wise self if there is a name you should use when consulting him or her and, if so, what the meaning of this name is. Also ask if your wise self is willing to help you journey back to the origin of the problem you are experiencing. If he or she says yes, prepare to travel.

4. With your wise self as a guide, slip backward in time. You soon find yourself in an earlier time and place.

5. At this earlier time and place, you are able to observe what happened. Noticing the persons or people involved in the damaging event, you are able to completely reexperience everything that occurred, including your emotional responses. You are also able to perceive the changes that occurred in your energetic field in reaction to the trauma.

6. If you are having a difficult time observing, seeing, or sensing what happened at that time—if you feel blocked in some way, receiving hazy or incomplete impressions, for example—ask your wise self to access the Akashic Records to review what happened and the Shadow Records to reveal what you *needed* to have happen at that time, but that did not happen.

7. Pencil and paper in hand, you now turn to the wise one at your side and ask his or her opinion about the following. You are able to write down what you hear or are shown, even as you are listening:
   - I was traumatized by this experience because:
   - Because of this experience, I decided to believe:
   - Because of this belief, I felt this way:
   - I decided that, to protect myself, I needed to:
   - To further protect myself, I developed this coping mechanism:
   - Whenever I am in an experience that makes me feel the same way, I react this way:
   - These reactions create the following problems for me:
   - What I really needed to have happen during and after the trauma was:
   - What I really need in order to heal is:
   - In order to be truly protected in my life now, my energetic boundaries should be formed like this:
   - I can remain both safe and loved this way:

8. After you ask additional questions of your own, you and your wise self look at the you that was injured by this past experience. Together, reach out your arms and hearts and hold this younger you. Reassure your younger self that everything is being put right.

9. Then, ask your wise self to reveal the knowledge contained in the Book of Life related to this event or experience. What is the *gift* of this event or experience that your wise self wants you and your younger self to receive? Sense how the recognition of this gift is a doorway to forgiveness and healing.

10. Magnetically drawn to the hearts of one another, your current, wise, and younger selves all merge together. The wise self transforms all wounds into wings of joy and all injuries into gifts of grace.

11. Take a few deep breaths, and record anything else you feel drawn to write down. Then return to a state of full consciousness. Know that you can engage your wise self for further information and healing any time you want.

REMOTE VIEWING: OBSERVATIONS THROUGH TIME AND SPACE

Remote viewing is a powerful yet simple process for accessing a distant place, time, or space for the purpose of gathering information. Although remote viewing is often described as a strictly science-based protocol (often used in military settings for gathering remote or hidden information), I have found it useful for laypeople as well. Imagine that you need to make a decision based on events occurring elsewhere. Why not journey there through remote viewing? Likewise, the cure for an issue might be secreted away in a laboratory or a healer's office halfway around the world, or it might lay in the distant past or far future. Remote viewing can be undertaken to access any time or any place.

The viewer—or voyager—employs their subtle energy senses to gather information. In terms of the chakras, remote viewing employs both the eighth chakra, also known as the shaman's chakra, located just above the head; the thymus and the heart chakra or high heart; and the visual intuitive gifts of the sixth chakra, which enable us to psychically envision someone, something, or a situation in the past, present, or future.

The voyager is fully awake and conscious throughout the session; they do not enter a hypnotic or meditative state. Different from a shamanic journeying session, where *interaction* takes place in the inner realms, remote viewing is an *observational* process. (See chapter 17 for information on shamanic journeying.)

Remote viewing is also not an out-of-body experience or astral travel. On the level of consciousness, the voyager stays in their body, accessing their heightened abilities to see, sense, and know through the safety and expanse of their own soul. Even though the voyager's soul doesn't actually travel anywhere, it is helpful to describe a remote-viewing session in terms of traveling, since the experience involves sensing intuitive information that isn't immediate to the voyager.

Voyager and guide. In remote viewing, it is preferable that a session be done with two people: a voyager and a guide. The remote viewer is the voyager and is supported by a guide, who is physically present. The guide helps the voyager to relax and ground, assists them as they travel, and notes the details that are conveyed through the viewing session. As you may choose to be both guide and voyager at different times, the basic outline that follows is written to clearly delineate both roles.

Focus and goal. At the start of the session, the guide may also help the voyager to determine where they want to travel—past, present, or future—and for what purpose. The voyager must have a distinct focus and a goal for their remote-viewing session. Where do they want to go and for what purpose? Having this clarity will allow them to paint their scenario as specifically as possible. Being precise and detailed is a key to remote viewing.

Grounding and centering. The guide helps the voyager to ground and center. First, the guide directs the voyager to take a few slow, depth breaths, drawing their breath all the way down into their feet. The guide can ask the voyager to feel the connection between their body, the chair beneath them, and the earth itself.

Choosing the departure point. When I guide a client through a remote-viewing session, I have them access their expanded senses through their eighth chakra. Containing the journey in the eighth chakra helps the client stay focused on the task at hand and keeps their energies wrapped within a boundary; as a practitioner, I don't need to focus so much on maintaining my own boundaries because my client's are contained. As well, all information across time is available through the eighth chakra, which enables my client to access the data needed. This energy center links with the physical body in the thymus area, located in the high heart area (just above the center of the chest), further ensuring that the voyager isn't misguided or misdirected by energies that aren't their own.

Moving in time and space. With the voyager's focus and goal as the catalyst, the guide asks the voyager to breathe their soul to the time and space that is their target, so that the voyager is able to see that time and space as if they were actually there. In fact, the voyager's soul remains in his or her body while observing this other time and space; as noted, this link to the physical body assures energetic safety.

Making intuitive observations. The guide now asks questions that assist the voyager in turning on their ability to see, hear, sense, and know that other time and space. By asking questions such as the following, the guide invites the voyager to engage their abilities of seeing and sensing in order to relate what they are observing.

- What are you seeing?
- Who is present?
- Where are you in relation to what is going on?
- What are you hearing?
- Who is talking?

As the voyager says out loud what they are seeing and sensing, the guide writes down the information. Additional questions can be added depending on the purpose of the viewing.

Tip: The guide should not ask the voyager to interact with the environment or situation they are viewing. In my own practice, I never tell a client what to do or what to interact with in a remote-viewing session.

Returning. Upon gathering the information they are able to view, the voyager returns the same way they began their travel—through the eighth chakra. The guide instructs the voyager to use their breath to bring their awareness back to the chair they are sitting in, back to their physical surroundings. With that, the remote-viewing session comes to a close.

THE VIVAXIS: YOUR EARTH-ENERGY BODY

In chapter 2, "Fields of Healing," you first learned about the Vivaxis, an energetic sphere that develops within us as a fetus and forever links us to our place of birth. *Vivaxis* is a term coined by Judy Jacka (and her teacher, Frances Nixon) and is described in detail in Jacka's book, *The Vivaxis Connection*.[1]

The central idea is that energy continues to flow between us and our place of origin (our birthplace) throughout our life, like a two-way umbilical cord of magnetic waves. When major shifts occur in the land, whether caused by natural or human alterations, we might experience similar effects in our own bodies. The Vivaxis is, therefore, an ideal energy body to assess if you or your client has symptoms such as fatigue, chronic inflammation, sudden-onset autoimmune disorders, or severe environmental allergies.

The following applications offer ways to address physical illness and emotional challenges, possibly transforming issues that have been resistant to other methods.

APPLICATION ONE: HEALING ILLNESS

I work with the Vivaxis whenever a client has chronic or acute physical conditions that don't seem to respond to allopathic or holistic care. You can diagnose a potential Vivaxis connection as the source of the presenting problems in two ways.

Research the place of birth. Ask your client to research his or her place of birth, specifically to uncover changes that have occurred in the environment since they were born, such as new construction, the razing of a building, or the addition of toxic waste, power lines or other electrical structures, or other anomalies. Then ask your client to sense how their body responds when you describe these circumstances back to them. Do their symptoms increase? Do they give a sigh of relief, as if the cause of their problems has been found?

Intuitive visualization of the birthplace. Conduct a guided visualization in which you help your client sense what is occurring at his or her birthplace now, exploring through intuition the connection between environmental shifts and their illness. (See chapter 15 if you would like instructions on leading guided visualizations.) Have your client imagine themselves traveling along their Vivaxis umbilical cord to the place of their birth. Note that the cord begins at the *hara*, the Japanese name for the portal located at the navel and considered to be the center of ki energy (also known in traditional Chinese medicine as the lower dan tien and the center of chi). For this healing process, it is important to know that hara is also the gateway to the etheric envelope surrounding the planet.

If the birthplace seems to be a source of your client's discomfort, encourage them to energetically pick up their Vivaxis and anchor it somewhere else. The new location could be their current residence, a favorite spot in nature, an element that suits his or her personality (see chapter 20, "Healing with the Natural World," for ideas), or even a place "off world," such as the spiritual site of heaven.

Then allow the energy of this new site to cleanse and clear your client's body and continue to replenish them for as long as necessary to heal the presenting condition. Know that your client might need to repeat this step every day for a few weeks in order to continue flushing the body.

APPLICATION TWO: GROUNDING INTO A GOOD LIFE

Some individuals feel very challenged by their life circumstances, so much so that they report difficulties with concentration, focus, decision making, and stability within their life. They might feel like they don't fit in or have a hard time negotiating normal life.

Similarly, as a healer you might feel frequently destabilized by your clients' issues or so sensitive that it's hard to remain centered in your work. Shifting a Vivaxis from a birthplace to a more life-enhancing site can often make a significant difference.

Following the steps in the application above, consider connecting to a new subtle energy residence—a place that creates the type of emotional and mental wellbeing that a client wants to feel (or that you want to feel). Again, this could be a place in nature, a vacation spot, or even an element that best supports your health and true personality (water, wood, air, fire, stone, earth, metal, light, ether, or star).

DISTANT HEALING

There are circumstances and situations where giving hands-on help is just not possible. This is when we can use *distant healing,* which involves sending or affirming healing energy long distance. Distant healing works at the subtle energetic level and is basically a way to reach out to people with your healing gifts. The exercises in this section are based on the work of my colleague Jack Angelo, author of *Distant Healing: A Complete Guide,* which is a thoughtful, clear, and immensely useful guidebook for learning to open to and send subtle healing energies to people, animals, environmental issues, and challenging situations.[2] The process described here can be used to send healing energy not only to a person, but also to a group or a situation, such as a place experiencing a natural disaster.

PERFORMING A DISTANT-HEALING SESSION

To get started, all you need is the name of the person you will be sending energy to. If they have come to you through an intermediary, such as a loved one who has reached out on their behalf, you will need to know whether the person has agreed to accept distant-healing help. Without this level of agreement, the healing energies may be unwanted, unnecessary, or ineffective. If you have a strong sense that the potential recipient would not want the healing energy, do not engage in a distant healing. Sometimes we don't know, however. In this case it is acceptable to send energy to a person's highest self or spirit, which can then determine how best to use the energy.

When people ask for your help, either for themselves or for a third party, asking them to give you a progress report engages them in the process and encourages them to take responsibility for their requests. Asking clients to join in can further empower them while also helping you, amplifying the healing energies through intention and attention.

Ideally, the recipient of the energy joins in the healing session at the same time as the healing is being sent, though this is not crucial. Remember, the energies travel outside of the space-time continuum. Invite the person to sit or lie quietly at the time you will be sending healing to them. Ask them to relax, breathe normally, and visualize a sphere of protective light around them. They should remain like this for fifteen minutes if possible. When people are able to participate in their healing in this way, they frequently sense the energies in all kinds of ways and are able to give you feedback about their experience, which may or may not coincide with your experience of their healing. In any case, their feedback will be interesting and informative, and it will demonstrate the many fascinating ways in which healing energy manifests.

1. As you begin, you may wish to light a candle as a symbol of the light of the Source (the Divine). If you do, dedicate the light of the Source to the work and to any helpers you might have in the spiritual realms. Give thanks that you have been given the opportunity to send out healing light (energy).

2. Bring your focus to your heart center (the fourth chakra). As you inhale, visualize this center filling with the light of the Source. With the next breath, the light fills your chest.

3. With the recipient's name written down in front of you, ask for the light to be sent out to that person, calling them by name. You can say aloud or in your mind, "I ask for healing to be sent to (name)." Pause and tune in to what is happening energetically.

4. When you feel energetically complete, give thanks. Rest assured that the person you focused on has received the healing they need. Sit quietly with your experience for a moment.

5. When you have finished, you can send out the light of the candle as you extinguish it. Pause for a moment before blowing out the candle and see if you intuitively feel where the light needs to go. This is usually the first place that comes to mind and could be the location of a specific person, a strife-ridden place, an environment under threat, or elsewhere. As you blow out the candle, say, "I send the light out to (name of the place)."

Once you have closed your session, you have handed over the name of the recipient to higher powers. It is time to stop thinking about the session.

14

HEALING MOVEMENT

May what I do flow from me like
a river, no forcing and no holding
back, the way it is with children.

RAINER MARIA RILKE

Remember childhood? For most of us, it was a time when we ran like the wind, climbed trees, rode bicycles, rolled around in the damp grass, jumped in puddles of water, and swam in just about any body of water we could, from blow-up kiddy pools to grand lakes. We may genuinely not *want* to climb trees now, but somehow we intuitively sense that we would be nourished and rejuvenated by more movement, the way we were as kids.

This chapter is devoted to the styles and types of healing movement that are exceptionally effective when working with subtle energies. In brief, we will explore yoga, acu-yoga, qigong, tai chi, mudra practice (for working internally with increased energy), and the unmatched wonders and joys of *walking*. Whether it is slow and subtle or fast and vigorous, each of the styles of movement outlined here has been chosen for its unique ability to open the chakras and meridians, clear the electromagnetic fields, and invoke and build up the life-force energy that heals. (Please consult your licensed professional if you have any questions before doing these or any other exercises.)

ACU-YOGA

Acu-yoga is the brilliant pairing of acupressure and yoga. Modified asanas (yoga postures) are utilized to gently stimulate specific acupressure/acupuncture points, meridians, and various parts of the body that are prone to holding tension. The postures, combined with breathing and relaxation exercises, are a form of physical self-therapy and practical tools for enhancing health. Acu-yoga is a subtle energy maintenance practice focused primarily on prevention of illness and imbalances.

As an adjunct to other holistic tools, the following are just some of the conditions that acu-yoga can help relieve:

- Chronic fatigue and nervous exhaustion
- Cold and flu
- Backache
- Hyperacidity and acid reflux
- Hypertension
- Heart disease
- Diabetes
- Obesity
- Depression
- Insomnia
- Impotence

ACU-YOGA ESSENTIALS: BRIDGE POSE AND WING LIFTING POSE

Two acu-yoga poses that are known for their overall rejuvenating effects are Bridge Pose and Wing Lifting Pose, outlined below. For maximum benefit, practice these two poses two or three times a day for one week, eventually establishing acu-yoga as a daily routine. Gradually increase the length of time spent in each pose. Most importantly, follow your practice with ten minutes of deep relaxation, lying on your back with your eyes closed.

Bridge Pose

This acu-yoga version of Bridge Pose is done with the arms overhead. The completed pose is shown in figure 14.1. Here's how to do it:

1. Lie on your back.

2. Bend your knees so the soles of your feet are flat on the floor.

3. Put your arms above your head on the floor and let them relax.

4. Inhale, arching your pelvis up. Hold for several seconds.

5. Exhale as you slowly bring your pelvis down to the floor.

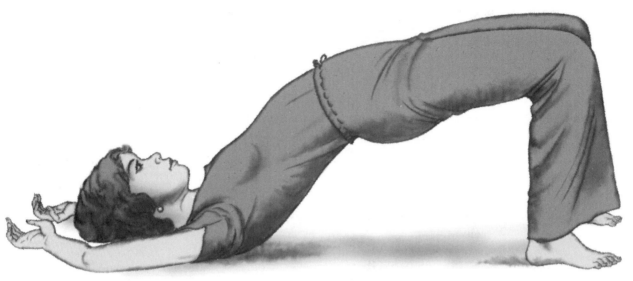

FIGURE 14.1
BRIDGE POSE

Lying on your back with bent knees and arms extended overhead, inhale and lift up your pelvis. Hold for several seconds, then exhale and lower.

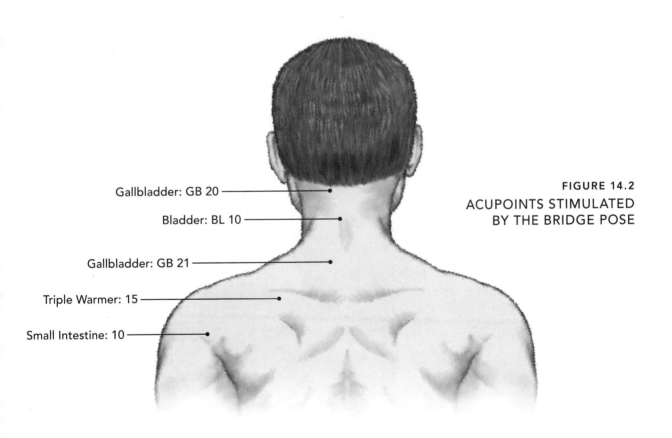

Gallbladder: GB 20

Bladder: BL 10

Gallbladder: GB 21

Triple Warmer: 15

Small Intestine: 10

FIGURE 14.2
ACUPOINTS STIMULATED BY THE BRIDGE POSE

6. Continue to inhale up and exhale down for one minute.

7. Remember to relax on your back with your eyes closed for a few minutes when you are done.

Another common version of this pose involves keeping your arms at your sides. While staying on the floor, lift your hips and torso while inhaling for several seconds. Exhale as you slowly bring your pelvis back down.

Bridge Pose provides benefits by stimulating the following acupoints, shown in figure 14.2, for healing effects:

Triple Warmer 15 (TW 15): Relieves stiff neck, shoulder and neck pain, and elbow pain.

Gallbladder 20 (GB 20): Relieves anxiety, shoulder and neck pain, rheumatism, eye tension, and excess heat and heaviness in the upper parts of the body.

Gallbladder 21 (GB 21): Relieves shoulder and neck pain, hyperthyroidism, and rheumatism.

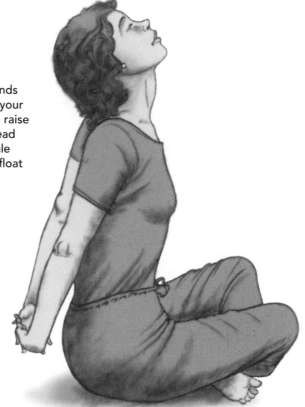

FIGURE 14.3
WING-LIFTING POSE
Sitting comfortably, with your hands clasped behind your back, press your shoulder blades together. Inhale, raise your shoulders, and drop your head back. Straighten your arms. Exhale and let your arms and shoulders float down. Repeat five times.

Bladder (BL 10): Relieves sore throat, neck spasms, and a feeling of fullness in the head.

Small Intestine (SI 10): Relieves muscular pain, numbness, swelling, and arthritis in the shoulder-scapula region.

Wing-Lifting Pose

This pose is demonstrated in figure 14.3. Here is how to do it:

1. Sit comfortably and clasp your hands behind your back, palms facing each other. You can sit on the floor cross-legged or with your legs extended. You can also sit in a chair.

2. Press your shoulders back so that your shoulder blades are squeezed together.

3. Inhale, raise your shoulders up toward your ears, and gently let your head drop back.

4. Straighten your arms and lift them away from your back and buttocks.

5. Exhale, and come to the resting position with your hands still clasped behind your back.

6. Repeat steps 2 through 5 five times. Work up to continuing the exercise for one minute.

DIAPHRAGMATIC BREATHING FOR QIGONG

DIAPHRAGMATIC OR YOGIC breathing is one of the most important aspects of qigong practice. It maximizes the healing and balancing potential of the movements by

- stimulating blood circulation,
- increasing oxygen to the brain and throughout the body,
- building internal strength by generating chi energy, and
- promoting relaxation and receptivity.

Simply breathe through your nose, with your tongue placed in a natural resting position against the upper teeth and palate, and with your lips pressed lightly together. When your tongue is pushing against the palate, it acts as a bridge that allows the chi energy to travel down from the top of your head and into your body.

When practicing diaphragmatic breathing, pause between your inhalation and exhalation to give the chi energy time to collect and build. (See chapter 18 for additional breathing techniques.)

7. Unclasp your hands and let your arms relax, and lightly shake your shoulders.

8. Remember to relax on your back with your eyes closed for a few minutes when you are done.

Wing-Lifting Pose is the go-to acu-yoga posture for preventing or alleviating hypertension (high blood pressure). Stretching and releasing the shoulders allows the physical and emotional tension that can contribute to hypertension to melt away. You can take the positive effects of the pose with you throughout the day by reminding yourself to breathe, relax, and open.

QIGONG

What is the subtle energy "secret" that more than sixty million people in China, and countless others around the globe, know about and practice? It is qigong, the ancient discipline that coordinates the movement of the body with deep-breathing exercises and mind-focusing disciplines. In other words, qigong is a form of exercise created to mentally generate and direct chi through movement. Qigong exercises often imitate the natural motions of animals, such as the crane, deer, or monkey, and are accompanied by simple breathing techniques.

Qigong can

- strengthen the connection between body and mind,
- enhance the nervous system,
- reduce stress hormones,
- ease depression and anxiety,
- boost the immune system,
- ease headaches and allergies, and
- facilitate deeper sleep.

QIGONG ESSENTIALS: TWO EXERCISES FOR EVERY BODY

Pulled from the treasure trove of qigong exercises, here are step-by-step instructions for two of the most useful and effective choices for personal and professional care — one for overall energy tune-ups and the other specifically for easing back pain.

Exercise 1: Ringing the Temple Gong

This is a simple go-to qigong exercise that you can do anywhere, any time, for both relaxation and an energy boost. For practitioners, Ringing the Temple Gong is an invaluable practice. Not only can you use it to increase your own energy and wellbeing, but you can also use it to prepare for your working sessions and can recommend it to clients when appropriate.

1. With your arms at your sides, stand with your feet shoulder width apart and your knees slightly bent.

2. Turn your torso as far as you can comfortably go to the right, allowing your arms to follow with a gentle swing. Then turn your torso and arms to the left.

3. Finding your own rhythm, keep turning right, then left. Gently build momentum until your hands lightly strike the abdomen and back at the end of each rotation. If it's comfortable, turn your head to look over each shoulder as you rotate.

4. Breathe normally throughout the movement, occasionally taking a deep breath to invite deeper relaxation.

Do this exercise for as long as you would like. After a few seconds or minutes, begin to gradually slow down, coming to a gentle stop. Allow yourself to stand still for a moment, consciously lengthening your spine and noticing the sensations of increased subtle energy throughout your body.

Exercise 2: Qigong Horse

Qigong Horse is a targeted, therapeutic exercise for easing back pain. To build up strength in your back, begin with the seated version.

1. Sit on the edge of a chair. Only your buttocks should be on the seat, not your thighs. Plant your feet flat on the ground, placing them shoulder-width apart with toes pointed forward and parallel to each other. Bend your knees to a ninety-degree angle. Keep your back straight, but not rigid, and your shoulders relaxed.

2. Notice the backs of your thighs, allowing any tension there to be released.

3. Lengthen your spine by visualizing a golden thread at the top of your head being gently pulled skyward. Raise your torso slowly and gently, until you are standing.

As you rise up each time, place your attention on the backs of your thighs and buttocks. If they are still tense, repeat the exercise from the sitting position on the edge of a chair. Repeat as many times as is comfortable.

Once you have built up strength in your back and legs, the standing version of Qigong Horse will increase the benefits of the exercise, bringing further relief to back issues.

1. Stand with your feet shoulder-width apart. The toes are pointed slightly inward. The knees are slightly bent. The crease at the groin area where your hip and thighs meet, known as the *kua* in Chinese, should be slightly indented.

2. Lengthen your spine by visualizing a golden thread at the top of your head being gently pulled skyward. Then tuck in your tailbone and imagine your torso and lower body sinking down, as if you were going to sit down on an imaginary chair. If you are standing in proper alignment, the backs of your thighs and buttocks will be totally relaxed.

3. Repeat as often as desired.

Practicing Qigong Horse frequently, standing and/or seated, will support the re-alignment of vertebrae and correct posture. This exercise can also help to relieve scoliosis and back injuries when practiced regularly.

TAI CHI: MOVEMENT AS MEDITATION

Tai chi chuan (more commonly called just tai chi) is considered an internal martial art, done solo for the purpose of improving one's internal self. Originating in China, tai chi promotes vibrant health and a long life through the cultivation of chi. In fact, *tai chi* means "the ultimate" and involves progressing toward the ultimate existence, in part through a series of movements that move chi through the body.

There are many different styles of tai chi, such as Yang, Wu, and Chen styles. The traditional tai chi routine of 108 postures (referred to as long-form tai chi) would typically take a student between one and three years to learn. Over time, short forms have been developed, from a 37-posture form to an 8-posture form.

In all forms of tai chi, practitioners employ a variety of stances and movements that stimulate chi. These postures are based on the meridians and serve as both exercises and parts of a therapeutic healing process. Tai chi is ideal for people who have limited mobility, whether temporarily or permanently, as the movements can be easily adapted for anyone. In this low-impact, slow-motion exercise, the movements are gentle and usually circular in motion. Muscles are relaxed, joints are not fully extended or bent, and connective tissues are not stretched. As you move, the focus is on breathing deeply and naturally and noticing any sensations in your body.

The benefits of tai chi include:

- Reduced pain and stiffness
- Improved flexibility and strength
- Improved coordination and balance (which means a lower risk of falls for older people)
- Enhanced sleep
- Increased sense of calm and wellbeing
- Greater awareness and spiritual clarity

TAI CHI EXERCISE: WAVE HANDS IN CLOUDS

The aim of this exercise is to combine hand and foot movements for a single, fluid, full-body movement. The movement takes you through a 180-degree turn in which you have your left hand raised as you face left and your right hand raised as you face right. Imagine yourself looking at a cloud that floats from one side of you to another, while you lightly follow the cloud with your arms, scooping water from the cloud on each side.

1. Begin standing with your arms at your sides. Your weight should be on your left leg, and your head is slightly pointed to the left. Your right heel is elevated off the floor.

2. With your palm facing outward, raise your left hand to shoulder level, extending it out from your side. Move your right hand just under your left elbow, palm facing up. Both elbows are slightly bent.

3. Flow from left to right in a circular manner, shifting your hands gently, until you are facing right, in a mirror image of your starting position: your right hand at shoulder level, palm facing out, and your left hand just under your right elbow, palm facing up. When facing right, your weight will be on your right leg and your head slightly pointed to the right. Your left heel will be elevated off the floor.

4. Flow back and forth, from right to left and back again. Conclude by resting your hands at your sides and taking a deep breath. Repeat the entire cycle three times.

CHAKRA MUDRAS: THE ART OF SUBTLE INTERNAL MOVEMENT

In the practice of yoga and other meditative forms of movement, there is an ancient complementary practice utilizing hand gestures known as *mudras* (a Sanskrit word meaning "sign" or "seal"). Mudras allow us to cultivate control of the flow of our energy or life force (prana or chi) and seal in that energy with specific hand positions that invite higher states of consciousness.

When we practice a hand mudra, intentionally connecting the fingertips, palms, and hands in specific ways, we activate, recharge, and redirect the subtle energy of our entire being. As each area of the hand corresponds to a certain part of the mind or body, using specific configurations between fingers and hands enables us to have an energetic conversation between the two.

In a sense, our relationship with the entire universe is represented in our fingers and hands. Each finger represents an element, a chakra, a planet, a body organ, an emotion, and the end point of a meridian.

The thumb represents willpower and logic and is connected to the fire element, the Lung meridian, and the planet Mars, the planet named for the ancient god of war. Use of the thumb restores equilibrium and creates order.

The index finger represents the mind, the power of thought, and inspiration. It is associated with the air element, the Stomach meridian, and the planet Jupiter, which represents the eternal nature of change.

The middle finger represents our spiritual path and is often called "the heavenly finger," in that it radiates to infinity. It is associated with the ether element, the Pericardium and Gallbladder meridians, and the planet Saturn, which is metaphysically compared to the gates of heaven.

The ring finger reflects vitality and health and is associated with the earth element, the Liver and Triple Warmer meridians, the sun, and Apollo, the god of healing and prophecy.

The little finger, which signifies communication, sexuality, and personal relationships, is associated with the water element, the Heart and Small Intestine meridians, and the planet Mercury.[1]

In traditional Hatha yoga, there are twenty-five mudras that are taught and practiced. Here we will focus on the seven chakra mudras as a way to activate the energy of the nadis and chakras and seal in the energy of each.

THE BASIC CHAKRA MUDRA PRACTICE

1. Start each chakra mudra session by energetically washing your hands. Simply rub your hands together approximately ten times, and then hold your hands in front of your second chakra (sacral chakra) for a few moments.

2. Sit with your back straight, either in a chair or comfortably on the floor with your legs crossed. Take a few slow, deep breaths to center.

3. Using the images and descriptions under "The Chakra Mudras" to guide you, place your fingers together as described for each mudra. Exert just enough pressure to feel the flow of energy (no need to press hard).

4. There is a suggested single-word Sanskrit chant correlated with each chakra mudra. As you hold each mudra, repeat the chants seven times each, or more if you would like. (These chants/words are included in the following descriptions.)

THE OM MUDRA

THE MOST WELL-KNOWN and frequently practiced mudra around the world, the OM mudra (figure 14.4), is one that we intuitively use to reconnect with our higher consciousness. It uses the same hand symbol used for the first chakra in the chakra mudra practice. The OM mudra is so universal, however, that we can elegantly and efficiently use it to connect us in entirety with body, mind, and spirit.

The thumb is considered the gateway to divine will (represented by the seventh chakra), and the index finger correlates to the ego (represented by the second chakra). Touching the thumb and first finger tip to tip allows the energy of heaven and earth to cycle through our systems.

As you do this mudra, chant *OM* (just as we do with the sixth chakra mudra) to further invite this reconnection. Or repeat the following affirmation: as you breathe in, say, "I am one with the Universe," and as you breathe out, say, "The Universe and I are one."

**FIGURE 14.4
THE OM MUDRA**

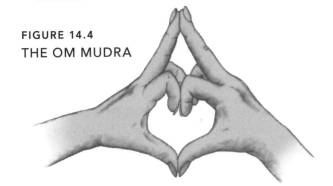

FIGURE 14.5
The Chakra Mudras

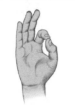

First Chakra Mudra

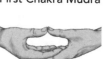

Second Chakra Mudra

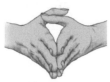

Third Chakra Mudra

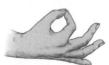

Fourth Chakra Mudra

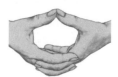

Fifth Chakra Mudra

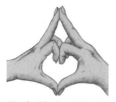

Sixth Chakra Mudra

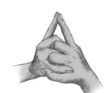

Seventh Chakra Mudra

You can further enhance your mudra practice by surrounding yourself with healing music, color, essential oils, or candles.

Tip: When focusing on activating and balancing the chakras, it is best to work from the first chakra upward (from root to crown), unless you are only working with one or two chakras at a time.

THE CHAKRA MUDRAS

See figure 14.5 for pictures of all the chakra mudras.

First Chakra: Touch the tip of your thumb with the tip of your index finger. Concentrate on your first chakra (root chakra) located at the base of your spine. At your own pace and volume, chant the sound *Lam* (pronounced "lum") and visualize the color red.

Second Chakra: Place your hands in your lap with your palms facing up, softly cupped together; your left hand is underneath, its palm touching the back of the fingers of your right hand. Lightly touch the tips of your thumbs together. Concentrate on the second chakra (sacral chakra), which is three finger widths below the navel. Chant the sound *Vam* (pronounced "vum") and visualize the color orange.

Third Chakra: Hold your hands in front of your solar plexus, between your heart and your stomach. With your fingers straight and pointing away from you, allow all of your fingertips to touch and cross your thumbs. Concentrate on your third chakra (solar plexus chakra). Chant the sound *Ram* (pronounced "rum") and visualize the color yellow.

Fourth Chakra: Place the fingers of both hands in the same position, with the tips of your index fingers and thumbs touching. Now place your left hand on your left knee, palm down, and your right hand in front of the lower part of your breast bone (slightly above the solar plexus). Concentrate on the fourth chakra (heart chakra). Chant the sound *Yam* (pronounced "yum") and visualize the color green.

Fifth Chakra: With your palms facing up, interlace your fingers on the inside of your hands, allowing your thumbs to be free. Let your thumbs touch at the tops and pull them slightly upwards to create a circle. Concentrate on the fifth chakra (throat chakra). Chant the sound *Ham* (pronounced "hum") and visualize the color blue.

Sixth Chakra: Place your hands in front of the lower part of your breast area. Point your straightened middle fingers forward and let the fingertips touch. Each of your other fingers is bent and touching at the knuckles. Your thumbs point toward you and touch at the tops. Concentrate on your sixth chakra (third-eye chakra) slightly above the point between your eyebrows. Chant the sound *OM* ("ohm") and visualize the color purple (or indigo).

Seventh Chakra: Place your hands in front of your stomach and let your ring fingers point upward, touching at their tips. Cross the rest of your fingers, with your left thumb underneath the right thumb. Concentrate on the seventh chakra (crown chakra) at the top of your head. There are two popular sounds to choose from: *Visarga* is often spoken as a breathy sound, like "ahhh." Other sects employ the sound "NG," which sounds like the end of the word "sing." While sounding, visualize the color violet (or the colors gold or white).

WALK THIS WAY

Walking is one of the most vital ways to reenergize yourself and clear your energy, if you convert it into a subtle energy practice through intention. Here are four steps for walking in a wise, healthy way that also bolsters your energetic system.

Step 1: Charge your breath. Before walking, stand still and take a deep breath. Allow this breath to charge every cell in your body with the vitality of life.

Step 2: Align your spine. Tense your body and then relax, allowing your shoulders to fall and your arms to hang loosely. Plant your feet about a shoulder's length apart and swivel your hips until they come to rest in a stable position. Lengthen your spine, draw your shoulders back, loosen your knees, and gently bounce up and down on the balls of your feet. When your body settles into a comfortable position, you are in alignment, and you are ready to walk.

Step 3: Walk from your navel. Your second chakra is the center of emotions as well as your lower Triple Warmer or Burner. It also contains the hara line, the Japanese center of your spiritual essence. Walk forward while concentrating on your navel, your legs swinging as if joined in the second chakra. Your emotions will flow in and through you as you move forward. Your soul's dreams arise from your navel and travel up your spine, entering your heart and continuing to journey to your shoulders and down your arms, which hang loosely. This same energy continues up your neck and into your head, opening you to the sunlight of enlightenment from above.

Step 4: Open to your body's wisdom. As you walk, let your mind flow to any places of discomfort in your body. Breathe into the tension while asking your body to uncover the greater wisdom that has been hidden under this blockage. Focus on each blockage until all tension has been released and you feel only joy or peace as you walk.

15

THE SUBTLE MIND
FROM MEDITATION TO SUBCONSCIOUS REPROGRAMMING

> You can shift your vibrations in
> the form of thoughts to those that
> are more harmonious with your
> desires, and you can then begin
> to take the small steps necessary
> for your inspiration to be sensed.
>
> WAYNE W. DYER

Whether you're new to the field or a long-time healing practitioner, you have undoubtedly experienced how the power of the mind impacts the subtle body. What and how we think has a profound impact on our emotions, and the ripple effect of this impact is mirrored in our physical bodies and reverberates through our energetic fields. In this chapter are a host of tools for working with and mastering the mind in all its magnificence. After learning about the various parts of the mind, you will learn how to open your mind through techniques such as meditation and how to engage the mind for healing with techniques such as guided meditation. As you will discover, many of the techniques and processes outlined here can be used very effectively in conjunction with other tools throughout the book. And the starting point is the discovery of the mind-brain connection.

UNDERSTANDING THE LEVELS OF MIND

The mind is a collection point of thoughts, beliefs, and information. When we talk about intelligence, we're really referring to how we process and utilize those three potent elements.

In working with clients, as well as in pursuing your own path of learning and personal growth, it is useful to know differences between the levels of the mind and how each interacts with the brain. Your mind is bigger than your brain. Unlike your brain, which is located inside of your cranium and interacts biochemically and neurologically with your body, your mind is both local (or linked with the brain and central nervous system) and nonlocal, or networked beyond your physical self. While your brain's primary concerns are your own survival and needs, your mind is intricately linked to all minds across time. It can therefore draw upon energy that is much more vast than the energy accessed by the brain.

Many scientists say that there are actually three parts of the brain, each governing different aspects of our life. These three parts of the brain are called the *higher brain*, the *mammalian brain*, and the *reptilian brain*. Each is vital to our survival and ability to thrive. Each of these three parts of the brain also relates to one of the three aspects of our mind. Our higher brain, which manages intelligent learning and consciousness, is connected to our *higher mind*. This is brain function that separates us from other animals, that invites the developing of wisdom through experience. It compels us toward social harmony and altruism. Our mammalian brain equates with the *middle mind*. We share this brain capacity with our fellow animals, who, like us, commit experience to memory in order to assure tribal security. Our reptilian brain, which relates to our *lower mind*, controls the basic drive for personal survival. It regulates the parts of the body that give us those gut reactions when we feel endangered, such as the urge to fight, flee, or freeze.

Understanding the basic information about the three categories of your mind and brain will help you to locate the mental cause(s) of presenting issues and to clear life disturbances at the level at which they occur in relation to both your mind and brain.

The higher mind. The higher mind contains all of the concepts we need to fulfill our spiritual destiny. The higher mind, primarily through the pineal gland, runs our higher brain. The most conscious aspect of the brain, the higher brain, is the learning and teaching part of the brain; it includes all of the higher-learning organs and glands, including the temporal lobes and the pineal gland. The higher brain is capable of all forms of communication, including sensory, psychic, intuitive, and spiritual. Its function is the achievement of full consciousness.

Neurologically, the higher mind relates to our *amplification system*, which interconnects us energetically to everything else in the universe. This system is difficult to track in the human body. Its presence can usually be tracked only through the appearance of certain chemicals emitted from the right temporal lobe and the pineal gland, such as the molecule known as DMT (dimethyltryptamine).

DMT, a naturally occurring neurotransmitter found in humans, plants, and animals, is also known as the "spirit molecule." It appears to function to expand our awareness beyond our ordinary, day-to-day consciousness.

The middle mind. The middle mind governs relationships, emotions, and reasoning and is the primary link between the mind in general and the brain. It links to the mammalian brain, or the relational section of the brain, and central nervous system, which includes the limbic and the pancreatic endocrine system. The various glands in the mammalian brain control the storage of memory and beliefs and the connection between thoughts and feelings. It governs our unconscious, the aspect of the self that directs relationships. Neurologically, the middle mind dictates the *digital system*, which regulates many functions between the spine and brain, including the transfer of information as electrical impulses from one point to another.

The lower mind. The lower mind governs our physical survival through the reptilian brain. This is the fight-or-flight portion of the brain and includes the brain stem, parts of the hypothalamus, the amygdala, and our adrenal functions. The reptilian brain is connected to our subconscious, which governs our deepest and our inherited desires and behaviors. The subconscious runs the *analog system*, the neurological system that works in waves. More ancient than the digital, the analog system reacts to geomagnetic fields, controls growth and rejuvenation, and can help us achieve a hypnotic state.

OPENING THE MIND: MEDITATION

Sometimes we need a little help to bridge the gap between the visible and invisible worlds, which is one of the reasons why meditation techniques and awareness practices are so valuable to the healing practitioner.

Simply put, *meditation* refers to the method, path, or process by which one is guided from within to a center of calm awareness. A meditative practice can also serve to awaken intuition and receptivity to subtle energies.

There are countless types of meditation, from transcendental meditation to Zen meditation, from secular to spiritual. One of the most accessible forms, practiced by people of many philosophical and spiritual backgrounds, is mindfulness meditation.

MINDFULNESS MEDITATION: FOR EMOTIONAL BOUNDARIES AND EQUANIMITY

As a professor of medicine emeritus at the University of Massachusetts Medical School, where he was the founder and executive director of the Center for Mindfulness in Medicine, Health Care, and Society, Jon Kabat-Zinn, PhD, has been a pioneer in bringing mindfulness practices into the mainstream. As a scientist and the author of several books, including *Full Catastrophe Living: Using the Wisdom of Your Body and Mind to Face Stress*, his research has explored the effects of mindfulness-based stress reduction (MBSR) on the brain and how the brain processes emotions, particularly under stress.[1] MBSR has been found to have profound effects on women with breast cancer, men with prostate cancer, and others whose immune systems are chronically or acutely challenged; it has also been shown to positively affect those with other conditions.

Mindfulness meditation offers a way to quickly enter a state of calm and gain emotional sobriety. The following simple mindfulness meditation is one that I adapted from several mindfulness meditation exercises especially for establishing positive emotional boundaries.

1. In a quiet place, sit up straight, but comfortably (not stiffly).

2. Allow yourself to set aside stray thoughts about yesterday or tomorrow, and bring your awareness to the present moment.

3. Pay attention to your breathing, feeling every part of your belly, lungs, and mouth respond to your inhales and exhales.

4. Envision every thought or worry flowing away on your exhale. As you watch your own emotions float away on the ethers, also notice the emotions of others that you may be carrying as they, too, are released from your energetic field. Sense your emotional boundaries becoming more vibrant and clear with each breath.

5. Keep returning to the awareness of release and the acceptance of your natural feelings and true thoughts, allowing your focus to move toward love and worthiness. Invite these healthy feelings and thoughts back into your body and life with each inhalation.

6. Linger here for a while—releasing and accepting on your exhale, embracing what *is* on your inhale.

7. End this time with a sense of gratefulness for yourself and the Divine in your heart.

ACTIVELY ENGAGING THE MIND: RIDING THE BRAIN WAVES

The brain receives electrochemical signals via highly specialized cells called neurons, which are located throughout the body. Receiving sensory information like sounds, touch, smell, and temperature from all parts of the body, the brain processes this data with remarkable efficiency, sending signals through complex circuits, networks of billions of nerve cells, to glands and muscles, as well as storing information. The brain waves that are generated by these electrochemical signals can be measured by EEG (electroencephalograph) instruments. The results of EEG readings can indicate our state of health, consciousness, and brain activity. There are brain waves that are optimum for daily life, for meditation, for sleeping, and for achieving a healing state.

Brain waves are measured in hertz, or cycles per second. The lower the number of hertz, the slower the brain-wave frequency. The following table lists the characteristics and potential healing effects of each of the five brain waves.

HEALING WITH BRAIN WAVES

Brain wave (frequency)	Characteristics	Potential healing effects[2]
Gamma waves (40-plus hertz)	Involved in higher mental activity and the organization of information. Advanced Tibetan meditators produce higher levels of gamma before and during meditation. Associated with highly attentive states.	Increases ability to manifest and opens higher states of perception.
Beta waves (13 to 39 hertz)	Active, waking consciousness; eyes open. These fast waves occur when we are actively thinking, working, concentrating, problem solving, and interacting with people.	Increases concentration, focus, waking consciousness, and analytical thinking; assists with issues related to ADHD and hyperstimulation.
Alpha waves (8 to 13 hertz)	Relaxed, calm state of consciousness; eyes closed. Also associated with daydreaming with eyes open.	Enhances relaxation, creativity, problem solving, and intuitive thinking.
Theta waves (4 to 8 hertz)	Deep relaxation, drowsiness, and light sleep stages. Characterized by quiet mind, body, and emotions; also associated with hypnotic states.	Encourages quick learning, behavioral change, trauma release, and resolution of addictions and phobias. The state for lucid dreaming.
Delta waves (Below 4 hertz)	Unconsciousness and deep sleep. Also associated with sleepwalking and sleep talking.	Deepens sleep, physical healing, surgical recovery, and deep relaxation.

Note: Depending on the study, there are discrepancies in brain-wave hertzian measurements. Included in the table are the frequencies most commonly referenced in scientific studies.

When there is a disruption in optimal brain-wave patterns, common culprits may include:

- Stress and worry
- Exhaustion and fatigue
- Lack of exercise
- Negative internal dialogue
- Emotional distress
- Physical pain
- Alcohol and drugs
- Some prescription medications

THE POWER OF THETA WAVES

For subtle energy practitioners, accessing the subconscious is one of the greatest gateways to transformation and healing. It is there that we are able to work with the beliefs that underlie our waking realities, as well as the feeling states that are prompted by our beliefs. By shifting from the higher brain waves (beta and alpha) into the theta state, we enter the domain of deep receptivity that allows us to identify our limiting beliefs and alter them if we choose.

Since the mid-1990s, Vianna Stibal, the founder of the technique known as ThetaHealing, has been teaching people how to utilize the theta brain-wave state to change negative emotions and thoughts into positive, beneficial ones.[3] After experiencing a spontaneous healing from cancer, she was inspired to develop her technique, which focuses on thought and prayer to achieve a clear, focused state and to connect to the "energy of all that it is."

THE THETA DOORWAY:
A SUBTLE ENERGY VISUALIZATION PROCESS

For use in my own healing practice, I have created the following visualization technique for achieving the healing state of consciousness afforded by the theta state. I have based this process on what is known as the Schumann Resonance, the 7.83-hertz frequency that occurs at the border zone between the alpha and theta brain-wave states. This is the same cleansing and clearing frequency we experience in the atmosphere after a lightening storm. In fact, it's the resonant energy field we are referring to when we use the term "as above, so below."[4]

In this process, the Schumann Resonance provides a doorway into the theta state, where you can attune to your own higher consciousness. One of several earth-based magnetic fields, it is a resonance that we are designed to literally walk around on and be restored by, were it not for the interfering frequencies of modern life. The following journey is an elegant way to activate this frequency and rejuvenate, restore, and heal on every level.

1. Find a comfortable place where you can relax without interruption for ten to fifteen minutes.

2. Gently close your eyes and begin with the Spirit-to-Spirit technique (see chapter 9). Breathe into your heart, affirming that you are a full and powerful spiritual being. (If you are guiding a client through this process, affirm that they too are a fully developed, spiritual being. Sense the presence of their spirit and engage this awakened aspect of them.) Then call upon the presence of your higher guidance or the Divine—whatever aspect of higher consciousness resonates for you.

3. Breathe again into your heart, acknowledging that it is the largest magnetic field emanating from your body.

4. With your awareness, carry yourself up to your pineal gland, bringing your focus to this tiny, pinecone-shaped gland in the center of your brain (also known as the home of the seventh chakra).

5. Imagine or sense a doorway offering entrance into your pineal gland. When you are ready to enter this doorway, acknowledge it as the portal into the healing field of vibration known as the Schumann Resonance.

6. Once the doorway is open, stream the light energy from your pineal gland into your entire brain and throughout your body and mind. Allow that energy to flow, syncing your brain waves to this resonance.

7. With another slow, deep breath, acknowledge that you have put yourself into the theta state of inner clarity and open receptivity.

8. From here, identify a situation or condition in your life where you would like to make a positive shift. It could be on the physical, material, emotional, mental, or spiritual level, or it could be a combination of those. In what way are you experiencing constriction or resistance in your life right now?

9. Look at the *beliefs* you are holding about this issue or challenge. What do you believe about the situation, yourself, and others who may be involved?

10. Where limiting beliefs have partnered with various feelings, there will be blocked or stuck emotions. Allow yourself to *see the foremost belief* and *feel the feeling* that is causing any stagnation of emotions within you. Using your intuitive gifts, see, hear, feel, or otherwise sense which of the major five negative beliefs seem most accurate:

    - I am bad.
    - I am worthless.
    - I have no value.
    - I am powerless.
    - I an undeserving.

11. Ask your body to help you sense which feeling(s) might be stuck. Concentrate on the physical areas that are most uncomfortable and sense which of the basic six feelings are stagnated:

MUSCLE TESTING: A Mind-Body Communication Tool

CHIROPRACTORS, NATUROPATHS, THETA-HEALING practitioners, and many other subtle energy practitioners utilize muscle testing (also called applied kinesiology) as a method for accessing the subconscious. The reason that muscle testing works is because the subconscious mind and the body are interconnected. It could even be said that the body is a reflection of the subconscious. By administering a series of yes-and-no questions and watching for minute changes in specific groups of muscles, we can bypass the filters of the mind to discover the answers that the body can provide.

You can use muscle testing on a client by having them extend one arm outward, parallel with the floor, while they're in a standing position. Ask the client the pertinent question, then lightly but firmly press down on the top of the client's wrist. When the client's arm muscles hold firmly, and the arm doesn't move, the subconscious is responding positively. And when their muscles are lax or weak, the subconscious is responding negatively.

For example, you might ask, "Do you believe that you are worthy?" or "Is this belief adding to your state of health?" If the muscles of the arm are strong, this indicates an affirmative subconscious answer; the client does believe they are worthy or the belief in question is adding to their state of health.

Not only is muscle testing a tool for discovering subconscious beliefs, but it is also used by many practitioners to determine whether various remedies (such as herbs, homeopathic remedies, flower essences, and types of exercise) will be helpful and in what dosage.

- Happiness (usually because it has not been expressed)
- Sadness (sense of loss)
- Anger (violation of boundaries)
- Fear (lack of safety)
- Disgust (something or someone isn't healthy for you)
- Pain

You might also experience guilt, the sense of having done something wrong, or shame, the sense that there is something wrong with you.

12. Once you have identified the primary belief and the corresponding feeling, give yourself permission to change them. What is the life-affirming *new belief* and *new feeling* that you wish to put in place? If you don't know, you can always focus on the belief, "I am connected," and the feeling of gratitude, one of the many versions of happiness that is always healing and pertinent.

13. Breathing into the new belief and the new feeling, sense the free flow of your emotions on the subtle level.

14. When you are ready, slip back through the energetic doorway of the pineal gland and into your normal, waking consciousness. Know that you have renewed and recalibrated your entire energy field.

Tip: As a practitioner, this process is an excellent way to tune up in preparation for your client sessions, which will help you be a clear conduit for healing energies.

AUTO-SUGGESTION: AFFIRMATIONS FOR SUBCONSCIOUS REPROGRAMMING

Franz Bardon, the twentieth-century teacher of the spiritual tradition of Hermeticism, wrote eloquently about the connection between the mind, body, and soul. In his 1956 book *Initiation into Hermetics*, Bardon described how to access and reprogram the subconscious through the practice of *auto-suggestion*, a method for replacing limiting beliefs and addictive behaviors with life-affirming beliefs and behaviors.[5] What he referred to as "auto-suggestion" is more frequently referred to in our modern times as using affirmations. The following is a simple overview of how and why auto-suggestion works and how to formulate affirmations that really work.

The brain-soul connection. Normal, waking consciousness has its seat in the soul and is activated by the "large brain" in the body, the cerebrum (located in the front of the head). The subconscious is also an attribute of the soul and is located in the "small brain," or the cerebellum (located in the back of the head).

Disengaging the driving force behind what we do not want. The driving force or impulse of everything that is undesirable to us, such as our shortcomings, weaknesses, and addictions, has its origin in the subconscious. Therefore, a key to making positive change is through the use of well-crafted auto-suggestions (affirmations).

Formulating effective affirmations. To ensure that your affirmations are effective, formulate a positive phrase in the *present tense*. Also, formulate the words or phrases in the form of *an order*. For example, rather than writing what you won't do at a future date, as in "I will stop smoking" or "I will stop drinking," affirm who you are and what you are doing in present time: "I am a nonsmoker." "I am a nondrinker." By stating affirmations in the present tense, in Bardon's words, we "impregnate the subconscious with a wish, and we will find that only the positive part of the subconscious is coordinated with it."

The optimal time for auto-suggestion. When we sleep, our normal consciousness is suspended, and the activity of the subconscious takes over. Therefore, the best time for an affirmation to be accepted by our brain is that in-between state when the theta brain-wave pattern is dominant—when we lie in bed, feeling tired and ready to fall asleep, or immediately after we have awakened, when we are still in a half-awake state. Incidentally, the state of heightened receptivity at these times is why it's important to not fall asleep with thoughts of grief, sorrow, and distress. The subconscious continues to be influenced by the thoughts and states that are most active when we fall asleep.

WRITING YOUR OWN GUIDED VISUALIZATION SCRIPTS

In all likelihood, you have listened to, read, and recited many guided visualizations, but have you ever written one of your own? If not, and if guided visualizations are a part of your healing practice, for yourself or others, I heartily encourage you to give it a try.

The following outline is a general blueprint for building your own guided processes.

Purpose. The starting place for the guided visualization is determining your desired purpose and outcome. Is this process focused on self-healing, connecting with the sacred, changing beliefs, balancing the chakras, envisioning a positive future, stress reduction, forgiveness, balancing the subtle body, or perhaps a combination of goals?

The overall structure. With your purpose in mind, determine steps that will facilitate your intended experience. How would you like the progression of this visualization to unfold? What comes first? What comes next? How will you conclude the process? You may want to read through all of the steps below before beginning to write, in order to get an overview and to begin to stir your creativity. Above all, let it be simple. Allow your visualization process to serve a clear purpose (avoiding overly complicated steps or a process that is too long).

Timing. Timing and spaciousness are important. As you write your script, keep in mind that you will want to allow moments in between your verbal directions where the listener, be it yourself or your client, can access inner resources and guidance. (This guidance could come in the form of images and symbols, sensations, feelings, thoughts, insights, and more.)

The senses. When it's appropriate within the context of the script you're designing, encourage the listener to notice the sights, sounds, smells, colors, and/ or sensations that might be involved in a particular place or moment. Not only will this help the listener to activate and open their senses, but it will also support them in being in the now.

The relaxation phase. Ideally, this phase will be a few minutes in which you invite the listener to relax and where they can give themselves permission to let the thoughts and concerns of the day melt away. Most importantly, invite them to consciously connect with their breath. Throughout the guided visualization, connecting with the breath will be their greatest tool for relaxing, connecting with themselves, and accessing their inner guidance.

In addition to the basic relaxation process (breathing, relaxing one's body, letting tension float away), inviting the listener to turn their attention toward their heart can also be relaxing at an even deeper level. Turning toward the heart helps them to bring their attention from the outer world to their inner world, from their mind activity to their feelings and emotions.

Note: An induction technique that involves counting a listener down (for example, counting backwards from ten to one) is a hypnosis technique that requires additional training, due to the deeper states of consciousness that can be accessed in this way.

The internal environment. As your listener connects with their breath and enters a relaxed state, you will then guide them to an internal environment—often a place of tranquility and beauty that connects them with their inner guidance and supports the purpose of the visualization.

For example, you may invite them to enter a safe place in nature that they love or to surround themselves with brilliant golden light. Another, more specific example can be found in the Theta Doorway process outlined earlier in this chapter. As you will recall, the process involves entering the pineal gland (or third eye), in essence "carrying" the listener to the threshold of that doorway of their own awareness so they can access the theta brain-wave frequency.

The ally or guide. Depending on the type and the length of the visualization, you might have your listener meet and be accompanied by a spirit guide, guardian angel, or dear and trusted friend—someone whose presence will affirm the sacredness and significance of the experience, as well as add to the feeling of safety.

The journey. Whether brief and simple or intricate and involved, the journey you take your client on will have a beginning, middle, and end.

The starting point of the journey will depend on the internal environment that you have chosen and the purpose and goal of the process. In the case of the Theta Doorway, the starting place is the doorway to the pineal gland. Other starting places could be a safe place in nature, the doorway to a great mansion, the entrance to a grand hallway full of many doors, the chakras of the body—whatever appropriately facilitates the process.

Unless you are directing the listener to a specific experience, as the Theta Doorway technique does, you will simply allow the listener to choose where they go (which path in nature, which room in the mansion, which door in the hallway, which chakra).

Note: It's best to not ask the listener to tell you out loud where they are or where they're going. Simply allow them to be fully in their own process. Along the way, as they explore the terrain (again, the hills and valleys, the expanse of the vista, the rooms in the mansions, the various doorways), they can energetically prepare for the next step.

One of the simplest and most effective ways to support them is to invite them to again connect with their breath. Among other benefits, connecting with their breath encourages receptivity and clarity.

The opportunity. This is the apex of the journey, the moment that fulfills the primary purpose of the visualization. This is where the listener can receive the sign, find the gift, release the limiting belief, feel the emotion, deliver the withheld communication, see the future vision, forgive themselves or another, discover the answer, see the symbol, open to their higher guidance, or allow the healing. Often, the apex will be an invitation to do only *one* of these things, though in some cases, you might combine a few. For example, you might have the listener identify an emotion that has been stuck (such as shame, fear, or resentment) so they can acknowledge and release it. And then you might invite them to open to a new possibility for their future (a future vision), which they might not have had access to before allowing the emotional and energetic movement. Be sure to allow them the time they need to receive the gift that this point in the visualization can offer them.

The return. After allowing the listener suitable time at the apex, you will bring them back to the starting point of the journey, letting them know that it is time to begin returning to the everyday world. If they are being accompanied by a spirit companion or have encountered another person (or being) during the visualized journey, let your client know that they can acknowledge and thank that companion for the support they have provided (as a silent witness, a guide, a protector—whatever is appropriate).

Ask the listener to take another deep breath, and invite them to become aware once again of their physical body. You can also have them bring their awareness back to their physical surroundings—especially to the chair or other surface

TIPS FOR LEADING GUIDED VISUALIZATIONS

PRIORITIZE SAFETY AND COMFORT. Creating a safe environment is essential for allowing your clients to relax and receive the benefits that are available through guided processes. What does it take to create a safe and comfortable environment?

- A quiet and clean physical space.
- Comfortable room temperature. (Have a blanket available, if needed.)
- A comfortable and sturdy massage table or chair.
- Relaxing music played at a relatively soft volume.
- Relaxing fragrances, such as a naturally scented lavender candle (nothing too strong or perfume-like).
- For you, as the guide, to be relaxed and well-prepared.

See chapter 7 for more in-depth ideas on creating a quality workspace for your healing practice.

Use the breath. As described in the outline on how to write your script, begin your guided process with conscious breathing, the most potent tool you have for helping your clients relax and gain access to their inner world.

Modulate your voice. Although you will want to talk in a slightly softer voice and at a lower volume than you probably use for normal conversation, do allow yourself to speak in a relatively normal voice. You don't want to speak in a way that seems too affected and is therefore distracting to your client. Simply relax, trust yourself, and allow yourself to connect with the highest good of your client. In doing so, your voice will be perfectly attuned!

Be aware of the pace. Allow time for your client to relax in between guided statements or directions. If you engage in the process along with them (rather than simply reading the script), you will naturally find the pace that best serves the process, neither too fast nor too slow.

Offer encouragement. Keeping in mind that some clients are more visual, some more auditory, and others more kinesthetic, you can occasionally encourage them to visualize in a way that feels good to them. For example, while one client might see a vivid landscape unfold before them, another might feel a warm, loving presence envelop them. Yet another client might hear a message from their higher guidance. Simply affirm their particular way of sensing and receiving information, encouraging them to trust the process and trust themselves.

VISUALIZATION IN ACTION:
Four Popular Applications

VISUALIZATION CAN BE used for both seeking information and as a means for changes in the subtle energy field. Here are four simple ways of using visualization. You can use these mini-practices when working on self-healing, or you can guide your client to do them during a healing session.

When you're dealing with a problem or an issue:

1. Visualize yourself in a safe place, seeing yourself surrounded by healing beauty (such as the beauty of nature, light, or color).

2. Now ask the Divine to send you a helper. This helper holds a gift that, when unwrapped, helps you better understand your problem or provides you with a tool for dealing with it.

When you're trying to figure out the lesson contained in a difficult life challenge:

1. Request a messenger to assist you in uncovering insight. Go right to the Divine and ask for a personal guide who can offer instruction and perhaps even ongoing teaching. Fully picture your guide in whatever form they appear.

2. After establishing a rapport with this guide, you can begin to ask questions that serve your goal. Questions that can help you (or your client) uncover the reasons for life difficulties include:
   - What is the lesson to be learned from recent events?
   - What action do you need to take to complete the learning process?
   - What action do you need to take to integrate the learning?
   - What will your life be like when the learning is complete?

3. Receive your answers to your questions. They may come as images, sounds or words, physical sensations, or inner knowing. If you don't understand the answers or information you receive, ask for clarification or more details. You can also ask for the answer to be repeated in a different form. For example, if the first answer you receive is a puzzling visual image, ask your guide to explain in words what it represents.

4. Now ask if you need to focus on anything specific to aid in healing, such as a specific shape, color, symbol, image, smell, sound, tone, or any other extrasensory input.

When you're experiencing body pain or illness:

1. Ask your gatekeeper to help you visualize the disease or stricken body part in symbolic form.

2. Now hold a dialogue with this image. Allow the image to show or tell you the message it holds for you and what action you need to take to clear up the problem.

beneath them and to any sounds in the environment. Encourage them to take their time and to open their eyes when they are ready.

Afterward, if it is appropriate and if there is time, you could encourage your client to jot down a few images, thoughts, or feelings that arose for them during the guided visualization—to capture these details while they are fresh. Alternately, you could encourage them to journal about their experience later, when they are at home.

Tip: When developing your guided visualization, you can refer to chapter 22 for additional ideas. Chapter 22 covers questions to ask in order to receive guidance through visual intuition and ways to incorporate color into your visualization script.

16

THE SUBTLE SPIRIT
PRAYER, CONTEMPLATION, AND COMMUNING WITH SPIRITUAL FORCES

> Great men are they who see
> that spiritual is stronger than
> any material force . . .
>
> RALPH WALDO EMERSON

In the field of subtle energy medicine, which is based more on what *cannot* be seen with the eyes than what *can* be, the influence and impact of the spiritual realms on healing is widely embraced. Patients and clients who are drawn to subtle energy healing, either in conjunction with conventional methods or as their sole approach, are usually open to or already engaged in spiritual practices such as prayer and meditation. As a subtle energy practitioner, you might very well have certain rituals and practices for opening to Spirit and inviting it to guide you in your work with others and to enrich your overall experience. Many practitioners find that subtle energy healing methods are often more effective when they are combined with spiritually focused tools and techniques, such as the essential energy techniques from chapter 9.

In this chapter, our primary focus is on the power of prayer, contemplation, and communing with a higher being, which we will call Spirit in this chapter, and other spiritual forces and beings to aid in the process of healing. While these three spiritual activities are interconnected, they are different. The differences and interplay between these three ways of spiritual communication are described under "Receiving Answers and Assistance," as are ways to receive insight and revelation.

With a discussion on prayer comes the inevitable question: who or what are you praying to? I think the answer to that question shifts and changes from time to time. At one moment, we're talking to God; the next we're talking to a beloved family member who has passed over; the next we're talking with our own higher self or consciousness. For subtle energy practitioners, Spirit and spiritual forces are some of the best allies. Therefore, the remainder of the chapter discusses angels and spiritual beings, our soul and our spirit, and other aspects of self that we can call on for direction, clarity, and guidance.

The beauty of prayer and other modes of spiritual communication is that anyone, practitioners or lay people, can successfully employ them for the purpose of healing.

RECEIVING ANSWERS AND ASSISTANCE

Many subtle energy practitioners rely on spiritual insight during a session, whether they are working on themselves or others. We can use three distinct, but related, forms of spiritual communication—prayer, contemplation, and communion—to obtain answers to questions, healing energy, or revelations that will help us understand the true nature of a dilemma.

These three forms of communication work this way:

Prayer is speaking to Spirit.
Contemplation is basking in the presence of Spirit.
Communion is opening to receive information and energy from Spirit.

Prayer can be done at any time and in any way. Many of us were taught to pray on our hands and knees, in a place of worship, or before a meal. These prayer rituals remind us that we can always lean on a greater presence for love, hope, and blessing. But we can also utter a prayer when driving to work or sitting in the movie theater, and we can encourage our clients toward understanding that there are no rules about prayer. Prayers can be shared with others—aloud or silently, through song or dance—or simply held inside the silent place within our hearts.

If our clients are comfortable with prayer, we can ask them what they prefer to call Spirit, and we can then pray for or with them. It's vital that we honor our clients' beliefs, however, or the prayer can feel judgmental or imprisoning. We can also pray privately and internally for spiritual assistance for our own work as a practitioner.

Contemplation occurs in hundreds of different ways, but they all share this in common: they acknowledge the presence of Spirit or spiritual forces and seek a peaceful unity with them. I encourage clients to take time during their day to simply sense Spirit, with no agenda. This clearing of the mind and soul is refreshing and can often lead to communion, or the receiving of assistance and healing.

During client sessions, I employ contemplation through the Spirit-to-Spirit technique (see chapter 9). I pause after each of the three steps and allow myself to embrace the sacred holiness of my own spirit, of others' spirits, and of the higher Spirit. I then ask Spirit to hold me in a state of oneness with its limitless power. When I feel stuck during a session, I stop, breathe, close my eyes for a moment, and then ask Spirit to remind me of its presence. This bonding moment is often all I need to know what direction to take.

How do you receive answers to the questions you are looking for? This is the point of communing, or opening to revelation.

During sessions, I often commune with Spirit to receive intuitive insights in the moment. My client asks a question; I see a psychic image in my head, hear words of knowledge in my ears, or am struck with flash of understanding through my body-self. These intuitive signs lead my client and me further down the road of understanding or healing.

Sometimes answers and healing energy don't come right away. I might then suggest that a client set an intention to enter a state of communion in their everyday lives. The key is to dedicate a specific period of time in which Spirit will respond. That time frame can involve more than a few minutes or an hour to several days or weeks. I often suggest that a client set their intention to receive guidance, then give Spirit days, if not weeks, to send them what they're seeking.

Living everyday life in a state of communion means paying attention to the types of signs and omens received intuitively but also through mundane reality. Signs might include dreams, visions, or intuitive flashes, but could just as likely involve reading an insightful book or being given a message from a friend. I once had a client learn everything he needed to about recovering from an illness watching a kid's television show while he was communing for a week. The key is to be willing and open; Spirit will do the rest.

These three spiritual communication processes can easily be blended in different ways. You might enter a contemplative state to acknowledge the presence of Spirit, then pray for assistance, and then move into communion to await an answer. You might pray and then contemplate so as to receive a revelation—or receive an insight and then pray for its explanation.

Note: Setting an intention to commune with Spirit could be considered a form of prayer. Any of the ten Prayers for Healing, discussed in the next section of this chapter, can be used as the opening to a period of communion.

PRAYERS FOR HEALING

There are ten types of prayer for communicating with Spirit and spiritual forces for the benefit of others and yourself. I call them Prayers for Healing. Knowing the distinctions of each type will help you craft a prayer that is ideal for your circumstances and healing goals. Know that you can conduct these prayers for yourself or others; before, during, or after a session; silently or loudly; and/or through speaking, writing, or singing—any means of expression you can think of, really.

When doing healing work with others, you can either pray aloud with them or suggest a type of prayer for them to say aloud or internally. Prayers don't have to start with a "Dear God," but they can. You can name the Divine as you and/or your client understand it, or simply breathe into your heart using the Spirit-to-Spirit technique (chapter 9) and formulate the type of prayer that would best suit the other person's needs.

To use prayers for self-healing, consider creating your own book of prayers in a special journal, jotting down the words, phrases, and ideas that come to you based on the ten different types of healing prayers described below. In fact, the time you spend writing down your prayer ideas can actually *be* little moments of prayer.

As you read the descriptions, allow yourself to sense which ones you find most inspiring right now.

MEDITATION: A Form of Communion

MEDITATION IS ONE of the most well-known processes for clearing the mind and quieting the body. This stillness often helps open the doorway between the Spirit and ourselves so revelation and healing can be ushered in. A meditation can involve sitting in the traditional lotus posture (cross legged) of yoga or deep breathing, but you can just as easily meditate while walking, chanting, or even cooking.

Meditation is a form of communing or communicating with Spirit. While prayer is reaching upward and outward, meditation closes the loop on our communication with Spirit. It asks Spirit to respond and respects the fact that we are worthy of receiving. Even the thought of receiving insight, assistance, and hope from Spirit heals the unworthiness issues that so many of us hold deep inside and that often prevent the movement and effectiveness of subtle healing energy.

For more on meditation, including its additional benefits, see chapter 15, "The Subtle Mind."

PRAYER OF DECISION: SECURING A CLEAR INTENTION

When there is an important decision to be made, we can sometimes find ourselves languishing in a state of confusion, avoidance, or doubt. A Prayer of Decision is an opportunity to make a statement of what we *need* to have happen—whether or not we are yet certain that it is the "right" or perfect situation, solution, or choice. Stating our need opens the door to even greater clarity. The purpose of this prayer is to decrease doubt and increase faith by securing a clear intention.

For instance, a client with cancer might wonder if she should use radiation, chemotherapy, herbal treatments, or all of these practices. She might frame a Prayer of Decision that says, "Spirit, I am willing to do what I need in order to heal, and I am open to all paths. I ask for clarity about which treatment most aligns with my healing desires." She could then spend an entire day praying for clarity around the use of radiation, making the statement, "Spirit, I am open to radiation as the highest solution for this illness," and see how this decision fits within her body and soul. She can then make the same declaration of Prayer of Decision for chemotherapy and herbal treatments, each on different days, and then finally evaluate the results to come to a final decision.

PRAYER OF PETITION: INVOKING HIGHER WILL

There are times when we sense that the solution to a problem or the optimal outcome to a situation is not necessarily what we might want or would choose on our own. Not finding the answer we seek through our mental or even intuitive capacities, we may know in our heart that the moment calls on us to invoke a higher will—to request the support of the Divine. The purpose of this prayer is to ask for the willingness to have our prayers met in a way that serves a higher order rather than our personal will.

PRAYER OF FORGIVENESS: RELEASE AND FORWARD MOVEMENT

We can feel it in our bones when it is time to release ourselves or another from a perceived offense and the hurt associated with it. Whether the incident or moment that left us feeling betrayed or abandoned happened thirty years ago or last week, we sense when it is time to lay down the righteous anger or bitterness that can accompany emotional pain, and to take a stand from higher ground, claiming, through prayer and divine support, that it is time to move on. In doing so, we open to a new path, a new way to move forward. The purpose of this prayer is to fully release ourselves or others from any such perceived offense, hurt, failure, or disappointment.

PRAYER OF SURRENDER: WILLINGNESS TO WAIT FOR A SIGN

There are those moments when we have tried to find solutions to issues by relying on our own thought process, deductions based on past experiences, and familiar belief systems, but we have not found the relief or resolution we need. Those are the moments when this prayer may be the solution. When we say something along the lines of, "I am willing to release everything that may be in the way. Assist me in surrendering to the forces of my highest good," we have employed the prayer of surrender. This prayer puts us in a place I call "the pause point"—the potent place of waiting. Waiting for help. Waiting for a response. Waiting for a sign. What makes this interim time of waiting especially potent is that woven into the request for surrender is the handing over of our burdens to a higher power.

PRAYER OF COMMITMENT: THE PROMISE OF ACTION

The prayer of commitment is the most overtly interactive of all the prayers. In a sense, it is where sacred communion meets life coaching. As you call on Spirit to support you in finding a solution, resolution, or healing of any kind, you simultaneously commit to doing *your* part. Just as you make the request for help, you also commit to getting clear about the actions you need to take in the matter, as well as when and how you take those actions.

PRAYER OF FREEDOM: WILLINGNESS TO STAND IN THE BEAUTIFUL UNKNOWN

The prayer of freedom may be one of the most radical of the Prayers for Healing, in that it is a communication with Spirit in which you state that you are willing to stand on new ground in your life. You're willing to discover yourself and life anew, even if you have backed away from doing so a million times before. At the heart of this prayer is the sincere proclamation that you are completely willing to be free of the underlying causes of presenting challenges and problems. You are willing to be free of negativity, old beliefs, toxins, other energies and entities, cords, influences—anything that is keeping you from living your highest expression.

PRAYER FOR GUIDANCE: A REQUEST TO BE OF SERVICE

Although each prayer involves a request for guidance in some way, this prayer holds a very specific purpose. It is the prayer to Spirit in which you ask to have guidance come through you in the way that makes *you* most effective, knowing that you are uniquely wired—fully equipped with your own perceptions, talents, skills, and gifts. This is the prayer in which you are asking to be of service and to make a difference. You ask the divine forces to provide the guidance that will allow you to have the greatest impact you can, based on who you are.

PRAYER OF COMPASSION: CLEARING THE SELF FOR THE BENEFIT OF ANOTHER

The prayer of compassion can be used when someone or something outside of us is in need of our help. Whether that person is a family member, friend, client, or a stranger on the street, this is the prayer to ready us—in a holy instant—to be available for another.

Not to be confused with pity, compassion is a sharing of love and support with discernment and respect. Compassion invites us to be clear and clean of distractions and personal agendas. Compassion occurs when we care for ourselves and others simultaneously, embracing the self-love and self-honor that enable us to truly show up for another and coming to the situation with the boundaries and discernment that are necessary in order to authentically help another.

The prayer for compassion aligns us with our higher selves and enables us to meet another and their situation with clarity and presence. From this place, we won't attempt to do for another what they can do for themselves. Instead, this prayer will lead us to the correct action and attitude needed to help the other person with an open heart.

PRAYER OF JOY: AN EXPRESSION OF SPONTANEOUS GRATITUDE

Rather than a request for guidance or an invocation of healing and assistance, we now express gratitude to the source of all life. Whether you direct your communication to your soul, your spirit, your higher self, your guardian angel, or simply God, the prayer of joy is an opportunity to express the appreciation, praise, and thanksgiving that occasionally bubble forth. The prayer of joy is a prayer of celebration—for the blessings of your life. As it arises spontaneously from the depths of your heart, you will know exactly what to say and when to say it.

PRAYER OF INTERCESSION: PRAYING ON BEHALF OF ANOTHER

The prayer of intercession is a sacred opportunity to request highest order. It is a chance to be a spiritual proxy, praying on behalf of another when they cannot pray for themselves. A beautiful gift that another may never know you gave, it is an absentee prayer for those who are very sick, in a coma, very young, or in some other way, for some other reason, unable to reach a hand to Spirit on their own.

SPIRITUAL SOURCES OF ENERGETIC SUPPORT

There are countless spiritual sources that can help us achieve our healing goals. A few of the most well known of these are briefly discussed in this section.

You can connect with these sources via direct prayer. For instance, you can ask for a certain type of angelic assistance through intention. In my own practice, I also ask Spirit to send me the spiritual forces or guidance that would best suit the situation at hand. That way I always know I am working with the most helpful sources of healing and inspiration.

THE REALMS OF SPIRITUAL SOURCES

There are four basic realms or worlds from which we receive spiritual support: Spirit and spirits, energy, nature, and humanity. We can draw on any of these to help heal others and ourselves.

The realm of Spirit and spirits is the least concrete, but often the most powerful. It is centered in the Divine or Spirit, the "one before all others." Surrounding Spirit is a pantheon of helpers that have never incarnated and yet serve humanity, seeking to help us mature and evolve. The angels are the most well known of these groups.

The energy world consists of spheres of beings that operate in various dimensions and zones. These primarily interact with our energetic systems. They might include a fifth-dimensional being that is capable of expanding our thinking or a former sorcerer who now exists on a different plane, one more heavenly than earthly. Possibilities can also encompass beings from other planets or universes that operate at a different frequency than humans do.

Healers have long excavated the natural world for assistance and healing energy, starting with the environment around them. In the everyday beauty of nature we find herbs, flowers, minerals, and foods that serve as everything from antidotes for illness to sacred medicines that bestow visions. There are the companion animals that provide unconditional love, and the elements, such as water and air, that we need for survival. Many natural objects, forces, and beings are also infused with their own individual spirits, which healers have traditionally called upon for assistance. For instance, a shaman of yore might summon the overarching spirit of owls for wisdom, or turn to the elemental force of fire to burn an infection out of a patient's body.

Finally, we can turn to the human realm for love, kindness, and healing, starting with the people around us. When we turn to another, or even ourselves, for healing, we are engaging with the very real power of love for a higher purpose. When we serve as a subtle energy practitioner, we are bearing witness to someone else's healing process. As well, we have various parts of the self that assist with our healing endeavors, such as our own soul or spirit, which are described in this chapter.

Not everyone within the human world is obvious, or even concrete. This sphere also encompasses the spirits of the deceased who still linger on earth, such as our ancestors; saints and avatars; and religious beings, such as the Buddha, Kwan Yin, and Christ, who remain on earth to provide continual teaching and healing.

Following are descriptions of a few of the types of beings in these different realms. Those described are the ones that most subtle energy practitioners find as useful in their personal or client work. Additional sources of spiritual forces are described in many of my other books.

ANGELS: MESSENGERS FROM THE SUBTLE REALMS

Jews, Christians, and Muslims believe that when creating heaven, God brought forth the heavenly hosts of angels, which makes angels older than humans. In the Old Testament, angels are said to be attendants at the heavenly court; their job is first to worship God and second to convey God's will to earth. The word *angelos* means "messenger," but the Israelites also assigned the concepts of servants, ministers, hosts, holy ones, and watchers to these beings. Their power, love, and guidance seem to be truly nondenominational.

In addition to general angels, there are several specific types of angels that are ready to partner with us in our journey as human beings and healers.

Cherubim, according to the Israelites, support God's chariot and act as guardian spirits.

Seraphim are the angels that surround God's throne and sing; their name comes from a word meaning "to burn."

Warrior angels fight in the army of God and include the Archangel Michael.

Thrones are angels thought to oversee justice in heaven.

Dominions are considered to be celestial housekeepers, carrying out the duties assigned them by Spirit and delegating tasks as they see fit. They also make sure that all the other angels are fulfilling the tasks assigned them by Spirit.

The virtuous angels work miracles and dispense the virtues, energy that encourages spiritual qualities such as integrity, courage, and grace.

Principalities are occupied with the welfare of nations or groups. Certain principalities are also called upon by God to create miracles for individuals. These miracles are performed so the individual concerned can better fulfill a destiny that will help many.

Archangels are the chief angels. Some, like the well-known Archangel Gabriel, deliver significant messages or healing from God. (General angels deliver lesser messages.)

The Thunder Beings and **Cloud People** are particularly forceful archangels, delivering power to earth.

The Nephilim, another type of archangel, could also be called *earth angels*, because they inhabit the material planes. The Nephilim are split into two factions: those that assist humankind and those that serve personal and selfish ends. The latter are often called *fallen angels* or *dark angels*.

Note: Almost every religion and shamanic tradition speaks of dark forces, the dark angels, or other troublesome entities that can be involved with people who are dealing with a far-flung variety of emotional, mental, physical, relational, and spiritual conditions. Refer to chapter 7, "Energetic Boundaries," for recommendations on clearing and protecting yourself and your clients when working with interfering energies or beings.

THE FORMS: ANGELS OF HIGHEST IDEALS

Forms are beings that have become so brilliant at their dedicated craft and purpose that they have actually transformed into a representative of that ideal. The idea of the Forms comes from Plato, who described a cave in which ideals like Justice and Truth dwelled, far from the living. Here are the most common Forms:

The Powers protect humankind from evil.

The Shining Ones bring heaven to earth and grant wishes and dreams.

The Ancient Ones assisted God with the creation of matter and continue to do so.

Archetypes have evolved into representative types or ideals and model these types or ideals for others.

The Muses provide heavenly energy for different and inspired ends, such as art, writing, or music.

Ideals exemplify standards we all try to achieve, such as the ideal of mercy, mothering, or kindness.

SPIRIT AND SOUL

Although many spiritual traditions and holistic systems define *the spirit* and *the soul* differently, we can agree that they are extensions of the divine mystery that some refer to as God. And by all accounts, it appears as though we exist in human form as extensions and expressions of our soul and our spirit.

While our spirit gives us perspective from the mountaintop of life, reminding us of what lies beyond our physical experience, our soul walks with us through the valleys, forests, and flower fields of living, privy to everything that holds personal meaning for us. In connecting with our spirit and our soul through prayer, contemplation, or stillness, we might recognize their messages and signals by attuning to the feeling that accompanies the transmissions. In essence, our spirit

LIFELONG SPIRIT GUIDES:
Guardian Angels and Other Spiritual Helpers

MANY SPIRITUAL PHILOSOPHERS believe that we have spirit guides that assist us throughout our lives. These invisible beings protect, teach, guide, and love us.

Based on my cross-cultural studies of various sacred scriptures and legends, I believe that we are each born with two lifelong spiritual guides. These might include an individual we knew in a past life, an ancestor from our this-life heritage, a saint or other religious figure, or even an animal spirit. And one of our guides might be an angel.

Even before the Bible proclaimed the existence of personal guardian angels (in the book of Matthew), the idea of personal angels was already well established throughout the ancient Semitic world, and it continues to be popular today. Through my client work, I have determined that if someone has two lifelong spiritual guides of the nonangelic variety, they are

also watched over by an angel. Thus, we really do have guardian angels that can be called upon when we need help. If serving as a practitioner, we can also encourage clients to seek assistance from their guardian angel, as angels deliver the highest form of spiritual help we can receive, alongside that which Spirit provides.

We receive additional guides as our life goes on. Some of these invisible helpers show up to help during a stage of life, say, our teenage or elderly years. Others assist us with a particular concern, such as healing an illness or attracting a mate. These guides can be culled from any of the realms of existence discussed at the beginning of this chapter, which means they can include spirits as well as energetic, natural, and human beings.

comes calling with the energies of clarity and passion, while our soul comes calling with the energies of closeness and compassion.

For a deeper perspective, the following descriptions of the spirit and the soul will provide you with distinctions and nuances that you may find useful as you source them for your own guidance and for working with your clients.

Spirit. The spirit is the purest expression of self that is composed of creative Source energy and enlightened or illuminated consciousness; the whole self that mirrors the Divine and expresses an eternal truth.

Overspirit. The overspirit, the most unified aspect of a spirit, manifests in material reality through three main parts:

The **seed of destiny** is a concrete energy that encodes the spiritual genetics into the body through the subconscious. While physical genes are composed of chemicals and amino acids that link in chains to determine psychological and physiological characteristics, the spiritual genetics fashion geometric shapes forged from spiritual energies like faith, truth, and hope. You can access these spiritual genes to serve as a template for healing, asking for aberrant physical genes to match the spiritual genes.

The **spirit star** connects one's personal spirit to the unfolding divine plan and is opened once the seed of destiny is unfolded. This energetic body can be opened or intuitively read to assist someone with finding his or her purpose and life plan.

The **spirit body** is the etheric coating within and around a materialized spirit and is responsible for connecting the spirit with the energy system. This energetic body can serve as a template to shift any part of the energetic anatomy to a higher level.

Soul. The soul is the aspect of the eternal self that moves through time and space, generating learning and love. There are several parts to the soul, including:

Soul fragments, individual and often independently operating parts of the soul. A soul might fragment due to trauma.

Oversoul, a parenting body that usually wants to unify the soul fragments.

Soul etheric body, a charged casing that protects a soul, but also connects each fragment to each other. The etheric body of a unified soul, a soul that has never fragmented, can separate from the soul and hold the soul, mind, or spirit's consciousness and thus travel through time and space.

Note: As profound and majestic as the soul is, sometimes there is trauma, shock, and unresolved pain that leaves a soul fragmented and damaged for a period of time. In these situations, the soul becomes something that needs to be healed rather than a source of guidance or healing for the rest of a person. Soul healing and integration can take place through a *soul retrieval,* in which a shaman finds and retrieves the lost part(s) while both the shaman and the client are in a meditative state. You can also serve as your own shaman and search and find your own missing soul part(s). When soul healing and integration has yet to take place, the spirit is always available as a clear source of healing, guidance, and inspiration.

LIGHT AND LOVE: THE HIGHER ASPECTS OF THE SELF

Although the emphasis in this chapter is the guidance we seek through prayer and communion, it could be said that every source of guidance is potentially a source of healing as well. That is certainly the case when calling on the forces of the *higher self* and *higher heart.* It's been said that we are spiritual beings having human experiences, and as the word *higher* implies, these are the higher aspects of our spiritual selves. They are our ever-present connections with Spirit while living our physical lives, helping us to integrate Spirit into our body, mind, heart, and soul.

Maybe there are times when, in your desire to talk with Spirit or send out a request for help and care, you want an approach that feels more familiar somehow, less mysterious. You may not feel the call to reach out to the angels or to Spirit. Instead, you might find yourself seeking to connect with the higher aspects of the self you know as *you.*

In the ancient Huna healing tradition of Hawaii, *higher self* is the term used interchangeably by the kahunas (shamans) when speaking of our unique spirit (see chapter 17). This part of us works with light. As shared in many religions and spiritualities, as well as science, we are made of light. To heal we have only to repair the rips in the various parts of ourselves, such as our soul or mind, that are causing us to lose light.

Your *higher heart* is the part of you that knows and shares only love, to the point that it can perform healing service for yourself and others with love as the only tool. We are made of light, but light is made of love—of bits, pieces, and streams of divine love—which is always available for service.

In a nutshell:

The higher self speaks the language of light. The higher self is a reflection of our spirit or our soul's view of our body. It can access guidance and healing when needed, especially when gaining clarity of vision, purpose, or intention is in order.

The higher heart speaks the language of love. The higher heart links love-based concerns and relationship matters with spiritual truths, changing the actual rhythm and function of the heart to support health.

The distinction between light and love is subtle. Light is made of love, but just as a son reflects his father, he is also different. Love is the more encompassing of the energies and always creates more of itself. To open to love or the higher heart is to invite a personal interaction with the source of all love—Spirit. Light is a more technical energy that accomplishes the tasks assigned it. It can be used methodically for an established outcome. To access the higher self is to assure that the protocol or procedures of love are enforced.

You might open to love if you aren't sure of what needs to be accomplished; you must then be willing to trust in the process that unfolds. You can apply light if you believe that you know the desired outcome and simply want the right protocol followed.

To clarify whether your higher self or higher heart holds the guidance and healing you're seeking, you could ask yourself this question: Given the nature of my prayer or concern, do I need light right now, or do I need love? The answer will be just the quality of aid that you most need and want.

17

HEALING WITH THE ANCIENTS

Modern physics is describing what
the ancient wisdom keepers of
the Americas have long known.
These shamans, known as "the
Earthkeepers," say that we're
dreaming the world into being
through the very act of witnessing it.

ALBERTO VILLOLDO

Many healing modalities and techniques of ancient cultures around the world are still being used by energy healers today. For this chapter, I've winnowed the thousands of available offerings to those I've found most effective and doable in my career as a healer. I think they are both powerful and accessible, and many are not taught in modern classes, making them refreshing and unusual tools for your healing kit. In this chapter you'll find details about shamanic journeying and unique approaches to the Vedic, Hebrew, Incan, and Egyptian traditions. Included also is a special shamanic practice involving the assemblage point, a central cluster of energy threads affecting the auric field.

SHAMANIC JOURNEYING

Shamanic journeying involves shifting your brain-wave frequencies and state of consciousness into resonance with spiritual, nonordinary realities to receive helpful knowledge and healing power for yourself and others. Nonordinary realities are those that exist beyond the third dimension or what we call "concrete reality." These are supernatural or spiritual realms and are sometimes called *the other dimensions, the spirit world, the other side, zones, the astral plane, planes*

THE TRAVELING SHAMAN:
How a Shaman Journeys

SHAMANS ARE ABLE to free their consciousness from the anchors of the concrete world in order to travel to other dimensions and interact with otherworldly spirits. This nonlocal traveling, which can include visiting other planes, dimensions, realities, and time periods, is standard protocol for shamans, who understand that the answers to here-and-now dilemmas might lie out of the here and now. The burning question for practitioners who seek to employ ancient shamanic methods is, what part of the shaman is traveling?

There are many ways that a shaman can travel, but they all have one thing in common: they involve the shaman's soul. The soul is the axis mundi of the shamanic practice. Traditional shamans, who are steeped in age-old shamanic philosophies, consider themselves to be soul healers. They connect with souls from the beings of nature, the human sphere, the energy realm, and other spiritual realms, in order to help heal a client's soul. And they most typically journey through their own souls, or a part of their souls, in order to accomplish their goals.

The soul has many parts that can be used as a traveling vehicle. The soul can journey in its entirety into any time and space, with full conscious awareness of where it is and what's happening. When it does this, it leaves the body, which continues to function but without consciousness.

This phenomenon of soul travel is not as fantastic as it might seem. During nighttime, most of our souls exit our body to visit other worlds, meet with our spiritual guides, or converse with the souls of our loved ones in order to gain insight and healing or to work out our issues. Usually we don't know that our souls have gone elsewhere, except when we feel it returning—when our soul drops back into our body (and we literally feel a jerk) as we awaken in the morning. Shamans, however, are able to direct their souls during their nightly (or daily) sojourns.

Shamans can also project a part of their soul into the spirit world while keeping part of it in their body. When they do this, they often remain conscious in two places at once: in the body and in the new locale. They can separate out a part of the soul itself or form a capsule out of the soul etheric (the soul's outer wrapping) and use these as vehicles for soul travel.

The problem with any of these options is that they can leave the body unprotected and unguarded, and therefore, open to psychic interference. So many shamans call on spirit guides or an apprentice to protect their body while they perform this out-of-body travel.

The traveling soul can also be vulnerable. Continually exiting their subtle energy field can poke holes and ruptures in the field, creating places where energy can leak out and foreign energies can sneak in. For these reasons, I encourage subtle energy practitioners to establish a gatekeeper and use the Spirit-to-Spirit technique (see chapter 9) to protect their souls and bodies before they embark on a shamanic journey. Any of the techniques in chapter 11 can be used to repair damage our personal energy fields incur through our journeys.

of existence, and *additional levels of reality.* They can include eras from the past, potential futures, and the parallel present. A parallel time is one that is occurring simultaneously with this one, although we are unaware of it. For simplicity and clarity, I will primarily use the term *spirit world* when referring to these nonordinary realms.

During a journey, a shaman voyages into the spirit world to perceive "invisible" potentials and possibilities as vivid, colorful, harmonious shapes and symbols. The shaman then returns to this world, or ordinary reality, to dance, sing, tell, and otherwise act out these healing, transforming spiritual energy patterns, releasing them into new life on earth.

Most shamanic journeying could be considered a form of *soul retrieval,* or gathering and reuniting the fragments of a soul in order to heal the wounds of that soul. (See chapter 16 for reasons souls might become fragmented.)

The following are some of the types of significant issues that can be addressed through shamanic journeying:

- Illness, including physical, mental, and emotional
- Loss and grief
- Depression
- Trauma and shock
- Addiction
- Sexual, emotional, and mental abuse
- Navigating big life transitions
- Clarifying life purpose
- Connecting with loved ones and ancestors

THE SHAMAN'S WORLDS

The spirit world comprises multiple worlds or levels. In a shamanic journey, you will generally travel to one or more of the following realms:

The middle world. This is the nonordinary mirror of the ordinary world. Shamans visit this realm to search for information that applies to life in the physical world. The shaman enters this world by asking to perceive what is really occurring in this world, under the surface.

The lower world. The lower world is populated by animals, birds, and fish. It is the realm of nature—forests, meadows, mountains, streams, oceans. All of these aspects of the natural world can offer us assistance, clarity, direction, and healing. This is where shamans go to meet their power animal (or animals) and other spirit guides from nature. It is entered through a descending opening in the middle world, such as a hole in a tree trunk or in the ground.

The upper world. The upper world is where shamans meet with spirit guides that most often appear in human, angelic, or godlike form. It is entered via the middle world through an opening in the heavens, such as where rays of sunlight are streaming through.

POWER ANIMALS: THE SHAMAN'S ALLIES AND GUIDES

A key feature in shamanism is power animals, spirit guides that appear in the form of animals. They specifically help a shaman with journeying, but can also help in everyday life, often increasing specific powers that are needed in important situations. They usually represent the highest qualities of the animals whose form they take and often infuse shamans with the particular attributes that they embody, such as courage, strength, wisdom, or vision.

Power animals come from the lower worlds, although they can appear in the other two worlds. Power animals can be mammals, reptiles, birds, fish, or other natural forms of life. It's common for shamans to connect with one or two particular power animals at first and then to receive new ones as life unfolds or when journeying for a particular purpose.

Sometimes the point of a shamanic journey is to meet a power animal. Other times, power animals simply show up as needed to provide aid. They might lead a shaman through unknown territory of the spirit world or show the way to another spirit guide, for example. The laws of ordinary reality don't apply to power animals; they can communicate with shamans through words, telepathically, or through their facial expressions and actions.

In working with power animals, it's beneficial to analyze their attributes in order to figure out what that animal is providing you. For instance, bears often represent strength. If you are met with a bear on a journey, you might consider where in your life you need strength.

A SHAMAN'S JOURNEY: ENCOUNTERING NEW FORCES OF HEALING

If you have never embarked upon a shamanic journey, the following active, guided meditation will give you an opportunity to get acquainted with this subtly textured yet exceedingly powerful spirit world. And if you are already a seasoned shamanic traveler, you might want to take this opportunity to reconnect with the guides and forces of nature that are behind the scenes, always available to help us navigate the physical world.

As with all guided processes offered in this book, you can use this outline creatively—reading it and then going through it based on inspired memory, recording it for yourself, having someone you trust guide you through it, and/or using it to guide your clients into this state of consciousness.

Begin by preparing your space, intentionally creating an environment that is conducive to journeying. You could light a candle, smudge the space with white sage, or spend a few minutes attuning to the subtle energies of the space by humming, toning, or singing along with a rattle or drum. You might play a CD or downloaded recording of indigenous music, such as Native American flute. Or you could play a recording of nature sounds, such as a mountain stream or a thunderstorm (if that's a positive sound for you).

When your setting is ready, lie down or sit comfortably in a chair and begin your journey, using the following process.

Breathe into every part of your body, and then place your attention on your heart. Turn toward yourself, look into your heart, and find your intention for this journey. What would you like to know, feel, remember, release, or perhaps realize? Write down your intention before closing your eyes and going deeper.

Breathe deeply again, close your eyes, and notice how your body feels. With no need to fix or change anything right now, simply be aware of the feelings, sensations, and thoughts that move in and around you.

Let yourself know that it's good to give yourself time during this journey; it's good to allow yourself to pause and breathe and let a different kind of rhythm pulse within you as you move through the experiences that await you.

Now, sensing that you can very easily get there from where you are, enter the middle world, the nonordinary mirror of the outer world you're so familiar with. As you arrive, you see that you're joined by a gatekeeper, one who is there to support you as you make passage to the other realms.

Together, you and your gatekeeper come to an opening that leads you downward, into the welcoming lower world that is alive with spiritual power. That entrance could be a doorway or an illuminated hole in a giant old tree trunk. Or maybe you step into a warm pool of water and are whisked down a slide. You might feel the energy of the lower world immediately, as you find your entrance.

As you and your gatekeeper find your way into the lower world, open your senses to what you see, hear, and feel.

Find a place to rest in the lower world, a place where you can do your healing work. Relax there, allowing yourself to be surrounded by rays of healing light. Your gatekeeper is there to watch over your boundaries while you open to earth and sky.

Ground into the center of the earth, imagining you have nourishing cords that extend downward from the bottom of both feet and from the base of your spine. Then connect into the bluest parts of the sky, imagining that you have an antenna extending from the top of your head up into the heavens.

Focusing on your breath, sense what is happening with those healing rays of light around you. Do they extend into the earth through your cords? Do they swirl upward with your antenna? What color are the healing rays?

Notice whether grounding into the deep earth and connecting with the lightness of sky have a particular effect on your mind or emotions. Is there something that you could easily release? A fear? A big decision? A doubt that has been weighing you down? If so, then take the opportunity to let that thought or feeling roll right off of you.

Cleansed and refreshed by nature, you move onward, ready to meet one of your power animals, the one that can bring you the greatest support at this time. From around a bend in the path, emerging from a cave, swooping down from a branch, or in some other way, your power animal appears in front of you.

Taking your time to get a sense of this power animal, let yourself know what it is that they reflect to you, about you. Let yourself feel the particular essence of power that this creature emanates. And then ask your power animal what message it is holding for you. Hear, feel, see, or sense what this animal guide is here to teach you or reveal to you.

Take your time, and remember to return to your breath as a way to remain present and open.

When it's time, your power animal will show you and your gatekeeper the way to the ladder or other passage upward to the upper world. Thank your spirit animal for its wisdom and guidance. And then make your ascent to the upper world.

In the upper world, you're going to meet a spirit guide who is eager to help you heal something in your life. No matter what the issue is, whether it is large or small, this guide will help you without hesitation if you ask for their assistance and are willing to receive it.

As you approach this spirit guide in the upper world, you can see that the healing rays you encountered in the lower world have been emanating from this guide. The healing streams seem to welcome you as you walk toward the celestial shaman who awaits you.

As you get closer and greet this spirit guide, notice that the rays of light change in color or feel. See how the light responds as you hold in your awareness the issue, illness, condition, or conundrum that your spirit guide is going to help you to heal.

WHAT IS A SHAMAN?

SHAMANS HAVE LONG been known as the priest-healers of their community. They are known by many names, depending on the area of the world: *medicine man or woman, sage, diviner, oracle, healer, witchdoctor,* and *brujo or bruja.* The word *shaman* is derived from the word *saman* and is used among the indigenous people of Siberia.

No matter what culture they're part of, shamans are magico-religious specialists who access the supernatural in order to perform healing or serve their communities. Most cultural specialists believe that shamans are spiritually called to their profession through dreams or signs and are then apprenticed to an existing shaman, although shamans can also inherit their gifts. One of the common perceptions of shamans is that they are "wounded healers"—that because of a crisis in their own lives, and the resulting compassion and activation of healing and intuitive gifts, they are able to minister to and heal others. Because they have personally crossed the threshold between life and death or wellness and trauma, they are released from the anchors of the daily world. Thus, they can journey or travel to other planes of existence as well as draw spirits to them to assist others. In presenting age-old shamanic techniques in this chapter, we are reaching back into the rich realm of a healing tradition that is truly universal.

Ask your spirit guide what limitation you need to release to allow the forces of healing to dominate in your life. Is it a limiting behavior or belief? Is it a situation or relationship that needs to be released? Is it a way of perceiving some part of your life that is limiting you?

Take your time and let your spirit guide speak the truth—the kind of truth that makes you feel more alive as you receive it.

If you are willing to release this limitation, let your spirit guide know this. If you are not, ask your spirit guide to help you figure out why not. Is there more to learn by holding onto your limitation? If so, what? How can you complete the lesson enfolded in the challenge? Is there an aspect of you that needs love, attention, compassion, or forgiveness? Do you need to provide any of these to another person or a family system?

If you desire, remain in the process of healing the block or limitation until you are ready to release it or can obtain information about how to better work on it while conscious.

Now ask your guide if there is anything else they want you to know before returning to ordinary reality. Listen with your whole being.

When you feel complete, thank your spirit guide for their deep honesty, courage, and love.

Heeding an inner call to return, you very slowly leave the upper world by the way you came. Down the ladder you go, back to the middle world, feeling energized, deeply relaxed, and fully whole.

As you thank your gatekeeper for accompanying you and providing their care, re-enter the room where you began, remembering everything that happened on your journey that is important for you to remember.

Take a slow, awakening breath, and open your eyes. Without delay, write down anything that you feel inspired to capture. Is there a feeling or realization you want to remember? Is there an action that you need to take to allow the healing channels of energy between you and your shamanic guides to remain open and clear?

As you go forth into your day or evening, and over the next three to seven days, watch for signs and signals from the shamanic realm in your day-to-day reality. Remain awake to and curious about the kinds of communication and healing support you might receive from your expanding council of protection and guidance.

THE VEDIC KOSHAS: EXPLORING YOUR FIVE LEVELS OF BEING

The ancient Vedic sages dedicated themselves to the realization of the self and exploring the unity of all creation. One of their many gifts is the knowledge of Pancha Kosha—the five sheaths or layers that address the five levels of the human being:

- The Annamaya Kosha: food sheath
- The Pranamaya Kosha: breath sheath
- The Manomaya Kosha: mind sheath
- The Vijnyanamaya Kosha: intellect sheath
- The Anandamaya Kosha: bliss sheath

An exploration of the five sheaths, the following Pancha Kosha meditation supports the unfolding realization of the unity between our true self and all of creation.

Find a comfortable place to sit or lie down. Close your eyes and take a slow, easy breath. Allow your breath to melt away thoughts of the day, sweeping away any tension and creating space for the openness of peace.

In the safety of your inner sanctuary, meet your gatekeeper, your spirit guide for the journey ahead.

Travel back to the time of ancients, and venture with your guide deep into a lush, tranquil forest, walking a well-worn path to the hermitage where an old guru lives. There you can smell incense wafting and feel quiet truth in the air.

Ask the guru, "What is God?"

The wise one tells you, "God is food."

God is food. What does that knowledge evoke within you? Allow your first images, words, thoughts, or feelings to arise. What do you sense? What is your relationship with food right now in your life?

You then sense the question bubbling up again from your seeking heart, and you ask the guru, "What is God?

The wise one tells you, "Prana is God; breath is Brahman."

God is breath. What does that knowledge evoke within you? Allow your first images, words, thoughts, or feelings to arise. What do you sense? What is your relationship with your breath at this time in your life?

Taking another slow, deep breath, you notice the inquiry is still stirring within you, and you ask the guru, "What is God?

The ancient one says, "God is mind."

God is mind. You sense the expanse of that knowledge. God is mind. Allow your first images, words, thoughts, or feelings to arise. What do you sense? What is your relationship with your mind at this time? As you sense the magic and mystery of consciousness, what does "mind" mean to you right now?

Taking another easy breath, and sensing the power of food, breath, and mind in the layering of your being, you ask the guru again, "What is God?

The old one says, "God is intelligence."

God is intelligence. Allow your first images, words, thoughts, or feelings to arise. What do you sense upon hearing these words? What is your relationship with intelligence at this time? How does intelligence serve you? How is it expressed in your life?

Sensing that your time with the guru is almost complete, and knowing that you can return to the hermitage any time you wish, you feel there is one more level to this inquiry. Taking another slow, deep breath, you allow the words to come forth again, asking the guru, "What is God?"

With a smile, the guru takes a deep breath, emanating a joyful peace. Leaning toward you slightly, the old one says, "God is bliss."

God is bliss. Allow yourself to feel and sense this truth in your own unique way. God is bliss. Allow your first images, words, thoughts, or feelings to arise. What stirs within you? What is your intuitive perception of bliss? Where is the radiance of divine realization alive within you? In your body? In your heart? In your thoughts? In your spirit? In your relationships? In your creative expression?

Thank the guru for sharing his wisdom, placing a gift at his feet; it could be a flower, a piece of fruit, a crystal, or something from nature that honors that which is sacred within you and all beings.

Travel with your guide back to the present moment, then thank this being of light for journeying with you as you unravel the mysteries within.

When you are ready, open your eyes. Take a few minutes to write about your experience with the guru and your encounter with the five sheaths of Pancha Kosha.

THE ASSEMBLAGE POINT

The *assemblage point* is the epicenter of the human energy field, the central point that gathers and actually helps create our energy field.

Every atom and molecule in the physical body vibrates with energies that enable interaction and communication between them. There are a lot of other energies in the body as well, all vibrating at different frequencies. Yet these energies harmonize like instruments in an orchestra, and all of their vibrations form a central point or vortex, which unifies these vibrating energies. According to assemblage-point theory, our aura radiates from this epicenter.

The assemblage point penetrates the front of our body in an area approximately one centimeter in circumference. It looks like a single point with a cluster of energies around it, and it is often quite tender to the touch when you find it on your body. Ideally, we'll find the assemblage point near the center of our chest, although it actually pierces through the chest to also run up and down our spine. Front and back, energy radiates as beams from the assemblage point and fans out as our auric field, surrounding us in 360 degrees. The extending energy is more than strings of energy. Its final form is a luminous egg, a cocoon of our life force, which is visible in infrared imaging.

Data about the assemblage point stretches forward from the mists of time. It is a known commodity in many shamanic traditions and referred to by Carlos

Castaneda, author of the mythic series of books about a Yaqui shaman named Don Juan.[1] In Don Juan's teachings, the energy fields gather to form a luminous ball around the physical body and all our energetic fields, and within that ball is a point of brilliance—the assemblage point. To Castaneda, the assemblage point was a shaman's portal to "the place of silent knowledge," and shifting the point made it possible for the shaman to perceive an entirely different world than the one we normally perceive, but a world that is just as real. Shamans would go to this world to gather energy, power, or solutions to problems that may seem unsolvable within the limitations of ordinary reality.

The assemblage point, the physical body, and the human energy field (the auric field) exist and interact in a cyclical dynamic:

- The place the assemblage point enters the human energy field and the angle at which it enters dictate the shape and distribution of the human energy field.
- The shape and distribution of the human energy field are proportional to the biological/physical energy and activity of the organs and glands, as well as the quality of the body's emotional energy.

In other words, the way we feel and behave, our state of illness or wellness, and our ability to recover from illness are all reflected in the location and entry angle of our assemblage point. When we shift the assemblage point's location or angle of entry, we relieve symptoms and restore harmony.

The ideal position for the assemblage point is near the center of the chest, and the ideal entry angle is ninety degrees, or perpendicular, to the body. When the assemblage point is in its optimum location and entering the body at the ideal angle, we are in good health. But it can shift, and when it does, we become ill and suffer physically, emotionally, or mentally.

Gross misalignment of the assemblage point location is present in many serious illnesses, such as depression, drug and alcohol addiction, Parkinson's disease, cancer, autoimmune syndromes, and multiple sclerosis. Someone with chronic fatigue, for example, might have an assemblage point that has dropped down to the liver area, despite medications they're taking or other healing methods they've employed. Unless their assemblage point is addressed, it isn't likely to return to its optimum location; as a result, their physical energy will remain depleted. Low biological or physical energy levels, in turn, can inhibit or prevent full recovery.

The good news is that we can shift the assemblage point's location and entry angle back to their optimal positions, closer to the center of the chest. In doing so, we restore balance to the overall energy field, greatly enhancing the potential for healing and the return of wholeness. I have discovered that shifting the assemblage point is highly effective in dealing with chronic conditions that haven't responded to other treatments. The relief from physical symptoms can buy time to work on deeper issues. I've also shifted assemblage points when someone is experiencing acute situations, such as a reaction to surgery or emotional trauma. The resulting calm is almost immediate.

The following information and techniques are based on the extensive research and teaching tools of author and researcher Jon Whale, PhD, and will show you how to find the assemblage points on your clients and yourself, and how to realign assemblage points with ease.[2]

ASSEMBLAGE POINT LOCATIONS

In both women and men, the assemblage point is located in the chest and passes through to the upper back, to the right of center, from where its energy operates in the spine. Think of the point on the chest as the entry point and the point on the back as the exit point, with energy passing through your chest. A woman's assemblage point will often be located approximately two or three inches above the right breast. And a man's assemblage point is typically two or three inches lower than a woman's point, off center from the sternum. (See figure 17.1.) Women's assemblage points are usually located at a higher point than men's because of women's higher vibrational sensitivities.

In clients who are experiencing anxiety or excessive mental energy, the assemblage point has usually shifted upward, and the entry angle has elevated. Depressed clients will often have a low location and descending entry angle. Figure 17.2 gives an overview of common locations the assemblage point can shift to and the conditions that can result.

How to Locate a Client's Assemblage Point

Ask your client to stand up and look straight ahead. You will stand facing the right side of your client.

Form your left hand into a shallow cup shape. You will use your left hand to feel for or sense the location of your client's assemblage point on their back, around the area between the shoulder blades. At the same time, gently squeeze the fingers and thumb of your right hand into a tight, concentrated point, shaped like a bird's beak. You will use the fingertips of your right hand to intuitively feel for the concentration or cluster of energy lines entering your client's chest. You might be able to feel the flow of energy between the assemblage point entrance at the front of the chest and the exit in the back.

FIGURE 17.1
HEALTHY ASSEMBLAGE POINTS

This energy of the assemblage point enters through the chest and exits through our back, at which point it runs along our back. Shown here are the healthy entrance and exit points and angles for women and men.

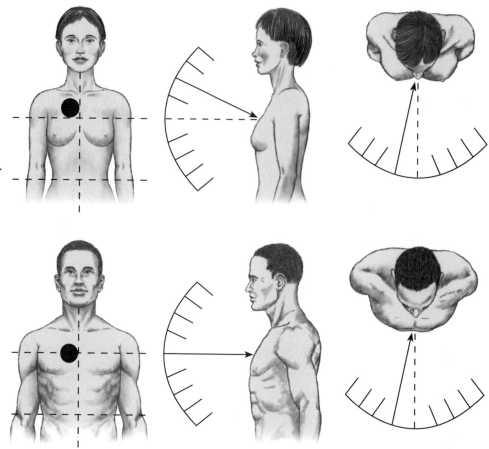

FIGURE 17.2
EMOTIONAL ENERGY AND DISLOCATED ASSEMBLAGE POINTS

Various conditions can result when the entry point of an assemblage point shifts up or down, right or left, from its ideal location near the center of the chest.

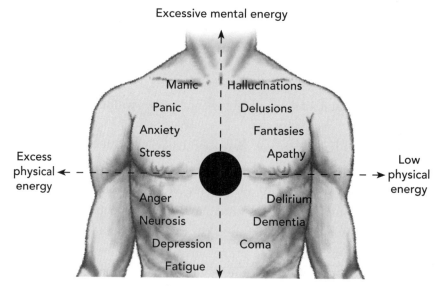

Excessive mental energy

Manic	Hallucinations
Panic	Delusions
Anxiety	Fantasies
Stress	Apathy

Excess physical energy ←   → Low physical energy

Anger	Delirium
Neurosis	Dementia
Depression	Coma
Fatigue	

Low physical and mental energy

With your arms fairly wide apart, hold your left hand behind your client (at their back) and your right hand in front (at their chest). Standing in a relaxed and grounded position, close your eyes and bring your awareness to your physical sensations. (You might choose to look away rather than close your eyes.) Moving both of your hands in a slow circular motion, slowly bring them toward your client's back and the chest. With the fingertips of your right hand and in the palm of your left hand, feel for the maximum energy disturbance or potential.

Distinguishing the difference in energy potential along the collection of energy lines of the assemblage point is generally easy. The energy lines tend to be concentrated and stronger close to the chest. When your cupped left hand and the fingers of your right hand are lined up with your client's cluster of energy lines, you will feel an energy surge passing along your arms and through your chest between your shoulders. Allow your client's energy lines to register in your arm muscles.

Allow your hands to touch your client's back and chest at the points of maximum energy concentration and connection. Move the fingers of your right hand back and forth across the energy lines of the assemblage point. As you do this, most clients will feel a pulling sensation deep inside their chest.

Once you have located the assemblage point, use small, Post-it-note-type adhesive labels to mark the front and rear positions.

If your client is unwell, you can expect the entry and exit points to differ from the optimum entry and exit points. For example, if the front position is two inches too low, the back position may also be two inches too low. But the entry angle can be off, too. For instance, people with clinical depression will have a low entry-point location and a descending entry angle, which puts their exit point lower than the entrance point. Individuals with a bright, happy personality might have a higher entry location and an upward entry angle, putting the exit point a bit higher than the entrance point. By looking at the difference between the entrance and exit points, you can figure out if the incoming angle of energy is ascending and uplifting or descending and depressing.

How to Locate Your Own Assemblage Point

In a relaxing and warm environment, stand up and look straight ahead.

Using the tip of your index finger of your left hand, press somewhat firmly into the tissue of the right side of your chest. If you're a woman, press just right of and two or three inches above the center of the chest. If you're a man, press just right of the center of the chest.

Remove your finger and press firmly again in a close adjacent spot. Repeat this until you have covered an area approximately four inches in diameter. You'll know you've found your assemblage point because it will likely be very tender or even painful. You may also intuitively sense it because of its great concentration of energy. Sometimes the sensations you feel upon finding the precise spot will extend deep into your chest and through to your back.

REALIGNING THE ASSEMBLAGE POINT: THE SLIDING SHIFT

Shifting and realigning the assemblage point is best done with a special quartz crystal. The stone should be as clear as possible, although it could be an amethyst or rose quartz. It must have a well-defined point. The point should have at least three perfect triangles among its six facets. You will shift the assemblage point by sliding the crystal from one location to another in the following manner.

1. With your client standing up and looking straight ahead, locate their assemblage point as described earlier.

2. Stand facing your client's left side. Hold the crystal in your left hand and place the domed end of the crystal on your client's entry point. Move the palm of your right hand around their back and find the exit point.

3. Ask your client to take three slow, deep breaths through their nose and out through their mouth.

4. On the third breath, when their chest is expanded on the inhale, ask your client to do the following three things simultaneously for a period of five to ten seconds:
   • Hold their breath in.
   • Contract their sphincter muscle and the other muscles in genital area.
   • Swallow and close the throat at the same time (with their head up and still looking forward).
   These actions effectively close the upper and lower exit and entry gateways to the body, loosening the energy field from the physical body.

5. Using the crystal, slide the front point of your client's assemblage point to the center of their chest. Use the palm of your right hand to move the rear location into the center between their shoulder blades. See figure 17.3 for examples of the movements to use to shift the rear point back to center. *It's important to never shift in a diagonal direction.*

6. In front, turn the crystal half a turn and remove it from their chest. Simultaneously, ask your client to breathe normally while you tap them lightly on the top of their head with your right hand.

Sometimes a client will let their breath go or forget to swallow. When this happens, the shift may be lost. If that happens, simply locate the assemblage point again and repeat the steps above.

THE SEVEN PRINCIPLES OF HUNA: HEALING WITH THE SUBTLE ENERGY OF ALOHA

The spiritual art and science of the ancient Hawaiians, now called *Huna*, was originally called *Ho'omana*. *Ho'o* means "to make," and *mana* means "life force." Mana is equivalent to *shakti* in Sanskrit, *chi* in Taoism, and *ki* in Japanese martial arts. In essence, the word *Ho'omana* means "empowerment"—to be empowered by spirit. The *kahunas* are the shamans who carry on the power and the beauty of the Huna traditions.

In the tradition of Huna healing and prayer, you carefully form thoughts that clarify what you are ready to release and that call forth what you want to manifest. Creating a clear picture in your mind, you increase mana and send the new thought forms along your *aka cords*, the etheric cords that connect everything and everyone through love to the lower self (the subconscious mind, known as

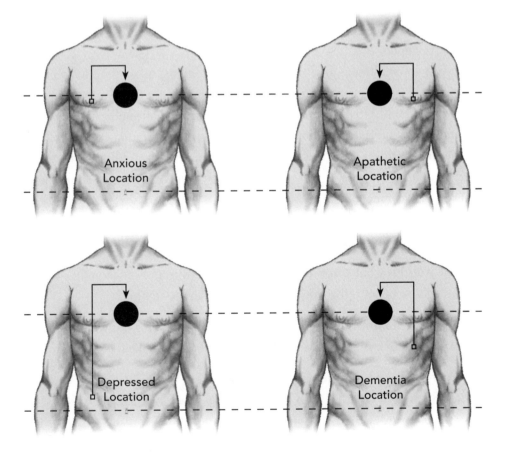

FIGURE 17.3 SHIFTING ASSEMBLAGE POINTS

When moving the entry point of an assemblage point back to its ideal location near the center of the chest, make sure to always move it at right angles, as shown in these examples.

unihipili). The lower self then carries them along the aka cords to the higher self (the *aumakua*). In addition to the higher self, *aumakua* refers to the "family gods," our spiritual ancestors that act as guides and healers. Often appearing as animals, such as owls, turtles, and sharks, their presence and counsel is sought during times of crisis and celebration.

Inspired by the kahunas' tradition of clarifying thoughts, the following exercise is a meditative journaling process based on the seven principles of Huna:

- *Ike:* The world is what you think it is.
- *Kala:* There are no limits; everything is possible.
- *Makia:* Energy flows where attention goes.
- *Manawa:* Now is the moment of power.
- *Aloha:* To love is to be happy with.
- *Mana:* All power comes from within.
- *Pono:* Effectiveness is the measure of truth.

CLEARING THE PATH: A HUNA PROCESS

This exercise can help you access your inner wisdom. As you move through the questions, write down the answers in a journal as they arise. Remember to breathe as you do so.

If you are guiding a client through these questions, allow time for their answers to emerge. You may want to gently repeat the questions a few times to evoke the responses that will help to clear the path internally and externally—for healing, for manifestation, or for personal and spiritual development of any kind.

Finding stillness. Find a quiet place where you can be undisturbed for ten to twenty minutes. Ask your higher self to quiet the voices of fear, guilt, or shame so that you may be free to heal and transform.

The questions. Reread each of the Huna principles in turn, then ask the questions pertaining to each, allowing answers to arise from a deep place within.

The world is what you think. If the world is a mirror of my thoughts, what thought or belief is the world mirroring back to me right now?

There are no limits; everything is possible. In what area of my life am I experiencing limitation? And what possibility would I like to open up to?

Energy flows where attention goes. Where am I placing the majority of my attention right now? How do I feel about the effect that placement is having on my energy flow?

Now is the moment of power. In what area of my life or in what specific situation do I need to reclaim my power? Where do I need to activate my power?

To love is to be happy with. What am I most grateful for right now? Where in my life is the light of love shining brightest?

All power comes from within. What aspect of my internal power is calling on me to embody it more fully or to own it?

Effectiveness is the measure of truth. What truth is reflected to me in the part of my life where I'm most *ineffective* right now? Where I'm spinning my wheels or experiencing failure? And what truth is reflected to me in the part of my life where I'm most *effective* right now? Where things are unfolding in a harmonious way?

Closing prayer. After you read through the answers, say a prayer of thanks, affirming that the honesty and power of your answers are now clearing a new path for you, making room for the arrival of new experiences, new opportunities, and new heights of love. Know that the spirit of aloha is caressing your life at this very moment.

THE LUMINOUS GOLDEN THREADS: A MEDITATION WITH THE ANCIENT INCANS

Within the exquisite cosmology of the Incans, each of us has a luminous energy field called a *popo*, which surrounds our physical body. Composed of light, it transfers information in and out of the body. The *popo* has four layers: the causal, the soul, the mind, and the physical body. The nine chakras of the Incan system are known as *pukios*, meaning "light wells." Because our personal and inherited memories and traumas are stored in the popo, it serves as a template for how we live our lives.

The following brief meditation will help ensure a beautiful flow between you, the natural world, and the divine world by unblocking and balancing your popo. You can use this meditation on your own or guide your clients through it.

1. Begin with Spirit-to-Spirit (see chapter 9), affirming that you (or your client) are a full, powerful, and loving spiritual being. Breathe into your heart while making this affirmation, and feel the resulting shifts in your energetic fields. Call on a spiritual guide, angel, or master to be present to love and assist you as you continue.

2. Notice your luminous energy field, your popo. Allow your awareness to flow with it down into the earth about one foot and up over your head about one foot.

3. Breathe deeply into the core of your heart. From here, notice luminous threads emanating from your heart pukio, as well as the other eight pukios.

4. See divine energy emanating from the core of your heart through the luminous threads. Allow this healing light to unfurl, unblocking and clearing any of the pukios that are obstructed or undeveloped.

5. With all of your energy centers clear and humming, allow yourself to *feel* your connection with all of nature through the five sources of energy that sustain human life:
   - Plants and animals
   - Water
   - Air
   - Sunlight
   - Biomagnetic energy
   Open your popo only to nourish and be nourished by these natural forces.

6. Now move your awareness to the eighth chakra or pukio—called *wiracocha* in the Incan language—a luminous globe just above the physical body. This is where your soul connects to the Creator. Feel the subtle energy radiating from this center, and open to receiving a message from your soul. That message may come as an image, a symbol, a word or phrase, or a sensation.

7. Notice the refreshment and balance you now feel, as your soul, through your eighth pukio, accepts the message, even while it basks in the forces of nature shimmering inside and around you.

8. Breathe into the ninth pukio—*causay*—your sacred connection to the Creator. This energy center lies outside the luminous energy field and extends through the cosmos. Having never entered the river of time, it can renew your sacred connection with the Divine. With your awareness on this eternal field, ask for an insight that you need at this time. Breathe deeply, in and out, allowing yourself to receive the insight as a gift from the source of all love.

9. With deep gratitude, affirm the loving assistance of the guide who appeared at the beginning of this meditation. Accept in return its appreciation of your unique personality and contribution to this world.

For detailed information about the Incan energy model, the popo, and the pukios, refer to *The Subtle Body*.

EGYPTIAN ENERGY BODIES: A MEDITATION FOR MANIFESTATION

The ancient Egyptians envisioned several different energy bodies. Though these bodies were separate, each interacts with the others. All nine bodies are described in *The Subtle Body*.

The following meditation is a compact, yet powerful inner process that provides quick access to two of the most potent energy bodies of the Egyptian system: the *ahk* and the *ren*.

1. Begin with Spirit-to-Spirit, affirming that you (or your client) are a full, powerful, and loving spiritual being. Breathe into your heart while making this affirmation, and feel the resulting shifts in your energetic fields. Call on the presence of a spiritual guide, angel, or master, who is there to love and assist.

2. Bring your awareness to the *akh*—your higher self. To the ancient Egyptians, the *akh* referred to the higher aspect of you that is forever the "shining one," the "luminous one." The *akh* is the energy body that oversees the healing of the physical self, whether that healing is physical, emotional, or mental. Think of what you would like to have assistance healing, and ask the *akh* to show you what needs to be known, opened to, or understood for healing to occur right now.

3. Now bring your awareness and focus to the *ren*. This is the part of you that makes things real. The word *ren* means "name," and in many cultures, naming is considered an important manifestation process, whole unto itself. *To name something is to manifest it.* What do you want to manifest in your life right now? What needs to be named so that it may be brought forth? Tell the *ren* in words, written or spoken, what you want to call into being— naming it specifically—and ask that it be according to divine will.

4. Turn to your guide and ask if there is anything else you need to know or be shown to complete the manifestation process in everyday life. Thank this guide and Spirit for the love and assistance that have led you this far and will carry you forward in light. Breathe deeply and return to your natural state of consciousness.

HEALING WITH THE ANCIENT TAOISTS: ENGAGING SUBTLE FORCES TO HEAL THE BODY AND EMOTIONS

As discussed in chapter 3, traditional Chinese medicine practitioners pay special attention to the interrelationship between emotions, organs, and meridians. By engaging the subtle forces of your own intuitive nature, you can gently and quickly assess which of the primary seven emotions of the five-phase model are seeking attention, as well as the meridians and organs that correlate to these emotions.

With this exercise, you will be journeying through the seven meridians that pertain to the seven main emotions. Because this exercise is meant to encourage intuitive knowing, you won't need to remember the exact flow of each meridian. Simply trust the information that you receive as being exactly what you need to know.

Find a comfortable and warm place to lie down, and begin to take slow, deep breaths. Take a few minutes to tune into your physical body and your emotions. What do you feel? What do you sense? Are you experiencing any physical pain or tension? Are you aware of a particular feeling or mood that is predominant in your emotional field? Simply notice what you sense, without judgment.

Place your attention on your heart and the Heart meridian, noticing the flow of energy through the three branches of this channel: one going to the small intestines; another running upward past the tongue to both inner eyes; and the third branch crossing your chest and traveling down your arms to the top of your little fingers. Do you sense a clear flow of energy or a blockage? Do you feel any particular physical or energetic sensations related to this channel? When you think of the word "joy," what thoughts or feelings arise?

Now move your attention to your liver and the Liver meridian, noticing the flow of energy that starts at the top of your big toes and moves up along the insides of your legs to connect with your liver and gallbladder before making its way up to your eyes. Do you sense a clear flow of energy or a blockage? Do you feel any particular physical or energetic sensations related to this channel? When you think of the word "anger," what thoughts or feelings arise?

Bring your awareness to your lungs and the Lung meridian, noticing the flow of energy that begins near your navel, moving up your chest to your shoulders, and traveling down your arms to the tip of your thumbs. Do you sense a clear flow of energy or a blockage? Do you feel any particular physical or energetic sensations related to this channel? When you think of the words "worry" and "sadness," what thoughts or feelings arise?

Bring your attention now to your spleen and the Spleen meridian, sensing the flow of energy that starts at your big toes, traveling up the insides of your legs until it reaches your armpits. One branch of the channel runs inside your body to the spleen, also linking with the stomach and heart. Do you sense a clear flow of energy or a blockage? Do you feel any particular physical or energetic sensations related to this channel? When you consider that excessive thought might be depleting to Spleen chi, what comes up for you? Have you been thinking too much by working long hours or trying to think your way through an issue or challenge?

Lastly, place your attention on your kidneys and Kidney meridian, sensing the flow of energy that begins at the center of the sole of each foot, traveling up the insides of your legs until splitting into two branches at your kidneys. These branches pass through your chest, intersecting at the Pericardium meridian, and traveling up to the base of your tongue. Do you sense a clear flow of energy or a blockage? Do you feel any particular physical or energetic sensations related to this channel? When you think of the words "fear" and "shock," what thoughts or feelings arise?

Wherever you sensed a constriction, disharmony, or depleted chi energy, ask Spirit to clear the particular channel (or channels), allowing Spirit to be your invisible, subtle energy acupuncturist. As you sense Spirit moving energy to restore balance to your body, mind, and soul, affirm the higher wisdom employed by Spirit. Everything inside and outside of you is now established in its right place, allowing you to breathe deeply and rejoin with the everyday world.

After completing the meditation, take a few moments to review what you learned. How was the flow of your Heart, Liver, Lung, Spleen, and Kidney meridians? What emotions stood out for you as needing to be balanced, whether soothed or boosted? If you discovered any meridians that need balancing and nourishment, refer to the following three sections that offer traditional Chinese medicine remedies:

- The "Body Clock and Chi Cycles" section in chapter 3.
- The section on "Food and Emotions in Traditional Chinese Medicine" in chapter 19.
- The Chinese herbs section of "The Herbal Kingdom" in chapter 20.

18

HEALING BREATH

The breath must be enticed or cajoled,
like catching a horse in a field, not
by chasing after it, but by standing
still with an apple in one's hand.

B. K. S. IYENGAR

The breath is the greatest ally for all living beings, connecting us to life in every moment. The breath is also one of the subtle energy practitioner's great tools, connecting us to the pulse of energy within ourselves and our clients.

In all of the great world traditions, the words for *breath* and *spirit* are one and the same. The Latin word *spiritus* means "breath." The Greek word *pneuma* refers to both breath and spirit. And the Hebrew word *ruah* speaks of spirit and the divine breath that animates all life.

Placing attention on our breathing is like inviting a small miracle. In subtle energy healing, consciously bringing awareness to the in-breath and the out-breath establishes a foundation for all healing to take place—whether that healing is emotional, physical, mental, or spiritual. Following the trail that breath leads us on, we discover where in our physical body and or subtle energy body there is tension, openness, pain, energy, fear, excitement, and countless other sensations, feelings, and thoughts. Without us needing to identify, name, or articulate our experience, the breath can *reach* us, bypassing the intellect to connect us with the pure experience of what is occurring in body, mind, and spirit. In this way, the breath connects us with the truth of our felt experience.

You can acknowledge the profoundly intimate connection between spirit and breath with each of the breathing techniques in this chapter, which you can effectively use for both yourself and with your clients.

A BRIEF HISTORY OF PRANA: THE BREATH OF LIFE

In the traditional Hindu system, *prana* is the most basic type of energy. The root word of *prana* is *pra*, which means "to fill." Present in all things, prana is essential life force; it is the upward-moving current in the body that fills the entire universe.

As the root of the Hindu energy system, prana is cultivated and utilized in the science of breath known as *pranayama*. While prana represents the infinite life force, *ayama* means "to increase, stretch, or control." Therefore, pranayama is the practice of consciously filling oneself with the breath of life.

In practice, pranayama is a set of breathing exercises designed to bring more oxygen to the brain, activate the subtle energy system, and control the life energy of the body.

THE CIRCLE BREATH: SEVEN BY SEVEN

The core technique of the ancient yogis, the Circle Breath is the most fundamental of all pranayama practices. Since the 1960s and 1970s in the United States, this form of pranayama has been at the heart of transformational breathwork systems such as Rebirthing (developed by Leonard Orr) and Holotropic Breathwork (developed by Stanislav Grof, MD, and Christina Grof, PhD).

The Circle Breath benefits our subtle energy system in the following ways:

Opening the chakras. Breathing in seven times and out seven times is a potent way to open all of the in-body chakras. This breath can be done whenever needed throughout the day. You can use the short version while performing subtle energy work on yourself or another, using this breath to support healing and encouraging clients to do the same.

Relieving anxiety and moving out of shock and trauma. When you're addressing high levels of stress, anxiety, or an acute trauma, or when working to resolve an old trauma, the short version of Circle Breathing is extraordinarily helpful. The seven in-breaths and seven out-breaths move, soften, and soothe various energies, emotions, and thought forms with unparalleled elegance.

There are two basic Circle Breath practices: the long and the short. Both versions can be incorporated into any type of meditation practice.

The Circle Breath Long Practice

For advanced practice, set aside twenty minutes and find a quiet, comfortable place to relax. Softly close your eyes. Starting slowly, breathe fully into your belly through the nose. Picturing your breathing as a continuous cycle, breathe in for seven seconds, and then breathe out for seven seconds. Do not stop at the top or bottom of your breath.

After about ten minutes, speed up your breathing so you are taking only two seconds to breathe in and two seconds to breathe out. Cycle into a slower breath for the last couple of minutes to readapt your breath to everyday reality. (Some individuals perform the long Circle Breathing for an hour, increasing their breathing tempo at the twenty-minute mark, then spending their last five minutes slowing down their breath.)

The Circle Breath Short Practice

The long practice is not always feasible or even necessary. Simply breathing in and out seven times without ceasing—without pausing between the inhale and exhale—can be grounding, centering, and clearing. The key is to do so with awareness.

CHAKRA-BALANCING BREATHING EXERCISE

Derived from the Yoga Sutras of Patanjali, this breath control technique, originally known as *Anuloma Viloma Pranayama*, is an exercise in alternate nostril breathing. It is designed to purify the psychic channels (nadis) through which prana and kundalini energy flow. In this way, this exercise opens, activates, and balances each of the in-body chakras, as well as the out-of-body chakras incorporated in many chakric systems.

Running through the spinal column is the *sushumna nadi*, the central master channel. Running alongside and intertwining the spine are the *ida nadi* (the channel of feminine, passive, cooling, mental energy) and *pingala nadi* (the channel of masculine, active, hot, physical energy). As the flow through these channels is harmonized, as it is with this exercise, prana and kundalini activate and balance each of the seven chakras.

As this practice activates prana and kundalini energy and awakens the chakras, it has a far-reaching, positive impact on the body, mind, and spirit. Some of the benefits include:

- Strengthening and soothing the nervous system
- Improving respiratory system function
- Purifying and oxygenating the blood

- Calming the mind, increasing inner peace and tranquility
- Cultivating meditative states of consciousness
- Creating balance, harmony, and rhythm in the entire body mind system
- Preparing the system for more advanced pranayama practices

THE CHAKRA-BALANCING BREATHING EXERCISE: STEP-BY-STEP

1. Sit upright in a comfortable position. If you can, sit cross-legged (*sukhasana*). Gently close your eyes.

2. Lift your spine upwards, elongating or lengthening your neck. To align the spine with the back of your head, bring your chin back and slightly downward.

3. Fold the index finger and middle finger of the **right hand** into the palm, so that only the thumb, ring finger, and pinky are extended.

4. Bring your attention to your breathing and take five slow, deep breaths though your nose.

5. With your **right thumb,** gently close the right nostril and breathe *in* slowly and completely through the left nostril, counting from one to four in your mind.

6. Gently close the left nostril with your **right ring finger** and **pinky** and release the right nostril. Counting from one to four, breathe *out* through the right nostril.

7. Next, breathe in through the right nostril, keeping the left nostril closed with your right ring finger and pinky. Again, count from one to four.

8. Finally, close the right nostril with your thumb and breathe out through the left nostril only, counting silently from one to four.

Note: As with any practice, do this exercise only for as long as you are comfortable. Start slowly and build up at your own pace. If one nostril is blocked, temporarily refrain from doing this exercise.

RAISING CHI: THE NISHINO BREATHING PRACTICE

A breathing method developed by Japanese chi expert Kozo Nishino is proving to raise the levels of chi as well as inhibit the growth of cancer cells, among other benefits.[1]

The practice is simple: you relax, stretch, and twist or rotate any part of your body while standing, taking a series of slow, deep breaths at the rate of one cycle of breath per one to two minutes. To achieve this breathing pattern, start by reducing your breathing to twelve to sixteen breaths per minute and then to six breaths per minute. But never push yourself beyond your capacity or to the point of dizziness.

If you want to use this practice with a client, both you and the client stand across from each other, facing one another, and extend your hands. Allow your hands to touch your client's hands, right hand to right hand, left hand to left hand, palm to palm. Breathing slowly, take turns sending chi to each other several times through your hands.

You can use this practice to actually help the chi move more fully through a client's body. Know that in Nishino's practice, the chi grows so strong that a practitioner can actually push a client over. You don't want to push your chi that hard in a client session.

ONEIDA BREATHING TECHNIQUE

The Oneida Tribe, one of the Native American nations of North America (also known as the People of the Standing Stone), offer a simple breathing exercise that is immensely powerful in its ability to renew, rebalance, and regenerate the body and mind with vital earth energy. Using this exercise allows you to

- release and recycle toxic energies, whether physical, mental, or emotional;
- discharge electromagnetic frequencies (EMFs) picked up from computers, cell phones, and other everyday electronic devices; and
- reconnect with the natural world.

To perform this breathing technique, plant your feet firmly on the ground. Take a slow, deep breath in through the nose, allowing all tension and stress to roll down the length of your body, out through your feet, and deep into Mother Earth. Note that your in-breath presses your problems downward, the breath doing the work for you. Release all of your concerns, worries, fear, or pain to the Great Mother, resting assured that she is happy to relieve you of any burdens and recycle the energies in beneficial ways.

Now open your mouth, and while you exhale, imagine pulling fresh, nourishing energy from Mother Earth up through the bottom of your feet, seeing it move all the way up through your body and out the top of your head. Allow this vital earth energy to cleanse and refresh you on every level.

Do this exercise in a round of four breaths—four in-breaths through the nose and four out-breaths through the mouth. For maximum benefit, you can use this technique throughout the day.

19

FOOD AS VIBRATIONAL MEDICINE

> We don't want to *eat* hot fudge
> sundaes as much as we want
> our lives to *be* hot fudge sundaes.
> We want to come home to ourselves.
>
> GENEEN ROTH

In almost every culture, food has long played a dual physical and spiritual role, and with that, many rules have been handed down. The Jewish tradition forbids eating pork, the Hindus forbid eating beef, and many Native American tribes prohibit eating foods that are not sacred. Conversely, there are foods that bestow spiritual power. Indigenous ceremonies are often based on stringent rules regarding what foods to serve. While conducting two weeks of shamanic ceremony in Peru, I was put on an *icaro*, or medicine man's purification diet. Refraining from salt, sugar, and heavy meats, I was given foods known for creating a healthy body and open psyche.

What each of these examples demonstrates is that food is powerful medicine. Sometimes the remedy lies in what we *take in*, and sometimes it's dependent upon what we *leave out*. The question is, how do we know what to eat or drink and what not to?

In the midst of too many (often conflicting) choices, there is the still, small voice within each of us that knows the answer to our question. It's the voice of our intuitive selves, the part of us that is innately connected to our deepest truth and always attuned to what we need in body, mind, and soul. Our intuition reminds us to slow down, listen, and pay attention to the messages and signs that our bodies are continuously delivering. These messages can be transmitted in a variety of ways, such as genuine hunger, cravings, addictions, allergies, good and bad moods, energy levels from high to low, physical discomfort, and pleasurable sensations.

The purpose of this chapter is to teach you how to pay intuitive attention to what your body needs right now, drawing on a number of energetic perspectives of food. If you are a subtle energy practitioner, the tools and information contained here can also be used with clients when you deem it appropriate.

The actual work is centered on the Intuitive Eating seven-day journaling process provided in the beginning of this chapter. This journal will help you or your clients connect the dots between specific emotions, beliefs, and food cravings. Then the rest of the chapter will supply you with ideas for using food as a subtle energy healing tool, such as foods that can balance the chakras and flavors (in the five-phase theory of Chinese medicine) that can balance the internal organs.

INTUITIVE EATING: THE SEVEN-DAY JOURNALING PROCESS FOR VIBRANT, WHOLE-BEING HEALTH

The Intuitive Eating Worksheet, a journaling and tracking tool, will help you tune in to the interconnection of emotions, thoughts, food choices, and the subtle body.

FOOD, MOOD, AND MIND

The following list of connections between food, emotions, and beliefs can be used as a stand-alone reference or in concert with the Intuitive Eating awareness process and journaling worksheet.

Cravings are important memos from the body and are its way of telling us about our emotional needs. They can also provide clues as to the limiting beliefs or negative self-talk that might be contributing to an emotional upset, whether that disruption is a minor, temporary state or a chronic, debilitating pattern.

The food and feelings connections outlined here can shed some light on the interplay between certain thoughts, feelings, and emotions that may be seeking your attention. Following are examples that we can all relate to.

THE EMOTIONAL MESSAGES OF FOOD

Using this list can help you begin to perceive your cravings and food choices through a lens of self-acceptance, self-respect, and kindness. For instance, if you find that you've primarily been eating crunchy foods, such as popcorn, celery, and chips, you might guess that you are angry. Take some time to figure out what or who you are angry with, and perhaps what subtle energy boundaries you believe have been violated or that you are violating in others. If your journal page is full of gooey, sticky breadstuffs, you are probably seeking comfort in all the wrong places—in food instead of relationships. By taking stock of your diet, you can get in touch with your inner heart and respond to your deeper needs in more self-loving ways than literally feeding your feelings. If you change your attitude and behavior, your food cravings and dietary habits will also become healthier.

Crunchy foods: anger. Crunchy foods help us act out our anger in a safe way, providing us an outlet so we don't have to deal with the people or circumstances causing us to be angry.

Salty foods: fear. We crave salty foods because we want to have more "spice" in our lives but are too scared to take a risk.

High-gluten or wheat products: comfort and safety. What's more comforting than a warm cinnamon roll, mashed potatoes, or a bowl of pasta? Gluten products give us the comfort and safety we need in a nonthreatening way. Has a cinnamon roll ever rejected you?

Sugar: excitement. When we can't provide excitement for ourselves, sugar does it for us; if we're unable to allow someone else to share joy with us, we can use sugar as a substitute playmate.

Dairy (milk, ice cream, fatty cheese): love. Our first food was milk—mother's milk. Rich, sugary, and/or fatty dairy products represent the unconditional love we received—or were supposed to receive—during infancy. We crave dairy products and foods when we desire unconditional love and protection and can't find it in our everyday lives.

Chocolate: sexual drive. We're all sensual, sexual beings. Eating chocolate is a safe way to feel sensual when our life lacks romance. It's also a substitute for the sex and physical love we need but might be too frightened to obtain.

Alcohol: acceptance. If you don't feel accepted for who you really are, or worse, if you were punished for being yourself when you were young, alcohol can provide the illusion of self-acceptance. It can also protect you from the perceived dangers of intimacy. The sugar in alcohol can serve as a substitute for excitement. The corn in alcohol can buffer feelings of failure, and grain alcohol can give us the warm feelings we might lack in our relationships.

INTUITIVE EATING WORKSHEET

Day # _____ (date):

My primary goal today in relationship to food (e.g., healing, regeneration, weight loss, vibrant energy):

My deepest desire today in relationship to food:

The feelings I'd like to encourage today would suggest I eat the following (see this chapter's section on "The Emotional Messages of Food"):

Foods to avoid so I can better deal with my emotions include the following (see "The Emotional Messages of Foods"):

Foods to avoid so I can better deal with my mental states include the following (see "The Mental Messages of Foods"):

Foods to enhance a certain chakra include the following (see "Food and the Chakras"):

Flavors to choose to shift my emotions include the following (see "Food and Emotions in Traditional Chinese Medicine"):

Ways to incorporate seasonal dietary needs include the following (see "Eating Seasonally with Ayurveda"):

Based on my *dosha* (see "The Food of the Yogis") I can incorporate the following *rasas*, or tastes, to enhance my body type (see "The Rasas, or Six Tastes"):

TUNING IN TO YOURSELF: QUESTIONS FOR BUILDING AWARENESS

What I ate today:

What I *wanted* to eat (if different than what I did eat):

When I ate today (specific times):

Where I ate today (the setting or environment):

Whom I ate with:

My emotional state just before eating:

My emotional state after eating:

My predominant thoughts while eating (my inner dialogue):

My predominant thoughts after eating:

My energy just before eating:

My energy after eating:

Did I receive intuitive, inner guidance prior to eating at any point today? If so, what was the message(s), and did I follow the guidance?

Intuitively, which chakra did I sense needed nourishment today?

Did I give this chakra the foods or nourishment that it needed? And is there a particular food that I could include tomorrow that will support, feed, and balance this energy center?

Special healing focus: To deal with my current illness or condition (whether acute, chronic, or life-threatening), I intuitively sense, or a professional practitioner has suggested, that I could add or eliminate the following from my diet:

Concluding notes (additional insights, observations, feelings, or thoughts):

Corn: success. We all want to be and to feel successful. Eating corn or corn products can not only momentarily imbue us with a sense of professional success, but also cushion us from deep-seated feelings of insecurity and failure.

Fatty foods: shame. Fatty foods hide our internal shame. They also cocoon us in a bubble of shame (fat) so we're safe from other people. After all, letting someone in close might make us feel even worse about ourselves.

THE MENTAL MESSAGES OF FOOD

In the table on the next page are common limiting beliefs and negative internal messages related to certain foods. When you review your Intuitive Eating worksheet, notice what types of foods appear most frequently, as well as in what circumstances. This information will shine a light on the unconscious beliefs that might be active in your subtle energy system.

FOOD AND THE CHAKRAS: EATING VIBRATIONALLY FOR THE SUBTLE BODY

You can strengthen a particular chakra by eating the foods and supplements that are energetically associated with it, provided you aren't allergic to those foods and don't go to extremes. All foods carry frequency-based messages and have the ability to change our vibration. On page 260, you will find examples of chakra-based foods and supplements and the energetic messages they provide.

THE FOOD OF THE YOGIS: AN OVERVIEW OF FOOD IN THE AYURVEDIC TRADITION

In Ayurvedic medicine, the best ways to eat and tend to your emotions depend upon your constitutional body type, or *dosha*. Doshas are determined by elements as well as physical and mental attributes. These are the basic principles behind the three doshas:

Vayu (also known as *vata*) is an impulse principle that manages the nervous system and is made of air and ether. **Characteristics of the vayu-dosha person:** tall and lean, talkative, shifting mind, earthy skin, hairy, prefer hot and oily dishes, tend to be constipated, love to travel, enjoy life, unsteady sleep.

Pitta is an energy principle that runs the bile, or metabolic, system and is composed of fire and water. **Characteristics of the pitta-dosha person:**

medium build, sweats a lot, pink skin, early baldness, impatient, fairly talkative, loves to eat and drink, brave and ambitious, average sleep.

Kapha is a body-fluid principle that regulates the mucus-phlegm, or excretory, system and is made up of water and earth. **Characteristics of the kapha-dosha person:** short and stout, sweats a lot, white skin, steady mind, can be silent, normal appetite and thirst, rests a lot, sleeps deeply.

MENTAL MESSAGES OF FOOD

Foods	Beliefs or Messages
Crunchy foods	Anger causes trouble.
	If someone is angry with me, they don't love me.
Salty foods	It's dangerous to be vibrant or enthusiastic.
	Being different causes rejection.
	Girls don't take risks.
	It's not safe to take risks.
High-gluten or wheat products	No one will give me what I really need.
	The world isn't safe.
	I can't rely on anyone but myself for love or comfort.
Sugar	It's not okay (it's evil) to have fun.
	I don't deserve to be joyful.
Dairy (milk, ice cream, or cheese)	I am unlovable.
	No one will ever love me the way I really am.
	Love is conditional.
Chocolate	Sex is bad.
	My sensuality is dangerous.
Alcohol	People will hurt me if I show who I really am.
	No one will accept my true self.
Corn	Success leads to pride.
	I am a failure.
	I will never succeed.
Fatty foods	I am a bad person.
	I don't deserve anything good.
	I am unworthy of love.

If you're unsure which of the doshas fits you, consider the following descriptions of imbalance and balance in each dosha. Which best describes you?

Vayu (or vata): When in balance, people with this constitution are vibrant, lively, enthusiastic, clear and alert of mind, flexible, exhilarated, imaginative, sensitive, talkative, and quick to respond. **When out of balance,** they are restless, unsettled, anxious or worried, sleep lightly, have a tendency to overexert themselves, become fatigued, suffer constipation, and be underweight.

Pitta: When in balance, these people are warm, loving, contented, enjoy challenges, have strong digestion, have a radiant complexion, concentrate well, speak articulately and precisely, are courageous and bold, have a sharp wit, and are intellectual. **When out of balance,** they can be demanding perfectionists; tend towards frustration, anger, irritability, and impatience; and have skin rashes, prematurely gray hair, or early hair loss.

Kapha: When in balance, these people are affectionate, compassionate, patient, forgiving, emotionally steady, relaxed, slow, methodical, stable, and optimistic, with good memories, good stamina, and a natural resistance to sickness. **When out of balance,** they are often complacent, dull, lethargic, possessive, overattached, and overweight, with oily skin, allergies, slow digestion, and a tendency to oversleep.

Based on your basic dosha assessment, you can review the following sections on foods for soothing your dosha, eating seasonally, and the importance of the six tastes (or *rasas*) of Ayurveda to see if there are one or two things you could change in your diet right now to restore the level or balance of energy you might be seeking. And remember to listen to the whispers of your intuitive voice as you go.

FOODS THAT SOOTHE THE DOSHAS

Vayu (or vata): Favor warm food with a moderately heavy texture, like wild rice soup or cream of wheat cereal; all oils; salt, sour and sweet tastes; and soothing and satisfying foods. Foods to avoid are red meat, corn, and rye. It's also good to limit the intake of certain astringent fruits, such as pomegranates, pears, cranberries, and apples (cooking them, however, works very well).

Pitta: Choose cool or warm, but not steaming-hot foods; moderately heavy textures; and bitter, sweet and astringent tastes. Go easy on fats and oils,

EATING TO NOURISH THE CHAKRAS

Chakra	Fuel	Spiritual Messages
One	Red foods, such as meat, beets, grapes, strawberries, and cherries	You deserve to be alive, safe, strong, and passionate.
Two	Orange foods, such as yams, salmon, sweet potatoes, papaya, and wheat	Your feelings are good, desired, and desirable.
Three	Yellow foods, especially corn, also grapefruit and squashes	You deserve success. You are intelligent. You can learn what you need to know.
Four	Green foods, such as vegetables and sauces	You are loved and loveable. You deserve healthy relationships.
Five	Blue foods, such as berries, as well as all spices, which stimulate the mouth	You can be honest and have integrity. You can manifest your needs. It is safe to communicate.
Six	Purple foods, such as grapes, and vision-inducing substances like wine, tobacco, and organic cocoa	You are acceptable as you are. You are made in the Creator's image. You deserve to make healthy choices.
Seven	White foods, such as parsnips, white asparagus, and fish; ceremonial substances like wormwood (used in absinthe), kava, salvia, wine and bread (as in communion); sacred herbs, including sage and lemongrass	You have a unique destiny. You are connected to the Divine. There is divine destiny.
Eight	Black foods (carbon based), such as alcohol, coffee, white flour, and sugar; past-life foods of meaning (often the foods that trigger issues); also colloidal silver	You can draw on the past for guidance and power. You deserve to be freed from the past. You can choose a new future.
Nine	Colloidal gold, bee pollen, honey; also foods symbolizing your soul	You are designed for greatness.
Ten	Earth foods: nuts, grains, potatoes, herbs, water	Your body is the meeting ground between the Divine and nature.
Eleven	Vibrational substances such as homeopathic tinctures, teas, and blessed water	Negativity can transmute into positivity.
Twelve	Minerals and vitamins; substances that benefit your unique physiology	You are fully human and fully divine.

and try to avoid salty foods and sour foods like pickles and sour cream. Salads, with their astringent greens and cool temperature, are excellent for balancing overactive pitta. Cold cereal, cinnamon toast, and apple juice make a perfect breakfast.

Kapha: Select warm and light foods cooked without much water. Add bitter (romaine lettuce and other leafy greens), pungent (herbs and spices), and astringent (apples, pomegranate, cranberries, pears, and legumes) tastes to most, if not all, meals. Consume a minimum amount of butter, oil, and sugar. Eating spicy food will promote better digestion and warm the body. It's hard, I know, but steer clear of all sugar except raw honey.

EATING SEASONALLY WITH AYURVEDA

Ayurveda recognizes six seasons rather than four, and each season involves general food and activity recommendations to support health and happiness.

March–April—*Vasanta-ritu*, spring. Eat lightly and sleep lightly.

May–June—*Grishma-ritu*, summer. Eat lightly and drink cold fluids.

July–August—*Varsha-ritu*, monsoon. Reinforce the appetite and eat hot foods.

September–October—*Sharad-ritu*, short summer. Eat cool, sweet, and astringent foods.

November–December—*Hemanta-ritu*, winter. Eat and exercise a lot.

January–February—*Shishira-ritu*, cold winter. As with Hemanta-ritu, eat and exercise, and also spend time in reflection.

THE RASAS, OR SIX TASTES

Diet is an important aspect of Ayurvedic medicine, as it is in traditional Chinese medicine, and food is intimately connected to the elements of nature within and around us. The beautiful alchemy of Ayurveda involves properly combining, avoiding, or increasing foods and spices of different natures. These natures are shown in the six basic *rasas*, or tastes, of Ayurveda.

Sweet: adds the elements of earth and water; nourishes, cools, and moistens; includes rice, wheat, and sugar.

Sour: adds earth and fire; warms and oils; includes acidic fruits.

Salty: adds water and fire; dissolves, softens, and stimulates; in all salts.

Bitter: adds air and ether; cools, dries, and purifies; in green vegetables and spices such as turmeric and goldenseal.

Pungent: adds air and fire; warms, dries, and stimulates; in ginger and mustard.

Astringent: adds air and earth; cools and dries; in honey, buttermilk, pomegranate, and spices such as turmeric (which is also bitter).

TASTEFUL HEALING

Rasa/Taste	Elements added	What it does for the body	Foods it's found in
Sweet	Earth and water	Nourishes, cools, and moistens	Rice, wheat, sugar, and root vegetables
Sour	Earth and fire	Warms and oils	Acidic fruits
Salty	Water and fire	Dissolves, softens, and stimulates	Salts
Bitter	Air and ether	Cools, dries, and purifies	Green vegetables, spices such as turmeric and goldenseal
Pungent	Air and fire	Warms, dries, and stimulates	Ginger, mustard, and cayenne pepper
Astringent	Air and earth	Cools and dries	Honey, buttermilk, beans, pomegranate, and turmeric

FOOD AND EMOTIONS IN TRADITIONAL CHINESE MEDICINE: The Five-Phase Approach to Soothing Heart and Mind

IN TRADITIONAL CHINESE Medicine, the five basic flavors in foods are frequently used to transform an emotion into fire in order to recalibrate the body. Foods can also be used to uplift and enhance important emotions, as well as to reduce troubling emotions and calm overstimulated emotions. Incorporating the five flavors into your diet supports the free flow of chi (vital life-force energy) and calms and nourishes shen (spirit and the psyche).

From a Western point of view, it can seem confusing to enhance so-called negative emotions such as anger, worry, sadness, or fear, or to reduce the seemingly positive emotion of joy. From an Eastern perspective, all emotions are considered normal, healthy physiological responses to stimulation, as long as they are kept in check and balanced. Too little or too much of any emotion, especially for a prolonged duration, will cause pathological damage to the organs and meridians.

For instance, too much joy will scatter the spirit and cause anxiety. This type of joy is not the sort that leads to deep contentment and peace, but rather overexcitement and hyperactivity. Lacking anger, our chi cannot rise, and we might fail to stand up for others or ourselves. If we're too angry, we become violent and cruel. If we don't worry enough, we might miss something important in our lives; we won't reach out and bond with others. Too much worry leads to despair and weakness. Sadness helps us feel love; this would be a shallow world if we could not feel loss. Too much sadness, however, will lead to being consumed by grief. And fear causes the chi to descend, helping us back down and take stock of a situation. If we are too scared, our mind becomes scattered, and we can't think or act correctly.

As you can see, every emotion is important when equalized and accessible.

Flavor	Meridians Enhanced	Emotions Enhanced	Emotions Reduced
Sour	Liver and Gallbladder	Anger	Thought
Bitter	Heart and Small Intestine	Joy	Sadness and worry
Sweet	Spleen and Stomach	Thought	Fear and shock
Pungent	Lung and Large Intestine	Worry and sadness	Anger
Salty	Kidney and Bladder	Fear and shock	Joy

Note: In traditional Chinese medicine, the body clock is a remarkable tool for supporting a particular organ and its corresponding meridian. Refer to chapter 3 to see the two-hour cycles of each organ.

20

HEALING WITH THE NATURAL WORLD

Nature's peace will flow into you as
sunshine flows into trees. The winds
will blow their own freshness into you,
and the storms their energy, while
cares will drop off like autumn leaves.

JOHN MUIR

The natural world offers an extraordinary bounty of healing remedies, restorative solutions to mend our bodies and soothe our souls. Often bursting with color and fragrance, these healing gifts arrive as textural wonders, their diversity ranging from robust leaves to soothing oils to stones of unbelievable beauty. While this chapter offers practical ways to utilize substances such as herbs, flower essences, essential oils, gemstones, and homeopathic remedies in your healing endeavors, it is simultaneously a celebration of the generosity of nature.

The party begins with a look at the essential elements that sustain us night and day.

THE TEN-ELEMENT WORLD

From Western allopathic medicine to shamanism, from every corner of the world, all healing traditions are ultimately based upon and derived from the elements. From the ground we stand on to the air we breathe to the stardust that is a part of our inherent makeup, we and the elements are inextricably united.

Having studied the indigenous healing traditions from every continent, I've compiled the following integrated, all-inclusive list of the elements. Every healing tradition, from traditional Chinese medicine to Ayurveda to the Cherokee

Tsalgi, recognizes different combinations of elements, and the ten elements listed below represent all of the elements that appear in various traditions. Once you read through the brief descriptions of each element, you can use the simple exercise that follows to assist a client or to work on yourself.

Water. Transmits psychic and feeling energies; soothes and heals; washes and cleanses. Water can be used to cleanse the lymph system or intestines of toxins and purify the body of old and repressed feelings.

Fire. Eliminates, purges, and burns away; builds energy, excitement, and new life; is the basis of the kundalini process and is important in healing. Fire can be used to purify the blood or lymph system of toxins. *Caution: Do not use fire intuitively on the heart or a critically inflamed area, as fire can enhance anger and inflammation.*

Earth. Builds, solidifies, and protects. Earth can be used to soothe any inflamed area and to repair and rebuild tissues, such as after surgery.

Air. Transmits ideas and ideals; allows the spread of energies from place to place or person to person; active when moving and directed; inactive, yet ripe with potential, when still. Air can be used to "blow away" negative beliefs or initiate helpful ones.

Metal. Protects, defends, and deflects. Metal can be used in the auric field to deflect harmful energies.

Wood. Adds buoyancy, adaptability, and a positive attitude; brings good cheer to a depressed state. Picturing trees or plants adds the wood element to the mind, which can alleviate depression.

Stone. Strengthens, holds, and toughens. Stone can be used to release toxic emotions; imagine putting all soul or subconscious issues or emotions, such as shame, into a stone and then throwing the stone into the ocean.

Ether. Ether is liquid gas. It is actually the "fifth element," the spiritual energy that scientists and metaphysicians have attempted to define for millennia. Ether holds spiritual truths and can be used to infuse any system, energy body, mind, or soul with such spiritual truths.

Light. Light is electromagnetic radiation of various wavelengths. "Dark" light is composed mainly of electrons that carry intelligence about power; "light" light is fashioned chiefly from protons that hold intelligence about love. Light can be directed, spun, fashioned, summoned, or eliminated to produce almost any desired effect.

Star. Star uses spiritual truths to form and purify physical matter. Star can be used to release negative misperceptions by formulating the truth.

APPLYING THE ELEMENTS

Here is how to use your intuition to draw out or call in elements to balance your subtle energy system.

Based on the presenting issue or condition, choose the element that you or your client will benefit from focusing on. Once the element has been identified, intuitively ascertain whether there is *too much* or *not enough* of that particular element. You can ask for higher guidance to assist you with figuring this out.

You can add the healing and balancing properties of an element to the physical body by energetically drawing it up into and through the body from the outside world. Then, using a healing stream of grace, you can then share the needed element with any energy system or bodily part requiring it. For example, if your client is experiencing financial distress and related fears of survival and security, their first chakra may benefit from the elemental force of stone, which can help them feel grounded and feel a sense of solidity beneath them.

You can subtract the characteristics of that element from any part of the body or any of the energy systems as well. For example, if your client has an inflammatory condition (fueled by the fire element) that is negativity affecting the Heart meridian, you can ask the spirit of fire to recede.

Another way to use the ten elements for healing is to call upon the spirits of the elements to conduct the diagnosis and healing for you. See the "Easy Natural Medicine" exercise in the next section, "Working with Natural and Elemental Beings," for complete instructions.

WORKING WITH NATURAL AND ELEMENTAL BEINGS

Shamanic traditions have long believed that everything in nature, from human to plant to mineral, has a spirit and that we can call upon these spirits to assist us in healing. The following is a list of some of the best natural sources for spiritual healing, along with the exercise "Easy Natural Medicine," a simple five-step process for engaging these helpful spirits.

Ancestors. Deceased ancestors can interact with us in many forms, including as entities, phantoms, ghosts, and spiritual guides. They can offer healing or hauntings, help or harm.

Forces of nature. Natural forces include the wind, storms, rain, sunshine, earthquakes, and any great natural movements of climate and the elements. Many cultures believe that spirits control these natural forces. Some imbalances within the physical and subtle energy bodies can be corrected by assuming the energy available through natural forces.

Local natural spirits. Natural spirits are usually associated with particular environmental features, such as volcanoes, streams, glens, or mountains. In most countries, special sites are assigned culturally specific names and called upon for beneficent purposes.

Nature spirits. These break down into the following basic categories:

Beings of the underworld or netherworld, which includes beings on the astral plane, such as dragons, and dwellers upon each of the post-death planes of light. (For more information on the astral plane and the planes of light, please see my book *The Journey After Life: What Happens When We Die,* originally published as *Illuminating the Afterlife.*)

Beings of the stars, such as extraterrestrials and beings from other planetary systems.

Beings of the faerie realm, like faeries and unicorns, as well as devas, whose name means "beings of light." These beings sometimes interact with the human realm to grant wishes and offer instruction.

The elemental beings, or spirits of each of the ten elements. Many shamanic traditions maintain that the elements are associated with spirits that convey the same properties as those elements. For instance, fire beings live in the center of the earth and are available to send fire energy for purifying and transmuting. Water beings are amoeba-shaped forms that dwell in wetness; they can be called upon for cleansing and renewal. Stone beings can deliver the healing properties of the gemstones they represent, and metal beings can often be called upon to establish armoring or protection, such as when we're establishing energetic boundaries.

Beings of earth, like plants, animals, and reptiles and their souls or spirits, often serve the human race. They can appear in 3-D form, in our dreams, or as spirit visitors. For instance, your companion animal might be living with you to mirror your healing needs back to you. They become sick right before you do or lick the area of your body that is coming down with an illness. The spirits of animals might appear in dreams or visions to provide you messages or warnings, to foretell an event, to share healing energy, or to symbolically present you the wisdom needed to solve a problem. Beings of earth include these specific beings:

- **Totems,** guiding figures that assist a particular family or clan
- **Power animals,** which can assist someone either for a particular task or throughout someone's life; different animals represent different types of messages (see chapter 17, "Healing with the Ancients")
- **Plant spirits,** the spirits of plants and trees, which can provide instruction on using the plant world for healing. For instance, the spirit of a particular plant can show you how to use its properties to provide physical or emotional healing or even send its vibrational qualities into you for healing purposes. The latter process can provide you the benefit of an herb, tincture, or plant without the side effects that might be involved with ingesting it.

Tip: *Spirit plant medicine* is the term for intuitively connecting with the actual personalities in the plant world, as well the personality of the plant world as a whole, in order to engage in a healing process (as outlined in the exercise "Easy Natural Medicine").

Note: *Familiars* are earth beings—animals, reptiles, or birds—that have been enchanted, entrapped, or manipulated so that their powers are available to the interfering person or entity that captured them. Plants, too, can provide divine or harmful guidance.

EASY NATURAL MEDICINE

This exercise opens you up to and invites the assistance of sacred beings from the natural world. You can access the spirits of different herbs or flowers, crystals or gemstones, as well as faeries, devas, or other beings of the natural universe, by linking to their healing frequencies. For instance, you might ask the deva of an oak tree to provide you strength during surgery, ask the spirit of an amethyst, a stone known for its protective qualities, to help remove an ancestral curse, or ask the spirit of a hawk, known for its clear sight and hunting ability, to spot details of a situation you might have missed. You can even access the spirits of a particular natural remedy or substance, such as the spirit of aloe vera for soothing a burn.

1. Use your breath to relax into a meditative state. Then use Spirit-to-Spirit to connect with the highest aspects of yourself and/or your client.

2. Based on the presenting issue, be it physical, emotional, or otherwise, call forth the natural spirit or being that would be most healing for the person or

condition. Your higher guidance can help you pinpoint the specific natural spirit that is needed or one that would carry the force or energy that will best assist your cause.

3. Ask the spirit to share its particular healing properties, directing them where they need to go.

4. Taking an easy, deep breath in, affirm with the nature spirit that your client is being infused with its vibration or energy of the substance it represents (e.g., the gemstone, element, herb, remedy).

5. Request of Spirit that the energy of the natural spirit and/or its substance remains with that person as long as they need it. For example, if you're working with the spirit of dandelions, the client may need its energy only for a month.

Tip: A complement to this exercise is "The Five Elements in Your Hands" found in chapter 12, which focuses on hands-on healing techniques.

THE HERBAL KINGDOM: INTUITIVE APPLICATIONS OF AYURVEDIC, CHINESE, AND WESTERN HERBS

Herbal medicine supplements can be as powerful as any drug in Western medicine. As such, it is safest to work with a professional herbalist or naturopath to decide what herbs to take medicinally and in what dosages. And it is always best to review your natural prescriptions with your allopathic physician.

It is safe, however, to use the exercise "Easy Natural Medicine" to call upon the spirit of a plant or herb for healing. The following is a list of a few of the top herbs in the Ayurvedic, Chinese, and Western natural systems that you can consider accessing for healing.

AYURVEDIC HERBS

Ashwagandha. In India, ashwagandha is considered a powerful adaptogen. This means that is has a normalizing effect on the entire body, helping the body adapt, in whatever way is best, to changes in the environment, as well as internal and external stressors. As a protector of the nervous system, ashwagandha is often used as a rejuvenator of body and mind. It can be used as a sedative, anti-inflammatory, or diuretic, and it can help increase physical energy and endurance. It's also beneficial for colds and coughs, diabetes, ulcers, insomnia, and Parkinson's disease.

Gotu kola. Gotu kola has been used historically for wound healing and to relieve congestion from upper respiratory infections and colds. It is also known for its ability to reduce fevers. Applied externally, it can be used to alleviate the symptoms of and aid in the recovery from herpes, sprains, fractures, and snake-bites. Long before "the Pill," gotu kola was widely used by women as a form of birth control.

Holy basil. One of the most powerful adaptogens in the herbal kingdom, holy basil is a supreme protector of the mind and body. It alleviates depression, stress, and anxiety, and it increases strength and endurance. It also promotes proper protein synthesis in the body.

Shilajit. In Sanskrit, *shilajit* means "destroyer of weakness," and this herb is considered one of the most important substances in Ayurvedic medicine. It has been used for thousands of years for longevity, as it promotes healthy brain function, bone healing, and the rejuvenation of the kidneys and spleen. It is also used for alleviating hypertension.

Turmeric. As a potent anti-inflammatory and antibacterial substance, turmeric is another powerhouse herb in the Ayurvedic system. The antioxidant known as curcumin is the active ingredient in turmeric, which is showing promising results in treating arthritis, skin and prostate cancers, psoriasis, cirrhosis of the liver, and more.

CHINESE HERBS

Astragalus. One of the most celebrated adaptogenic herbs in Chinese medicine, astragalus root increases energy and helps to expel colds, ulcers, diabetes, and general weakness. It strengthens the immune system and has remarkable anti-inflammatory, antiviral, and antibacterial properties. It also supports overall cardiac function.

Dong quai. Sometimes called the "female ginseng," dong quai is a woman's herbal tonic that has been widely used for over 2,000 years to balance hormones and blood. It helps to alleviate PMS, irregular menstrual bleeding, fibroid tumors, and symptoms of menopause. Dong quai also eases hepatitis, shingles, constipation, headaches, and allergies.

Ginkgo biloba. Ginkgo improves oxygen and blood flow to the brain, thereby promoting mental clarity and a vibrant memory. Ginkgo also helps to ease depression, prevent heart disease and strokes, alleviate tinnitus (ringing in the ears), and more.

Korean ginseng. Korean ginseng (panax ginseng) has been used traditionally to increase mental and physical vigor and reduce stress. As an adaptogen, it offers a wide diversity of healing actions, including alleviating digestive disturbances, strengthening the lungs and easing asthma symptoms, and improving circulation for better heart health.

Licorice root. Licorice root is one of nature's great detoxifiers. Another strong anti-inflammatory and antibacterial agent, licorice supports the alleviation of asthma, athlete's foot, baldness, body odor, canker sores, chronic fatigue, depression, colds and flu, dandruff, emphysema, gingivitis and tooth decay, and gout (a hyperacid condition).

Goji berries. OK, goji berries are technically fruits, not herbs. But their healing properties make them one of the most used substances in Chinese herbal medicine, so they qualify for this list on that account. Also known as lycium fruit or wolfberries, goji berries are rich in monounsaturated oleic acid, an important essential fatty acid. Increasing the suppleness of cell membranes, goji berries support the functioning of hormones and neurotransmitter and insulin receptors. They also support liver function, sexual function, eyesight, and overall longevity factors.

Gynostemma. Gynostemma is an adaptogenic herb that strongly supports overall health. Widely known for its longevity properties, gynostemma is known to prevent senility, improve sexual function, calm the nervous system, eliminate fatigue, and ease anxiety and depression.

WESTERN HERBS

American ginseng. As an adaptogen, American ginseng is an outstanding stress reducer and energizer. Although widely used to reduce fatigue, it also helps to alleviate colds and is showing promising results in regulating blood-sugar levels and easing diabetes.

Bilberry. Bilberry is rich in anthocyanin, one of the most powerful antioxidants known to exist. Anthocyanin is shown to improve the flow of blood to the nervous system, lower blood pressure, and reduce blood clotting. Bilberry also helps to prevent and heal macular degeneration, cataracts, and night blindness.

Black cohosh. Black cohosh has long been used for circulatory problems, rheumatism, and arthritis, as well as to reduce cholesterol. Now it is most well known as a powerful tonic for women of all ages. It is often used to treat symptoms of menopause, including hot flashes, vaginal dryness, and fatigue. Black cohosh has also shown to be very effective in alleviating PMS and menstrual cramps.

Burdock. Burdock is a potent blood purifier, often used to clear skin conditions such as acne, psoriasis, and eczema. A strong antioxidant, burdock is known to support liver and gallbladder health and is frequently used as a cancer preventative herb.

Echinacea. Echinacea is one of the best-known herbs for stimulating the immune system and promoting T-cell activation. Often used for colds, sore throats, flu, and upper respiratory infections, it is also known to support the healing of urinary tract infections, skin conditions, candida, and more.

Maca root. Also considered a superfood, maca is an endocrine-system adaptogen that appears to have a powerful rejuvenating effect in the hormonal health of both women and men. Maca aids in rebuilding weak immune systems, remineralizing the body, and increasing energy and endurance.

Valerian root. Known to calm and soothe the central nervous system, valerian root is considered generally safe to consume and has long been used to alleviate insomnia, nervous tension, anxiety, stiff joints, and stressed muscles.

HOMEOPATHY: VIBRATORY MEDICINE FROM THE KINGDOMS OF NATURE

Homeopathy is an advanced system of medicine practiced in many countries around the globe. It emphasizes treating all aspects of the person or organism, from the physical disease to the mental and emotional components that accompany the core set of symptoms. Homeopathy is based on three basic principles: (1) the infinitesimal dose, which means you need very little to make a difference; (2) the Law of Similars, which says that like cures like; (3) the Law of Cures, the progressive pattern of healing symptoms resulting from treatment.

Although its exact mechanisms are not yet understood, the healing action of homeopathic remedies is directed at the vital force, described by Samuel Hahnemann, the father of homeopathy, as the intelligent organizing quality within the person. The effectiveness of many common homeopathic remedies has been validated by several well-designed clinical studies. These remedies have been proven useful for conditions such as headaches, allergies, gastrointestinal disturbances, diarrhea, influenza, insomnia, and coughs.

HOW HOMEOPATHIC REMEDIES WORK

A homeopathic remedy is a dilution of a pure, natural substance that triggers the body to heal itself. It does so by mirroring the physical symptoms that the patient is experiencing, and by activating the emotional and mental landscape that underlies the disorder. For instance, a homeopathic doctor might recommend the remedy Allium cepa for watery eyes and a runny nose. By triggering the same symptoms, the remedy also activates the body's ability to heal the issue(s) causing the symptoms.

Homeopathic remedies have vibratory patterns that align or entrain with the vibratory patterns within us. When we're sick on any level—physically, mentally, or emotionally—our vibratory patterns are said to be incoherent, or out of rhythm and balance. The remedies' vibratory patterns create a more healthy interaction between the incoherent parts of us. They might align specific organs, tissues, meridians, and cellular and biochemical processes, and they also might align particular emotional and mental fields. Even when used for detoxification, or the release of physical and emotional toxins, the correct homeopathic remedies will create coherency, making sure that the entire body is balanced.

Any time we shift a physical, mental, or emotional process in the body, our chakras also change. For instance, a remedy might stimulate a muscular release in our hips. The resulting bone and muscular expansion might then open our first chakra, so we are now filled with more passion for life. You might take a homeopathic remedy for constipation, an issue that correlates with the second chakra. In the course of releasing the bowels, the remedy might also stimulate the second chakra to release fear, a common feeling underlying constipation, as well as related negative beliefs, such as "I am only safe if I'm tense."

Homeopathic remedies also interact with our meridians. As they release the stagnant chi related to a specific issue, the meridian unblocks, allowing the chi to flow freely. If a remedy releases the energy of the Lung meridian, for example, every place in the body that meridian touches also receives healing energy. And meridians are highly interactive. The Lung meridian, which is yin, links with all other yin meridians and partners with its "yang mate," the Large Intestine meridian. As one simple homeopathic remedy invites increased coherency or communication between all the yin meridians and the Large Intestine, its beneficial effects are shared throughout the body.

TAKING HOMEOPATHIC REMEDIES

Homeopathic remedies come in several forms, including liquids, creams, gels, pellets, or tablets. With pellets, the remedy is sprayed on the outside and can rub off in your hands, so they're dispensed from vials right into your mouth. They can also be crushed and mixed into water. Tablets are usually soft and made of lactose. Because they so easily melt in the mouth, they are usually considered the easiest form to use for children. Both pellets and tablets are placed under the tongue; you want to make sure you have nothing else in your mouth, so nothing interferes with the minute dose. It is best to take homeopathic remedies thirty minutes or more before eating or drinking; after taking them, wait an hour before brushing your teeth. Homeopathic practitioners might tell you to abstain from ingesting or using other substances, such as coffee and camphor, while taking a remedy.

Homeopathic practitioners will typically tell you how many pellets or tablets to take, in what strength, and how often. Usually the more often you take a remedy, the more effective and intense it is. Rarely do you take a remedy for several days in a row. For mild conditions, such as a twisted ankle or nuisance sore throat, you can dose every four hours until the symptoms start to improve. Then space the doses further apart, taking the remedy only if the symptoms start to return. If there is no improvement after four doses, you should choose a different remedy or consult a homeopath.

For moderate situations, such as a sprained ankle that can sustain weight or a persistent sore throat, you can dose every two hours until the situation improves. If there is no improvement after four doses, choose a different remedy or consult a homeopath. For anything more severe, it is best to consult a homeopath before taking any remedies. In really serious situations, such as when you are in shock, you can consider dosing a homeopathic remedy every fifteen minutes until you reach medical help.

For children, you should give no more than four doses every fifteen minutes, but the doses are often smaller than they are for adults, which is why it is wise to consult a homeopath or follow directions on a remedy package.

Note: A remedy may produce new or exaggerated symptoms if it is incorrect for the person or situation. When in doubt, consult a homeopathic professional to figure out your exact remedy and dosage needs, especially if you have been sensitive or reactive to homeopathic remedies in the past.

TYPES OF HOMEOPATHIC REMEDIES

Homeopathic remedies are typically prepared from items in the three major kingdoms of nature—plant, mineral, and animal—as well as a fourth category known as "the imponderables," which encompasses substances like electricity, radiation, light, and the magnetic fields of the earth. The sources can be either animate or inanimate natural beings or substances, and it is believed that the remedies are infused with the sources' characteristics. For instance, plants are rooted and stay in place, yet must remain sensitive to their environment in order to grow. Homeopathic remedies made from members of the plant kingdom lend us these features through their vibratory patterns, helping us become both more stable and "flowery" or creative.

COMMON REMEDIES AND THEIR USES

The following single-substance homeopathic remedies have been selected by my colleague James Mattioda, PhD, DHom (Med), one of the brightest lights in the field of homeopathy today.[1] All of the remedies listed are derived from the plant kingdom.

In general, these products are available at holistic stores and can be taken as prescribed on the bottle. Remedies come in different potencies, measured in centesimals, noted as a number followed by a C on the bottle; an average potency is 30C. To be safe, try a low potency or limited number of doses, and watch how you respond before taking the full round of treatment recommended on the bottle.

With a range of uses in healing, these particular remedies are not considered deep acting and are therefore safe in the recommended potencies for the conditions indicated.

Aconitum napellus, 12C to 200C potency, addresses anxiety and fear resulting from a sudden sense of danger; it also addresses the fear of death.

Belladonna, 6C to 12C, can be taken for headaches, coughs, or gastrointestinal disturbances. It is often taken to alleviate emotional conditions involving anger or furious excitement so strong it causes rushes of heat to the head. (Remember that homeopathic remedies mimic the very conditions they are addressing; therefore, taking this remedy may produce the same symptoms.)

Chamomilla, 12C to 200C, is a classic remedy for teething and irritability in children. Many homeopathic physicians recommend one 30C dose. You should see results in fifteen minutes. If you do, you can dose again in several hours or the next day. If there is no improvement, use a different remedy.

Ignatia amara, 30C to 200C, is nicknamed the breakup remedy. It is a grief remedy specifically for a prolonged sense of loss. This plant is also useful in relationships with jealousy and recrimination.

Staphysagria, 12C to 30C, works for those who need to stand up for themselves. It is often the remedy for victims of abuse, who don't seem to be able to overcome their indignation and who internalize their anger.

Fucus vesiculosus, Sodium alginate, Phosphorus, and **Strontium** are remedies for radiation protection.

AROMATHERAPY AND ESSENTIAL OILS: MULTIDIMENSIONAL HEALING TOOLS

Essential oils uplift the emotions, stimulate mental focus, encourage relaxation, relieve pain, improve blood circulation, cleanse the system of toxins, clear the respiratory system, move energy, and much more. Essential oils are living substances, and like any form of life, they have their own subtle energy fields, measurable in hertz and visually captured with polycontrast interface photography (PIP).

By applying high-frequency essential oils, we can increase the vibratory rate of our physical bodies and emotional states. When we apply essential oils to our bodies or inhale their aromas, we stimulate our electromagnetic fields, which in turn assists us in shifting moods, unlocking memories and stored emotions in our cells, and opening the door to healing on all levels. Essential oils can do all of these things on their own, but combined with intention, breathwork, meditation, subtle energy healing methods, or talk therapies, you can create and support a dynamic energy flow.

You can dab a dot or so of an oil on your skin. Many people select an oil particular to a chakra and dab the oil on their body in the chakra's vicinity. Before using an oil topically, first make sure you're not allergic to it by placing a very small dot of it on your skin and seeing if you react over the next few hours.

Note: Certain oils are irritating or dangerous to the skin. There are dozens that can cause inflammation and aggravation and should never be used topically, such as bitter almond, camphor, fig leaf absolute, horseradish, mustard, parsley seed, santolina, sassafras, savin, turpentine, verbena, lemon verbena, wintergreen, and wormseed.[2] It's important to do your research before you use a topical oil.

Oils can also be transformed into aromas with an aromatherapy diffuser or by dropping a few drops into boiling water on the stove. You can also call upon an oil's spirit by using the exercise "Easy Natural Medicine."

The subtle body practitioner can make good use of oils and aromas either in their office or as an assignment for their clients. I know a practitioner who commonly works with sexual abuse victims. If they can tolerate mandarin oil, which assists with healing the inner child, she recommends that they dab it behind their ears or diffuse it in their homes, especially when childhood emotions are triggered. Yet another practitioner I know uses applied kinesiology, or muscle testing (see chapter 15) to see if his clients would benefit from any particular oils. You can also spread an array of oils in front of a client and ask them to intuitively select the oils that might benefit them.

Tip: An aroma that is helpful to one person can easily trigger allergies in another. So it is best not to use essential oils in your office. Use them for yourself in your home or other personal space, and have clients do the same.

THE ESSENTIAL NINE OILS

Jodi Baglien, a certified clinical aromatherapist, offers the following list of nine of the most important essential oils for healing, plus two recipes for oil combinations that support energetic connection and opening.[3]

Angelica: Teaches us we are not alone. Brings us into conscious relationship with the angelic realm to receive its teaching. Promotes an alliance with our higher self.

Bergamot: Clears the fogginess of a heavy heart and weary mind. Offers a sense of completion, encouraging us to embrace all of life's experiences with joy in our heart.

Cedarwood: Provides clarity during times of spiritual confusion. Brings wisdom closer. Helps with grounding. Prevents the absorption of others' negativity. Clears, cleanses, and strengthens.

Coriander: Increases our confidence about the timing of healing. Offers a promise and signal of new life. Helps during times of change.

Cypress: Fortifies patience, strengthens, and comforts. Promotes wisdom. During the grieving process, cypress fragrance brings the angels to console us.

Eucalyptus: Helps with burnout and stress and when we're overwhelmed. Also helps with releasing anger. Shifts energy blockages, especially in the lung and upper chest and head.

Frankincense: Deepens our breath to help us move through emotions. Clears the mind and expands consciousness. Connects us with the Divine.

Mandarin: Connects us with our inner child and heals unhappy events from the past.

Rose: The oil of "compassion and wisdom." Teaches us lessons of love and helps ease sorrow. Symbolizes the divine feminine and invites unconditional love.

SPECIAL ESSENTIAL OIL RECIPES FOR SUBTLE ENERGY HEALING

When working essential oil recipes, keep the percentage of essential oils low—under 8 percent. Mixing your blend any stronger brings you into the physical field alone and makes it more difficult for your system to access mental or emotional energies.

Recipe for Spiritual Connection

2 tsp. fractionated coconut oil or other organic vegetable or nut oil

2 drops Angelica

2 drops Frankincense

1 drop Rose otto (a type of Rose oil)

Mix together in a 10-ml glass bottle. Anoint your third eye, heart, and bottoms of feet.

Recipe for Opening

2 tsp. fractionated coconut oil or other organic vegetable or nut oil

3 drops Eucalyptus radiata (a type of Eucalyptus oil)

3 drops Mandarin

1 drop Coriander

Mix together in a 10-ml glass bottle. Anoint your wrist creases and below the pad of your thumb.

ANOINTING WITH ESSENTIAL OILS

MANY SACRED TEXTS contain references to anointing. Probably the most well known is the biblical story of Mary Magdalene, who showed her love and devotion to Jesus by anointing his feet with "nard," or spikenard, before his crucifixion.

Anointing is a sacred ceremony for blessing and healing. The act of "touching with oil," combined with intention, ceremony, and right action, offers you a sacred space for your spiritual focus. Anointing enhances prayer and meditation, and afterward, it acts as an aromatic reminder of your stated intentions.

Here is a process recommended by aromatherapist Jodi Baglien for incorporating anointing into a meditation for spiritual guidance.

1. Create sacred space. Remove any "busyness" from the day. Incorporate any colors, candles, art, stones, and other spiritual objects you see fit.

2. Mist the space with your favorite aromatherapy spray, spraying it in the four directions (north, east, south, and west) to raise the vibrational fields.

3. Drop your awareness into your heart area. Ask for guidance or help from your spiritual sources.

4. Set your intention. Say it aloud, if possible.

5. Anoint your body with the chosen oil blend. For instance, anoint your hands if your intention involves action, the third eye to see more clearly, the heart area for healing, and back of neck for protection.

6. Open to guidance and listen with all your senses.

7. Add any prayers, blessings, or requests.

8. Close by giving thanks. Then draw the energy of the oil to your heart. Take a moment to reflect on the information you may have received and write it down.

BACH FLOWER REMEDIES

Flower essences, also known as flower remedies, are dilutions of flower material that are believed to contain the healing properties of the plant. In the 1930s, Edward Bach, an English physician and homeopath, developed thirty-eight different flower remedies to address thirty-eight different emotional, soul, or psychological issues. For example, the remedy Willow is indicated for someone who, when out of balance, feels resentful, bitter, and envious of others and adopts a "poor me" victim stance. When this person takes Willow, the issues underneath the psychological challenges clarify, and the person is better able to work through the underlying problems.

Bach believed that the dew found on flower petals holds the plant's healing energy and that that energy is especially effective for healing emotional and spiritual conditions. The typical remedy contains a very small amount of the flower material in a 50:50 solution of brandy and water. Bach believed that this dilution worked vibrationally.

You can select a Bach flower remedy for yourself or for a client by assessing the presenting challenges. Select the remedy based on not only the negative patterns, but also the positive, desirable qualities each essence leads to. You can also use applied kinesiology, or muscle testing (see chapter 15), to see if clients would benefit from particular essences.

BEYOND BACH: Other Flower Essences and Sources

THE TERM "BACH flower remedies" refers to the thirty-eight flower essences Dr. Edward Bach created in the 1930s. Because Dr. Bach lived and worked in England, his original essences are derived from plants native to the British Isles, and he felt that there would never be any need for more flower essences beyond his thirty-eight. Today, "Bach Flower Remedies" is a trademarked name held by a company called Directly from Nature, as is the name "Bach Rescue Remedy."

Yet many other companies produce flower essences using the same thirty-eight plants and natural substances Dr. Bach did and using methods based closely on his. These and other companies are also making and researching flower essences derived from plants around the world. The northern California–based Flower Essence Society (FES), for example, produces a wide range of essences using North American plants, from aloe vera to zinnia. Green Hope Farm in New Hampshire produces flower essences from plants native to not only New England, but also from Ireland, Spain, Italy, and the Caribbean. Desert Alchemy of Tucson, Arizona, specializes in flower essences made from desert plants.

The recommended dosage is traditionally four to six drops, taken under the tongue, four times daily. Usually each dose is taken fifteen minutes before or after a daily meal. It is best to listen to your body to determine how long to continue taking a remedy. Professionals often recommend anywhere between a few days and three weeks of treatment. Children are usually given lower doses, often four drops two times a day. For acute states, you can take four drops every thirty to sixty minutes, for up to a few hours or until your symptoms are relieved, although some remedies might need to be taken only once. Dr. Bach said that morning and evening doses are the most critical, because at these times, the human energy fields are at their optimum level of vibrational responsiveness.

You can also mix remedies in water. For short-term issues, put two drops of a selected flower essence in a glass of water, then continue drinking the water until you feel relief. For longer-term problems, sip from the glass throughout the day, but at least four times a day. Make up a fresh glass of water each day.

Other practitioners recommend that you use Bach flower remedies topically, putting them directly on the skin. You can apply them to chakra sites or meridian pathways, selecting the places that represent the greatest need to address with a specific remedy.

In order to keep the essence pure, you should not touch the neck of the bottle or the mouth with the dropper. You should also store your remedies away from electromagnetic fields.

The following is a brief synopsis of Dr. Bach's thirty-eight flower remedies. For each, the presenting challenge is given, followed by the desirable quality it promotes.[4]

Agrimony: anxiety to inner peace

Aspen: fear of the unknown to trust

Beech: criticalness to tolerance

Centaury: people-pleasing to healthy boundaries

Cerato: doubt to self-confidence

Cherry Plum: fear of losing control to spiritual surrender

Chestnut Bud: repetitive patterns to wise action

Chicory: possessiveness to respect

Clematis: avoidance to focused presence

Crab Apple: compulsiveness to inner clarity

Elm: overwhelm to effectiveness

Gentian: discouragement to perseverance

Gorse: pessimism to optimism

Heather: self-absorption to self-sufficiency

Holly: jealousy to gratitude

Honeysuckle: nostalgia to embracing the present

Hornbeam: fatigue to dynamism

Impatiens: impatience to harmonious flow

Larch: self-censorship to self-confidence and creative expression

Mimulus: apprehension (of the known) to courage

Mustard: gloom to joy

Oak: inflexibility to accepting limits

Olive: mental exhaustion to deep rest

Pine: guilt to self-forgiveness

Red Chestnut: worry to compassion

Rock Rose: panic to transcendent courage

Rock Water: self-denial to spontaneity

Scleranthus: indecision to inner resolve

Star of Bethlehem: shock to wholeness

Sweet Chestnut: despair to safety

Vervain: fanaticism to grounded idealism

Vine: dominance to service

Walnut: tribalism to individuation

Water Violet: false pride to dignity

White Chestnut: unwanted thoughts to tranquility

Wild Oat: confusion to conviction

Wild Rose: resignation to commitment

Willow: resentment to acceptance

Dr. Bach also created a five-flower combination essence, a "rescue remedy," ideal for immediate trauma recovery, as well as everyday stress relief.

YARROW FLOWER ESSENCE FOR THE AURIC FIELD

YARROW FLOWER ESSENCE is an outstanding companion to caregivers, healers, and helpers everywhere. Place a few drops of Yarrow in your water and sip throughout the day when you feel the need to:

- Knit together and strengthen your auric field so that you're protected from absorbing the feelings and thoughts of others.

- Create an energetic boundary with outside energies so that you can know your own thoughts and feel your own heart.

- Quickly shift your energy so that you can think and communicate clearly.

- Restore, rejuvenate, and turn on your energetic light!

Tip: One of the benefits of working with flower essences is that they are safe. While you can overdose with herbal supplements or homeopathic remedies, or select the wrong formulas, you cannot do so with flower essences. If you select the wrong essence, it has no affect on your body. This is why they can be great tools in your subtle body medicine kit.

GEMSTONES: STONES OF LIGHT

Gemstones have been employed for healing and divination since time began. Each stone carries within its crystalline structure specific frequencies and attributes that can affect the energetic fields near it. Thus, each type of stone carries a different set of vibrational qualities that supports our mental, emotional, physical, and spiritual health. The following list will help you select the stone or crystal that has the properties needed for healing yourself or a client.

Agate: Brings emotional security and spiritual insight. Alleviates inner turmoil. Supports the kidneys, spleen, pancreas, lymph system, colon, and circulatory system.

Aquamarine: Improves tolerance and patience. Supports the eyes, jaw, neck, and throat, and helps release retained water.

Amber: Brings serenity and emotional harmony while soothing and nurturing. Supports the brain, central nervous system, thyroid, and inflammation due to viruses. Draws pain out of the joints. Also said to help with tooth pain and to be helpful for teething babies. (Place the amber near the baby; do not let them chew on it.)

Amethyst: Enhances spirituality, calms the temper, and brings healing during sleep. Supports the endocrine system and stimulates all meridians. Expels negative energy.

Aventurine: Raises psychic perception and creative inspiration. Brings tranquility and optimism. Supports the alleviation of skin diseases.

Bloodstone: Raises consciousness and sweeps away heavy feelings and beliefs. Stimulates the immune system. Supports circulation and healthy blood. Helps relieve menstrual cramps, hemorrhoids, and anemia.

Carnelian: Sparks motivation and initiates transformation. Supports radiant life-force energy by warming, cleansing, and purifying the blood. Good for fertility issues.

Citrine: Energizes. Enhances creativity, self-esteem, security, and inner calm. Supports digestion and organ health by promoting physical activity.

Coral: Balances. Leads to acceptance of self and others. Good for children. Supports the heart and circulatory system. Alleviates anemia and varicose veins.

Diamond: Contains the entire color spectrum. Brings back a sparkle, strength, positive energy, and spiritual ecstasy. Clears negativity from the auric field and draws out toxicity from the physical body. Supports brain health.

Emerald: Excites greater insight, improves intuition and clairvoyance, illuminates dreams, and facilitates meditation. Balances the heart chakra and emotional energy bodies. Supports circulation and eases eyestrain. Good to wear near the heart.

Fluorite: Initiates spiritual awareness, solid foundations, and unconditional love. Helps to alleviate arthritis, osteoporosis, and tooth decay.

Garnet: Calls forth self-respect, imagination, courage, compassion, and success. Strengthens the heart. Supports blood circulation and health. Balances and enhances sexual energy.

Herkimer diamond: Provides direction, happiness, serenity, upliftment, and clarity. A good stone to use as a dowsing pendulum. Should *not* be used to treat cancer or circulatory issues.

Jade: Promises inner peace, tranquility, achievement, and integrity. Strengthens the whole body, and specifically supports the kidneys, liver, spleen, heart, throat, and fertility.

Jasper: Provides grounding and energizes. Invites patience, tolerance, and understanding. Stimulates access to past lives. Restores and reenergizes the physical body and etheric body after prolonged illness.

Lapis lazuli: Promotes self-worth, spiritual purity, direction, integrity, wisdom, and light. Supports the thyroid gland, bronchial passages, and throat. Beneficial near the fifth chakra.

Malachite: Promotes general wellbeing, spiritual maturity, and meaning in life. Supports the kidneys, spleen, pancreas, and eyesight. Helps to ease dyslexia, epilepsy, tumors, leukemia, colic, infections, and vertigo.

Moonstone: Strengthens intuition and accesses the divine feminine in all persons. Aids in dieting, alleviates stress, and helps balance women's hormones.

Obsidian: Absorbs darkness and converts it to white-light energy, transmuting anger, blame, judgment, and fear.

Opal: Aligns with the seventh chakra. Enhances psychic awareness, spontaneity, and sensitivity. Calms the emotions. Supports the pineal gland.

Pearl: Balances the fourth (heart) chakra. Soothes emotions. Eases stress and irritation. Helps to alleviate skin disorders.

Pyrite: Increases energy, mental capacity, focus, and confident communication. A tremendously grounding stone that balances the third chakra and supports the stomach and intestines, and the circulatory and respiratory systems. Alleviates depression.

PRECIOUS METALS TO COMPLEMENT HEALING GEMSTONES

LIKE GEMSTONES, PRECIOUS metals also carry particular vibrational properties that can be used for healing.

Gold: Encourages satisfaction and positivity. Eases the load when you're overburdened. Supports brain function, the circulatory system and blood, the nervous system, and digestion. Helps alleviate hormonal and chemical imbalances. Strengthens meridians. A high-level amplifier of subtle energies.

Silver: Has antimicrobial and protective properties and can be used to deflect negative energy. Can be worn to enhance your psychic abilities while protecting you from others' energy; also produces psychic dreams. Draws out your own negative energy and reflects others' harmful energies back to their higher self. Reinforces all energetic boundaries.

Copper: Helps the wearer amplify thoughts when sending and receiving psychic communication. Stimulates the flow of mental and physical energy and aids in overcoming lethargy. Bolsters self-esteem and releases mental burdens. Said to assist with healing arthritis, detoxifying the blood, reducing inflammation, and stabilizing the metabolism. Copper bracelets are often worn to create these physical effects, but they do leave a residue on your wrist.

Platinum: Known as the most pure metal, platinum is said to aid in the fight against cancer and to change DNA and RNA. Balances and harmonizes all levels of the body, mind, and spirit and promotes healthy tissue regeneration. Improves memory and mental alertness.

Quartz crystal (clear): Increases energy and reconnects us to life purpose. Dramatically enhances healing of the body, mind, and spirit. *Not* for use on cancer or extreme blood-related issues, as it might multiply cells.

Rose quartz: Brings peace after emotional pain; heals traumas of the heart. Supports equanimity of heart and mind; good for meditation. Protects us from negative energies, including radiation. Supports circulation.

Ruby: Sets a healing process in motion, brings strength and personal empowerment, and enhances intuition. Calms the mind and helps alleviate depression. Supports the heart, circulatory system, and large and small intestines. Stimulates chi throughout the meridians, especially the Heart meridian.

Sapphire: Assists with concentration, clarity of life purpose, serenity, and intense love. Aligns the higher chakras and the auric field; supports spiritual development, awakening psychic awareness, telepathy, and clairvoyance.

THE CHARGED WATER SYSTEM:
Crystals Creating "Informed Water"

JUST LIKE MANY people are now using devices attached to their water sources to cleanse their water, you can now harmonize and balance your energetic system with equivalent devices. Using a process called intrinsic data field (IDF), Tim Simmone, a radionics specialist and inventor, is creating programmed crystals that will balance your subtle body through water. The IDF process stores information in a crystal much like one can store data on a computer hard drive.[5]

This crystal, which "copies" the beneficial information into water, is programmed to attune your major and minor chakras, auric layers, meridians, spiritual points, and even twelve DNA layers, in addition to activating sacred geometric forms in your energetic anatomy for health and protection. The crystal can be placed in your water pitcher, glass, or bottle.

Healers have used crystals to encode and hold data, focus healing energies, and bolster manifestation for thousands of years. Crystals also have been used as information-storage vehicles for decades. And it's not only rock solid crystals that are being used this way; scientists have even recorded images in liquid crystals.[6] In fact, scientists have recently figured out how to use crystals to store one of the most challenging sources of information: quantum light, which, made of photons, has a tendency to disappear. This light-encoded information is now able to be stored in certain types of crystals, which actually share the information through an "echoing" of the original data.[7]

Good for opening fourth and fifth chakras during meditation, especially when used near pituitary gland.

Smoky quartz: Welcomes self-love. Aids in completion of life cycles. Anchors earth energy and supports the heart, nervous system, and reproductive organs. Helps to correct infertility and PMS.

Sodalite: Imparts youthful freshness and effervescence; relieves a heavy heart. Supports and strengthens lymphatic system.

Sugilite: Protects psychic centers; brings spiritual truth and enlightened energy. Can balance left and right brain, as well as the pineal and pituitary glands. Helps to alleviate dyslexia and symptoms of autism.

Topaz: Balances emotions. Activates third chakra. Improves appetite.

Tourmaline: Alleviates fear. Releases victim mentality and builds self-assurance. Strengthens the entire auric field.

Turquoise: A calming stone that calls forth courage, success, personal power, and strength of conviction. One of the main healing stones for the subtle body.

SIMPLE TIPS FOR WORKING WITH GEMSTONES

You can use the following techniques to access the qualities of these brilliant stones of light.

- For a continuous stream of healing energy, carry the stone with you.
- When meditating, hold the stone in your hand or place it in front of you.
- Wear jewelry with the particular stones that can strengthen your energetic boundaries, help you manifest your desires, or invite needed healing.
- Program your stone with an intention, using instructions in chapter 9, in the section "Using Intention to Bless an Object."
- Surround your bed with gemstones that will provide the assistance you are seeking. Know that single-pointed clear quartz crystals can be placed under your bed, with the points facing outward, to ward off negative energies or send unhealthy electrical energies away from you.
- When cleaning crystals and gemstones in water, avoid extreme temperatures. You can cleanse them with sage, incense, salt, saltwater, or sunlight.
- Remember to thank the spirit of your gemstone for its aid.

GEMSTONE ESSENCES

Gemstone essences are vibrational infusions, carrying the most potent level of the healing properties of gemstones and crystals. The frequencies and attributes of the stone, when blended with water and sunlight or moonlight, and then infused with your intention, create a potent, customized remedy.

Most often, gemstone essences, like flower essences, are taken orally. Drops can be placed on or under the tongue from a dropper. These essences also work well topically and can be absorbed through the skin by osmosis. Apply essences to any part of the body that is calling for healing. Additionally, gemstone essences are also good in baths and can be mixed with massage oils.

To make a gemstone essence:

1. Choose a gemstone that holds the appropriate healing properties.

2. After washing the stone, put it into a glass bottle of water.

3. Program the water with your healing intention or with the Healing Streams of Grace technique (see chapter 9).

4. For an essence that will heal presenting issues, place the bottle in the sun for two to four hours. For an essence that will heal subconscious issues, place it in the moonlight overnight.

5. After its time in the sun- or moonlight, the essence will be ready to use. You can leave it in the larger glass bottle or distribute it into small bottles with droppers.

Note: Moonstone should not be used as a gem essence.

Note: While gemstone essences are made from stones' subtle energies, gem elixirs typically incorporate actual ground stones. Elixirs should not be made without expert instruction and guidance, as ingesting some stones is dangerous.

21

SOUND HEALING

Each celestial body, in fact each and every atom, produces a particular sound on account of its movement, its rhythm or vibration. All these sounds and vibrations form a universal harmony in which each element, while having its own function and character, contributes to the whole.

PYTHAGORAS

Sound healing is a form of subtle energy medicine based on vibrational frequencies. Everything in the universe is made of energy that vibrates at its own unique speed or frequency, which means that *everything is sound,* whether it's audible to us or not.

A primary principle of sound healing—in fact, all subtle energy work—is that symptoms and suffering, whether physical, spiritual, mental or emotional, first occur in the human energy field, and the stronger this dissonant or chaotic energy becomes, the greater the impact it will have on the person. When we change the energy field or our corresponding chakras and meridians, symptoms and behaviors also change. Sound, a mechanical wave, is one of the two main ways to create these subtle changes. (Light and color, covered chapter 22, is the second.)

According to Kay Grace, renowned sound-healing practitioner and trainer, there are three ways that sound creates healing change:

- Sound can **dissolve** a block by matching its frequency, like an opera singer can shatter a glass by matching the frequency of her voice to that of the glass (destructive resonance).
- Sound can create pathways through or currents on which unwanted energy can be **released** from the body.

- Specific sounds and intention can bring you into a particular state of being, such as relaxed, focused, or energized. **Entrainment** is the term for how the powerful rhythmic vibration or sound of one object or person (through talking, singing, or an intense mental or emotional state) can cause the less powerful vibrations of another object or person to adjust to the more powerful vibration. Entraining our body's vibration to a healing vibration can restore balance and wholeness to our physical and subtle energy bodies.[1]

On the physical level, sound healing effectively induces a state of calm, slows and regulates breathing, lowers blood pressure, alleviates pain, and reduces stress, all of which boost the function of the immune system. Sound can take brain waves from a beta (active) state to an alpha state, as if one were meditating, or even into a theta state, where very deep healing often occurs just below the surface of conscious awareness. (See chapter 15 for more on the healing potential of brain-wave states.)

There are many ways to create healing sound. A few of these include using your own voice to create sounds; toning; nature-based vocalization, which occurs when you are mimicking the sounds of nature; instrumentation, using drums, rattles, tuning forks, Tibetan or Himalayan singing bowls, crystal singing bowls, chimes, bells, and more; and chanting or uttering mantras or phrases created with intention. Sound healers also employ culturally based syllables, such as the Hindu seed syllables, in order to work directly on the chakras. These Hindu seed syllables are the same as the sounds of the chakras listed in chapter 4, in the section "The Seven Hindu Chakras."

SOUND HEALING BASICS

Sound-healing professional Kay Grace shares her basic structure for a sound-healing session; an outline of sounds, Hindu syllables, and tuning-fork frequencies appropriate for individual chakras; plus tips for using the healing power of sound in everyday life.

When conducting a sound-healing session, Grace uses the following steps:

1. Breathe and ground. (See "The Five Steps for Grounding" in chapter 9, or use your own method of grounding your energy.)

2. Tune into the wisdom of your higher self and ask to be a clear channel for healing sound.

3. Set your intention for the session. If you're working with a client, work with them to establish and set their intention. Express your intention with conscious words of power, such as *certain*, *radiant*, *peaceful*, or *present*.

4. Assess your energy system (or your client's energy system) using voice, singing bowls, tuning forks, or other tools to scan your energy field. Allow your higher self to show or to tell you what tools or techniques to use.

5. Following that guidance, use sound to release or dissolve what's not working (e.g., blocks, pain).

6. Now fill the space vacated by what was released: combine sound and the intention set in the beginning of the session to bring in and anchor what you do want. Filling this space will restore the energy system to wholeness and harmony. You do not need to state an entire sentence, such as "I am certain," although you can. It is enough to say the power words out loud or mentally while making a sound.

7. Close the session with another round of grounding and by expressing gratitude. Also be willing to receive any higher-self messages, insights, or feelings that will help anchor the healing so you or your client can return to that state of being more easily.

APPLICATION OF THE BASIC SOUND-HEALING PRACTICE: LISTENING-BASED SOUND HEALING

One of the most important sound-healing skills we can develop is listening. We must hear what is off before we can figure out what sound can turn health back on.

The following exercise is an application of Kay Grace's basic sound-healing practice for chakra healing. It will guide your heart chakra so you can listen for the off, or discordant, sounds and then intuitively open to the sounds that will promote healing. You can adapt this process to respond to any chakra or auric field, meridian, or even a body part. The exercise is written so you can conduct it on a client, but you can use the same process on yourself.

You can conduct this exercise with a particular focus in mind, such as to heal cancer or financial issues, or for an all-purpose healing.

Step 1: Preparation. Use the Spirit-to-Spirit technique to establish your energetic boundaries. Tune into the wisdom of Spirit.

Step 2: Set your intention for the session. Restate the overall goal that you and your client have agreed on.

Step 3: Assess your client's energy field. Totally focus on your client's heart chakra. If they give permission and you are near them, put your hand gently on the upper part of their chest. Breathe deeply and be silent. Attune your verbal intuitive abilities to this chakra. Making a sound—such as a simple OM with your voice or a chime with a singing bowl—over the heart chakra can help you tune in. Breathe deeply, be silent, and pay attention to any sound that emerges in your inner ears. You are listening for sounds, noises, messages, words, tones, or other verbal indicators telling you what is off in this energy center. You might hear wheezing, hissing, clunks, or other sounds that indicate energetic damage. If you made a sound over the chakra, you may notice it changing tone or harmonic.

Step 4: Share your perceptions with your client. Ask if they relate to any of the sounds or messages you've found. Do they have any memories that account for the wounds or noises? What emotions are triggered in reaction to your information? Do they think of a particular person or situation that might be creating the difficulties symbolized by the sounds you are bringing forth? Continue inviting responses from your client until you both feel like you have arrived at a core issue.

Step 5: Swap healing sounds for unhelpful ones. Ask Spirit to help you intuitively hear sounds or messages that will heal your client's heart chakra and the revealed issue. These sounds or noises might directly address the aberrant ones. For instance, the dysfunctional phrase, "I am bad" might be replaced by "I am loved." A hissing sound, indicative of an energetic leak, might be overcome by the sound of a closing zipper. Review each of the sounds that were important to the client and state, sound, chant, or tone the healing sound—or ask the client to do it for themselves.

Step 6: Fill the remaining space. When you've finished substituting a healing sound for every aberrant one, ask Spirit for a final message, sound, tone, chant, or truth for your client. You can deliver it aloud, then invite your client to echo it. This final sound will fill in any remaining pockets in the heart chakra and protect it from additional damage.

Step 7: Close with gratitude. You and your client might decide to hum, chant, sing, or perform some other form of verbalization together in order to end the session with grace and love.

THE NINE-CHAKRA SOUND HEALING SYSTEM

Grace utilizes a nine-chakra system when performing sound healing. Her "Earth Star" chakra is the equivalent of the tenth chakra in the twelve-chakra system, and the "Soul Star" is the same as the ninth chakra. You can select a chakra to focus

SOUND HEALING: WORKING WITH THE NINE-CHAKRA SYSTEM

Chakra	Location	Vowel Sound	Hindu Seed Sound	Hz/CPS (tuning forks)	Issues or Challenges	Sound Placement	Conscious Words of Power (frequency you want to embody)
Earth Star	12–18 inches below the feet	Uh	OM	Otto 64	Ungrounded, fearful, scattered, disconnected	On or above pubic bone, in the energy field between the feet, or on the bottoms of the feet	*Reverence, certain, courageous, disciplined*
Root, 1st	Base of the spine, the perineum	Uh	Lam	Otto 128 (C)	Anxious, holding back, afraid to trust and let go	Base of spine/ tailbone, pubic bone/ pelvic floor	*Grounded, sovereignty*
Sacral, 2nd	Approximately 2 inches below the navel	Oo	Vam	136.1 Hz (earth frequency)	Sexuality blocked or destitute, inner-child wounds, creativity blocked	2 inches below the navel or sacrum	*Playful, pure, creativity, wonder*
Solar Plexus, 3rd	From just below the navel to bottom of sternum	Oh	Ram	256 (C) / 384 (G)	Imbalance of power: disempowering self or others; lack of belief in one's abilities or worth	Center halfway between the navel and the bottom of sternum	*Capable, generous, gracious, confident*
Heart, 4th	Center of chest	Ah	Yum	329.6 (E) / 440 (A)	Feeling unloved or unlovable, closed off from others, lack of forgiveness, grief	Center of chest; over the heart	*Loving, appreciation, allowing, kindness, happy*
Throat, 5th	Arc between base of neck and chin	Aye	Hum	256 (C) / 384 (G)	Throat blocked, difficult to speak truth, lying to oneself or others, unwilling to be true to oneself	Throat area, front and back (in energy field)	*Commanding, present, integrity, willing*

SOUND HEALING: WORKING WITH THE NINE-CHAKRA SYSTEM, continued

Chakra	Location	Vowel Sound	Hindu Seed Sound	Hz/CPS (tuning forks)	Issues or Challenges	Sound Placement	Conscious Words of Power (frequency you want to embody)
Third Eye, 6th	Center of forehead, between the brows	Aay	OM	288 (D) / 468 (A#)	Intuition is blocked or devalued; unwilling to see beyond the obvious or one's own blind spots	Center of the forehead	*Clarity, focused, willing*
Crown, 7th	Top of the head	Eee	Silent	2675 Hz Crystal Tuner	Disconnected from Spirit, blocked spiritual connection or expression	Top of the head	*Boundless, cherishing, reverence*
Soul Star	About 8 inches above head	Silent	Silent	4096 H2 Angel Tuner to open and close space around silence *or* an octave	Living a "divided life," disconnected from one's soul path and purpose	Above the head	*Radiant, peaceful, masterful*

on based on the chakra meanings and/or the chakra-specific issues and challenges listed in the chart "Sound Healing: Working with the Nine-Chakra System."

The same chart lists specific vowel sounds to balance each chakra and the Hindu seed syllable to open the chakra. During a healing session, you can intone or sing the appropriate syllable to the client while concentrating on the appropriate chakra. You can also encourage your client to join you in making the sound. The chart also lists what frequency tuning fork can be used in order to effect change in each chakra. You can use the tuning forks alone or in tandem with the vocal sounds. The combination of vocal sound and tuning-fork vibration is extraordinarily powerful. In your healing session, you direct your vocalization toward or place the tuning fork at the location noted in the "Sound Placement" column.

Tip: To activate a tuning fork, hold the stem and strike the fork on a block of hard rubber (a hockey puck works great) or a block of wood covered in leather or fabric. Strike so that only one of the two prongs touches the striking block, at 90 degrees to the block's surface.

Words also have frequencies. You have only to think or chant the conscious words of power related to each chakra to embody those frequencies and, thus, those characteristics.

TIPS FOR EVERYDAY SOUND HEALING

Kay Grace also offers the following tips for incorporating sound healing into our daily lives:

- Don't bite your lip or hold your breath if you're in pain. Instead, groan and make sounds to release it!
- Speak the truth with kindness and awareness and in a way that lines up with your core values.
- Sing often, whether you can carry a tune or not.
- To shift your energy quickly and easily, tone a simple vowel sound, like *ah*, *oh*, or *ee*; add your intention (such as, "to be peaceful," "to be capable," "to be confident," or "to be gracious"); and sing the chosen vowel sound for at least three minutes.
- Play music often, at least an hour a day. Choose music that feels good—calming, energizing, and peaceful.
- Pay attention to your sound environment, changing what sounds you can. For those sounds you can't change, try harmonizing with them by singing the same unpleasant tone or another tone that is in harmony with it.
- Your thoughts are inaudible sounds and have a very powerful effect on your whole being—physically, emotionally, and spiritually. So pay attention to them and weed out the thoughts that don't support you.

THE SIX TAOIST HEALING SOUNDS

Sound healing is an excellent way to work with the meridians, especially employing the six Taoist healing sounds. Each of these six sounds is associated with a set of meridians, an excess of a particular emotion, and an element. When uttering the related healing sound, you should inhale through the nose and exhale slowly

Element	Meridians	Excess Emotion	Healing Sound
Wood	Liver, Gallbladder	Anger	*Sh*—as though saying, "Hu*sh*, be quiet." At the end of the *sh*, form your mouth into a U shape.
Fire	Heart, Small Intestine	Joy (excitement)	*Ho*—identical to the sound of *hoo* in the word *hook*.
Earth	Spleen, Stomach	Brooding	*Hoo*—just like the word *who*.
Metal	Lungs, Large Intestine	Sorrow	*See-ah*—a barely audible prolonged chant.
Water	Kidneys, Bladder	Fear	*Chrooee*—a low chant.
Not applicable. There is no organ and therefore particular element associated with the Triple Warmer.	Triple Warmer (or Burner)	None	*See*—while making the sound, form your mouth into a smile.

through the mouth. The system shared here was developed by Ken Cohen, distinguished health educator, author, and qigong master.[2]

OTHER SOUND HEALING APPLICATIONS

TONES AND BOUNDARIES

We can use different Hindu syllables or octave notes to boost our energetic boundaries for protection. Each syllable or note entrains the chakra and its related auric layer to its vibration, dissolving blocks, freeing repressed feelings, releasing toxic energies, and inviting positive protective energy. The resulting cohesiveness strengthens energetic boundaries, but also invites healing into the parts of the body governed by the chakra and its auric field. (See chapter 7 for a review of the four types of energetic boundaries and the connection between these boundaries and the chakras.)

You can chant, sing, or say each of the syllables while focusing on each chakra, one at a time, or focus just on one chakra. You can do the same to clear and bolster each auric layer or heal a particular auric layer.

Sound can be silent as well. It is enough to internally chant a sound as a silent mantra while meditating or even when seeking to calm yourself under stress, such as during a business meeting or stressful relationship interaction.

You can also use a tuning fork with the appropriate octave note and apply it to the bodily area related to a chakra while chanting the Hindu seed syllable.

MAKING A MANTRA

A mantra is a word or series of sounds chanted or sung repetitively as an incantation or prayer. The easiest way to use a mantra is through vocalization. You can use the Hindu seed syllables or any other tone or note as a mantra, but you can also personalize a mantra for a personal need.

A mantra will help you to delve deeply into your consciousness to focus on your higher self. To create your own, select a life area that's disturbing you. Jot down how you're feeling or your state of mind, starting with the phrase "I am." For example: "I am stressed." Now write down the opposite: "I am at ease." If you want, create additional positive statements, making sure to avoid using the negative word; the brain can't distinguish between negative and positive statements.

Now write both the statements about how things are ("I am stressed") and how you would like them to be ("I am at ease") on an index card and vocalize them. Use whatever tone of voice you would like and let yourself sink into the tone and meaning of each statement. Use this mantra for however long you would like.

CLEARING CHAKRAS AND AURIC LAYERS WITH YOUR VOICE

Your voice is a built-in sound-healing tool. It is able to clear your own or another person's chakras and auric field, dissolving energetic congestion, releasing blocked energy, and even drawing desirable energy to you.

Choose your preferred words, octave tones, or Hindu syllables for each chakra or auric field, as per Kay Grace's chart ("Sound Healing: Working with the Nine-Chakra System") or the chart in "Tones and Boundaries." Start by vocalizing the tones related to the first chakra, knowing that you are simultaneously clearing the first auric layer. Continue through the upper chakras and end your clearing session with an OM, the most universal tone of healing.

THE BASIC REIKI DRUMMING TECHNIQUE

The following process is based on the work of Reiki master Michael Baird, and I have transformed it to use in my own classes.[3] It blends the subtle energy of Reiki with the shamanic power of drumming for deeply balancing and healing effects.

SOUND HEALING THROUGH OCTAVES

Energetic Boundary Type	Chakra and Auric Layer	Hindu Seed Syllable	Octave Note	Boundary Shift Results
Physical	1st	Lam (pronounced "lum")	C	Promotes physical health; encourages the release of addictions; attracts money, work, and positive primary relationships; strengthens our ability to be patient
Emotional	2nd	Vam (pronounced "vum")	D	Helps us feel our feelings, release them from our body, and mature them toward joy; promotes sensuality and creativity; promotes intestinal and sexual health; enhances the vibration of purity, encouraging a "return to innocence"
Emotional	3rd	Ram (pronounced "rum")	E	Enhances mental clarity; promotes success; increases mental and personal power; improves digestion; increases spiritual radiance and self-confidence
Relational	4th	Yam (pronounced "yum")	F	Attracts love and positive relationships; supports breast, lung, and heart health; leads to increased contentment
Relational	5th	Ham (pronounced "hum")	G	Enhances communication ability and the ability to speak our truth; attracts guidance; improves thyroid health; enhances hearing; enables us to control our eating and make healthy food choices; activates the power of unity in all life areas
Spiritual	6th	Om (pronounced with a long O sound)	A	Enhances vision and eye health; improves our connection with our higher self; enables us to see the future and possibilities; improves self-image; builds a spiritual foundation for all parts of life, physical and otherwise
Spiritual	7th	None	B	Helps us find and connect with our purpose; enhances our connection with the Divine; brings balance to all life areas; enhances higher brain functions, such as learning and thinking; encourages the embodiment of our spirit in everyday life

The following steps are written for use with clients, but you can easily cast yourself as the client.

You need a drum and mallet, but any drum-like object—a bucket and paint stick, or box and a wooden spoon—can stand in. Drumming is one of the most powerful ways to stimulate life energy. Don't *not* drum because you don't own a drum.

During the drumming, you will be using the Cho Ku Rei symbol described in "Healing the Reiki Way," in chapter 12. This symbol is ideal for opening and closing a sound healing ceremony, but can also be focused on for the entire drumming ceremony, as it invites higher healing. Decide if you want to use the symbol clockwise or counterclockwise. As covered in chapter 12, the clockwise spin brings energy to you, and the counterclockwise spin releases energy from you. You can always draw the symbol twice, in both directions.

Step 1: Set an intention. Help your client clarify the life challenge they would like to heal. This process can itself become a healing or a partial healing, because while digging to the core of our presenting problems, we often illuminate truths that immediately begin changing us.

Step 2: Assess willingness. It's important to ask the client if they are willing to heal the clarified issue. Sometimes we experience payoffs for holding onto an underlying belief, the emotions associated with a problem, or the physical symptoms impeding our lives. For instance, an alcoholic might not be truly ready to release their craving if the alcohol is allowing them to avoid feelings of worthlessness. If a client is in doubt, I ask them if they are willing to allow Spirit to override any unwillingness and to gently perform a healing anyway.

Step 3: Begin in gratitude. Gratitude is a form of happiness that assumes the best for all concerned. It invites Spirit to create a sacred space inside and around us. Ask your client if they are willing to feel grateful for the healing process regardless of the outcome and to hold yourself as the practitioner in the same holy attitude.

Step 4: Prepare the drum. With your hand, draw the Cho Ku Rei symbol over your drum. Ask Spirit to infuse the drum with the power of this symbol and to allow the meaning of the symbols to resonate through the drum's sounds.

Step 5: Prepare the client. Draw the Cho Ku Rei symbol over the front and the back of the client's heart chakra with your hand. If you are working on yourself, you can form the sign on the front side of your body and ask Spirit to do so on your back side

Step 6: Prepare the space. Most indigenous communities use some form of a medicine wheel to create sacred space during a ceremony and to call forth help from the spirit world. Pictorially, a medicine wheel is a circle with two intersecting lines inside of it, much like the symbol for a compass. The lines intersect the circle at four points that recognize the four cardinal directions: north, east, south, and west. The medicine wheel draws forth the "medicine" of nature, the vital force of love present in the earth. Each of the four directions is linked to a great and intelligent power that we can be turn to for assistance. We also have the equivalent powers within us, and the medicine wheel can help us cultivate them. I work with a version of the Lakota medicine wheel, which places warrior power in the north; visionary power in the east; healing power in the south; and shamanic power in the west.

To create your wheel, raise your mallet or your hand, and pray for assistance from the spirits in each of the directions. (In the Lakota tradition, we call upon Warrior, Visionary, Healer, and then Shaman.) Encourage your client to do the same.

Step 7: Drum. Start by drumming softly near your client's heart, first in the front and then in the back. Ask Spirit to energetically perform the drumming for you on your back side. You should drum each area for three to four minutes and from about a foot and a half away. Modulate the sound so it is comfortable for your client, and follow your intuitive sense of how fast or intensely to drum.

Then move your drum to spots on or around the body that call for attention. Move from the first spot of healing to others that call you, asking your client to guide you as they feel the need. If at any time the client wants to drum, invite them to do so.

While you're drumming, your client might feel the need to cry, shout, or speak. Memories might come up, as could visions or other intuitive insights. Continue to drum throughout your client's process until you both feel like the session is done or your time has drawn to a close.

Step 7: Closure. Return to the heart area and drum in the front and back of the heart. Then drum to each of the four directions before stopping. With your hand, draw the Cho Ku Rei symbol on the front and back of your client's heart to seal the healing.

HEALING YOUR INNER CHILD WITH SOUND

Our wounded inner child often believes that he or she is unworthy of love, and until we heal that child, it's hard for us to open to the flow of healing and grace that is always available. Sue Govali is a professional singer, songwriter, and teacher who helps individuals heal through sound and visualization, merging two powerful forms of healing. Following is Sue's exercise, which employs not only sound, but also visualization and color, for healing the wounded child within.[4]

PART I: PREPARING YOUR CHAKRAS

Sit in a comfortable chair with your back relaxed. Breathe in deeply. On your out-breath, move your attention to the center of your heart.

In your heart, imagine that you are reexperiencing the Big Bang, that moment when the universe started. Behind you is what is called the Cosmic Mirror, through which you can see the origin of all. Travel through the mirror to the true center of your heart. There, take a deep breath in, then completely let go of everything you've been holding.

Gazing around the center of your heart, you find yourself within a glowing river of energy that runs up and down your body. The liquid is gold and silver and moves slowly, lovingly. Within this river are balls of energies, or your chakras, located at the top of your head, the center of your head, your throat, your heart, your solar plexus, your sacrum, and your perineum or genital area. You also discover another island of energy in your chest, a meeting point for your internal organs.

See how much distance lies between the atoms in your heart. Now think of your atoms as your ego and the river of energy as flowing from Source or Higher Spirit. Travel through the ego into the deepest core of your heart by flowing along the river of spirit. Here at the core you spy a horizontal circle, the outer rim of which glows with a blue the color of natural gas. Land within the middle of this circle and be embraced by peace and silence.

From this center point, peer up and down the body. Every chakra holds a similar place of tranquility and quiet. Following your vision and the river of energy, you also discover a gold-colored chakra about a foot above your head and an earth-colored chakra below your feet. You are connected to the heavens and the earth through this source-flow.

Tone through each of the in-body chakras to connect with them and prepare them to heal your inner child. When toning, simply resonate the sound listed below into each chakra while imagining the related color. Feel the river of source-energy flow into the chakra and the respective area of your body, releasing blocks and relaxing the area. The chakras and the extra chest area are described in the table on the next page based on location.

Once you've reached the crown chakra, return to your heart chakra. Next travel to the gold chakra over your head and flow back down your body to the chakra under your feet. Now return to your heart chakra with the sound *ah*.

PART II: HEALING YOUR INNER CHILD

While remaining centered in your heart, watch the river of energy pass through the gold chakra over your head and into an ultraviolet light that flows up to

SOUND HEALING PHONETICS

Chakra Location	Sound (Phonetic)	Color	Function(s)
Perineum	*Uh*	Rich red	Feeling of safety
Sacral Point	*Ooh*	Rich orange	Creativity and openness
Solar Plexus	*Oh*	Daffodil yellow, gold	Confidence and power
Heart	*Ah*	Spring green, white gold	Love towards others
Center of the Chest	*Aaaa*	Silver	Awareness of here and now
Throat	*I*	Periwinkle blue	Wisdom; the speaking of truth
Third Eye	*Ay*	Purple	Far-seeing vision; truth of one's spirit
Crown	*Eee*	Lavender or white gold	Connection to the Divine

the heavens. Connect with the heavenly energy of the male Divine or Great Father. Now move your attention to the chakra below your feet, following the river of energy to infrared light, then darker and darker lights, until you experience complete darkness. Continue to flow to the center of the earth, protected and safe, and connect with the pearlescent wisdom of the female Divine or Great Mother.

Imagine that your chakras now turn upward like glowing cups, each similar to a champagne cup, receiving light from the heavens, which pours white light through every chakra to the center of the earth and the heart of the Great Mother, who purifies the energy and then sends purple fire up through every in-body chakra to the gold chakra above your head, back to the Great Father.

Return your attention to the center of your heart and now consciously connect with your inner child. If this child is lost, bring him or her back to the center of your heart. Surround your inner child with the love of the Great Father and the Great Mother, casting your inner eye to your seventh or crown chakra and tone an *ah*, the sound of the heart. Now focus on each chakra, one at a time, providing your inner child with a gift of energy from each of the chakras.

In your perineum, dip your inner child into the source-river of boundless healing energy. Your child-self is now completely safe.

In your sacral chakra, acknowledge the child's feelings and expansive creativity.

Through the solar plexus, emphasize the importance of this child's authentic self. Let him or her know it's okay to have boundaries and follow his or her own willpower.

Usher your inner child into the center of your chest, inviting him or her to join the source energies of the earth with that of the heavens.

In your throat chakra, speak the words your child has always needed to hear.

In the third eye, see this child the way the Divine would.

And through the seventh or crown chakra, ask the Divine to breathe into the soul of your inner child.

Then call your child back into a special haven in your heart. Your child is now gently placed in a place of peace at the center of the horizontal blue circle within the heart chakra. Bathed in sunlight and prisms of joy, your inner child has been reborn into love.

Take a deep breath in and tone a relaxed *ah* in the center of the heart and then make this statement: "I am that I am." By doing so, you are verbally announcing that you are unified within yourself and with everything outside of yourself as well.

Take another deep breath in and give yourself a gift of golden light coming from the back of the heart, passing through the center, and shining out into the Universe. Be here and now in the center of the heart for a moment or two, your inner child and you. Know that you can now be your full self, inner child and adult, and that you are safe and loved.

22

COLOR HEALING

The whole world, as we experience
it visually, comes to us through
the mystic realm of color.

HANS HOFMANN

Whether seen with our eyes in the outer world or sensed within the realm of our inner world, color energy is everywhere. We are enveloped in a spectrum of color that is born of light. Color generates or bolsters healing processes. Every color vibrates at its own frequency along the electromagnetic spectrum of light; therefore, each invites a specific type of change in the physical body or energetic anatomy. In essence, when we are healing with color, we are healing with light, and vice versa. When a color light is directed at a diseased part of the body, its frequency encourages physical and emotional healing.

Subtle energy practitioners can augment many of their techniques with the use of color. Just visualizing a particular color being applied to a part of the physical or subtle body is enough to access the healing frequency of that color, but color can also be applied literally. The following chromatic therapies are just some of the ways that color is used for healing and revitalizing the fields, chakras, and channels:

- Directing color into the auric field. By inserting the correct colors into the field, you release blocks and stagnation, fill holes and leaks, and open the field to manifest your desired reality. You can direct the energy with mindful intention, by placing your hands over the area requiring a color boost, or by shining colored lights into the auric field. You can also expose yourself or a client to colored light bulbs in your environment.

- Visualizing color being applied to the chakras to balance and open them.
- Applying color to acupoints, known as chromapuncture. While professional chromapuncture specialists use machines and instruments, we can place colored stones on acupoints, put colored paper over a small flashlight and shine the light on the points, or put our hands on the points and visualize the color we wish to send.
- Tapping into the natural partnership between color and the elements, such as using colored water and gemstones to affect change throughout the subtle body.
- Wearing clothing or jewelry in specific colors to boost energetic boundaries.

A PALETTE OF MEANING: A REFERENCE GUIDE TO COLORS

Subtle energy practitioners, especially those whose strengths include visual intuition (see chapter 6), can assess the condition of the subtle energy body by discerning which colors are present and in what hues, as well as what colors are absent. Particular colors in the auric layers or chakras, for example, can tell you

THE POWER OF LIGHT IN SUBTLE HEALING

SINCE THE INVENTION of lasers nearly forty years ago, low levels of visible or near infrared light have been used to reduce pain, inflammation, and edema; to promote wound healing; and to prevent damage to tissues and nerves. Such healing properties were originally thought to be peculiar to laser light (soft or cold lasers), but now we know that noncoherent light, the type of light emitted by LEDs (light-emitting diodes), also has such properties. Photobiomodulation and photobiostimulation are two emerging treatments that use low-level laser light to stimulate cellular function and tissue repair.

Some researchers are exploring the healing effects of full-spectrum light, like that provided by sunlight and specially designed full-spectrum lights. Full-spectrum light affects our sleep, mood, and our overall health. Contrary to popular belief, research is showing that proper exposure to the sun actually prevents certain types of cancer and major illnesses, rather than causing these diseases.[1] Light, it seems, is its own nutrient, promoting healthy levels of vitamin D, boosting the immune system, stimulating metabolism, lowering blood pressure, and more.[2]

which energies need to be released because they are causing congestion or blockages and which energies need to be absorbed in order to restore balance. The absence of particular colors can tell you what frequencies are needed for healing and balance.

The following at-a-glance reference guide offers a "palette of meaning" to help you make these evaluations and determine which colors or hues would be the most helpful for you or your client. Also see "The Seven Hindu Chakras" in chapter 4 to review the colors corresponding to each chakra.

RED—AND ITS HEALING HUES

The lowest vibrational color, red has the most tangible impact on the physical body and relates to the heart. Depending on various factors, red can either attract or repel money and material possessions, and impact our overall sense of safety and security. When out of balance, red relates to money worries, anger, anxiety, and obsessions.

Specific red hues in the subtle energy body translate to the following qualities:

Clear red: Powerful, energetic, competitive, sexual, passionate

Deep red: Grounded, realistic, active, strong-willed, determined, survival-oriented

Muddied red: Angry, irritated; internalized criticism or blame, which can be projected on others

Orange-red: Confident; creative power

Red for use in healing. Red increases our heart rate and improves our circulation, respiration, and blood pressure. It stimulates the appetite, boosts brain-wave activity, and nourishes the sexual glands. In general, red provides healing energy and warmth to counterbalance colds and flu and feelings of chilliness, fatigue, lethargy, and passivity. In its pure state, red can nourish a healthy ego.

PINK—AND ITS HEALING HUES

Pink combines all the energetic and spiritual qualities of red and white. The specific shade of pink in a subtle body gives you specific information:

Bright and light pink: loving, tender, sensitive, sensual, artistic, pure, compassionate, affectionate, romantic; can indicate clairaudience

Dark and murky pink: immature, shallow, dishonest

Pink for use in healing. Pink is used for healing grief, sadness, and a feeling of separation from the Divine. It helps to connect us with our feelings and can restore youthfulness. Pink can also be used to relieve tension (both muscle tension and stressful thoughts) and suppress an overstimulated appetite. Because of its soothing influence, it is often used in the decorating schemes of hospitals and healing centers around the world.

ORANGE — AND ITS HEALING HUES

Orange corresponds to the reproductive organs, sexual expression, emotions, and creativity. It is the color of vitality, vibrancy, vigor, and good health. It is the color of energy, enthusiasm, stamina, creative productivity, adventurousness, and courage.

> **Orange-yellow:** Intelligent, detail-oriented, perfectionist, scientific, creative

Orange for use in healing. Orange can be used to stimulate appetite and the digestive system. A color of warmth, cheer, and excitement, orange is useful for addressing apathy, melancholy, and depression. Orange also has a freeing influence on the psyche, alleviating feelings of shyness, introversion, and constriction, as well as relieving repression.

YELLOW — AND ITS HEALING HUES

Yellow is the color of positive life energy, inspiration, awakening, intelligence, action, play, optimism, and ease.

> **Light or pale yellow:** Hope and optimism; positive excitement about new ideas; psychic and spiritual awareness

> **Bright lemon-yellow:** power struggles and working to maintain control in a personal or business relationship; fear of losing control, prestige, respect, and influence

> **Dark brownish-yellow:** Mental strain, overanalyzing, mental fatigue and stress; "cramming" for a test or overworking to meet a deadline

Yellow for use in healing. Yellow energizes, improves memory, relieves depression, and stimulates the appetite. It helps to balance the nervous system and stimulate the mind (including the subtle energies of mind). In traditional Chinese medicine, yellow stimulates Spleen meridian chi.

Gold is related to yellow. See "Over the Rainbow: Other Important Colors in Healing" later in this section for details.

GREEN—AND ITS HEALING HUES

Green correlates to the beauty and healing capacities of nature. It is also the color of the emotional and spiritual heart. When seen in the auric field, green usually represents a state of balance or growth leading to positive change. It also corresponds to the love of others—people, animals, and nature.

Bright emerald green: Strong healing capabilities; a love-centered person

Yellow-green: Creativity stemming from the heart, heart-centered communication

Dark or muddy forest green: Jealousy, resentment, a victim mentality; blaming self or others; insecurity and low self-esteem; lack of personal responsibility; sensitive to perceived criticism and defensiveness

Turquoise: A wise healer, counsel, or therapist; compassionate; corresponds to the immune system

WHITE LIGHT HEALING: A Cosmic Energy Exercise

YOU CAN USE this exercise for yourself or guide a client through it.

1. Find a comfortable place to sit or lie down and turn off any potential disturbances. Close your eyes and take a few deep breaths, concentrating only on your breathing. Relax and let go.

2. Visualize, sense, or feel white, universal cosmic energy entering your head through your crown chakra. Invite and allow the white light to move down and spread to every part of your body—especially to any area where you have tension, pain, or disease. As it passes through each part of your body, notice your oneness with this energy. As you do, feel the specific part(s) of your body relaxing and opening.

3. Let the energy move down into and through your feet while simultaneously allowing it to flow down your arms out through the palms of your hands. Spend a few minutes feeling this energy flowing through both palms and feet.

4. Repeat steps 1 through 3 with a color of your choosing, noticing any sensations, images, or feelings that arise as you are working with this color.

5. When you are ready, and feeling blissfully saturated with color and light, gently open your eyes.

Green for use in healing. Green is relaxing and helps to alleviate anxiety and depression. It represents harmony with nature (inner and outer nature) and is deeply soothing to the body and mind. Green is useful in helping to relieve almost any physical ailment or emotional disruption. In addition to aiding the heart, green is also soothing for the lungs.

BLUE—AND ITS HEALING HUES

Blue is a cooling and calming color. It relates to loving care guided by intuitive sensitivity. Blue correlates to the throat and communication that integrates physical sensing with higher knowing.

> **Soft blue:** Intuitive, peaceful; clarity and truthfulness in communication

> **Bright royal blue:** Clairvoyant; strong spiritual nature; generosity; indicates that one is on the right path or new opportunities are coming

> **Dark or muddy blue:** Fear of the future; fear of facing or speaking the truth; fear of self-expression (especially verbal self-expression)

Blue for use in healing. The calming effects of blue can be used to decrease respiration, lower blood pressure, or cool fever and inflammatory reactions. Blue can help to relieve headaches, as well as to balance or heal the thyroid. The astringent nature of blue can help to break up congestion and lymphatic stagnation. On the emotional level, blue calms strong emotions like anger, aggression, hysteria, or general overwhelm.

Blue light therapy is used for a variety of issues, from healing acne breakouts to alleviating circadian rhythm disorders, like delayed sleep stage syndrome and seasonal affective disorder (SAD).

PURPLE—AND ITS HEALING HUES

Purple is the color of deep feeling arising from intuitive sensitivity. Correlated with the third eye and the pituitary gland, purple is the color of visual intuition and spiritual insight. It often represents positive and powerful transformation.

> **Violet:** Psychic power, attunement with the higher self, idealism born of vision, being a visionary; art and magic of a spiritual nature; relates to the pineal gland and nervous system

> **Lavender:** Imagination, intuitive vision, etheric energies, daydreaming

> **Indigo:** Spiritual philosophy, contemplation; increases subtle perceptions of psychic realities

Purple for use in healing. Inviting spiritual renewal and inner peace, purple is a potent color for breaking through delusion, denial, and addictions. Purple is also good for alleviating migraines and moving through sadness into empowerment.

OVER THE RAINBOW: OTHER IMPORTANT COLORS IN HEALING

Silver signifies the awakening of the cosmic mind. It is also the color of spiritual and physical abundance. Bright metallic silver indicates receptivity to new ideas based on intuitive sensing. Dark or muddy gray relates to blocked energies, guardedness, or a residue of fear that may have accumulated in the body and holds the potential for health problems, especially if gray clusters are seen in specific areas of the body.

   Gold is the color of enlightenment and divine protection. When observed within the auric field, gold indicates that a person is being guided toward their highest good. It is the color of the spiritual mind and intuitive thinking, inner knowing, and high wisdom. A bright and shiny metallic gold correlates to an inspired person whose energy is activated and whose power is awakened.

   Black is a transformative color, whether for the betterment or detriment of a person. It draws or pulls energy to it and, in so doing, transforms that energy. It captures light and consumes it. It can indicate long-held resentment and blame toward another, which can collect in a specific area of the body and manifest as a health challenge. If it appears in the ovaries, black can also correlate to unreleased grief from abortions. Also, it can indicate a past-life wound or an entity within the auric field.

   White reflects a pure state of light and the spiritual, transcendent, etheric, and nonphysical qualities of the higher dimensions. It relates to angelic qualities, such as purity and truth. It can also represent a new, positive, and not-yet-designated energy within the auric field. Flashes of white light or sparkles in the energy field indicate that angels are nearby. They can also signal that a woman is pregnant or will be soon.

   Earth colors and earth tones correlate to soil, wood, minerals, plants, and an essential groundedness. This palette of colors indicates a love of the earth and is often seen in those who work outdoors and live "close to the earth"— farmers, avid gardeners, construction workers, park rangers, for example. These colors are generally indicative of a positive connection to the natural world. But a dirty brown energy correlates to holding on to something out of a feeling of insecurity.

   Rainbows, in Hawaiian shamanism, signal the presence of the soul. Rainbow images in the energy body, such as rainbow beams streaming from the hands, head, or body, can signify a healer (such as a Reiki healer), a star person, or someone who is experiencing their first incarnation on earth.

Pastels, as unique blendings of color and light, represent sensitivity, sometimes on the emotional level and sometimes on an intuitive level. Pastel colors appearing in the auric field can also indicate the need for peace, serenity, and kindness.

HOW TO USE COLOR IN SUBTLE ENERGY HEALING

Equipped with the previous "A Palette of Meaning" reference list, you can intuitively examine the energetic anatomy (the fields or auric layers, the meridians, and the chakras), as well as the physical body, in order to assess the following:

- Regarding the chakras and auric fields specifically, are the appropriate colors present or not (e.g., red in the first chakra, orange in second chakra)?
- What is the quality of each color that you see (e.g., clear, healthy, strong, vivid, muddy, murky)?

Whether you're working with a client or on yourself, you can conduct a guided relaxation and visualization process to assess the colors and their qualities in the energy body. Once you have a baseline assessment of colors that are present or missing, ask the Divine or a gatekeeper the necessary questions to determine which colors must be released or applied. For example:

- What color is needed most right now?
- If you are working with a specific physical condition, like a broken leg or kidney disease, ask a targeted question: What color is most appropriate now to help restore balance to the leg or kidneys?
- The same applies if you are working with an emotional state: What color is most appropriate now to help release this anger/heal this hurt/feel more confident/find forgiveness?

Once you receive the requested insight and information, visualize the release of any congested, unhealthy, or negative colors and the inflow of positive, healthy, and healing colors. If you're working with your client, you can use your hands to help draw out the unhealthy colors and send the healing colors. Intuitively sense the unhealthy colors and the healthy colors that should replace them. Now aim one of your hands at the unhealthy area and ask Spirit to draw out the unhealthy colors. Don't pull the energy into your hand; rather, see it flowing over your hand to be disposed of by Spirit. Aim your other hand over the congested area, and while the unhealthy energy is being removed, ask Spirit to insert the healthy colors. This energy also flows around your hands into the area. You can also visualize (or direct your client to visualize) exhaling any stagnant, life-depleting colors and inhaling the appropriate healing, life-enhancing colors. As you inhale the necessary colors for healing, use your powers of visualization and intention to send the colors wherever they need to go.

In addition to this basic format for healing with color, some of the following techniques may be beneficial in specific instances.

COLOR HEALING MADE EASY: TWELVE TECHNIQUES

The following color-healing tips and techniques can stand alone or be used to augment a broader plan of healing for your client or yourself.

Transfer color energy from an object. You can perform healing with gemstones, colored water, or other natural substances that are the appropriate healing color. Hold the colored substance in your hand and energetically transfer negative energies into that substance; then energetically send the positive energies of the color into yourself or your client as a replacement for the unhealthy energies. See chapter 20 for a comprehensive list of gemstones and their healing properties.

Create gem essences based on color. Selecting gemstones with the appropriate healing properties and color, create a gem essence using the process described under "Gemstone Essences" in chapter 20.

Drink colored water. Use "solarization" to program drinking water with a color's healing frequency. Place a glass bottle of water over a colored paper, cloth, or piece of cellophane and expose both to sunlight for an hour. Drinking the color-charged water will imbue your energy body with the color's healing frequency.

Use colorpuncture. Visualize a needed color flowing into an acupoint while you press on that point. See the "The Ten Golden Acupoints" listed in chapter 12 for the top points to work with. Know that professionals often use various pulsations or oscillations generated by a machine that uses electricity and glass rods to produce the most beneficial effect.

Use a pendulum to find healing colors. Use a pendulum to determine what colors are appropriate for your healing situation (or that of your client). Pendulum work, also called dowsing, is described in chapter 23. Using yes-no questions, you can ask the pendulum to tell you if specific colors would be beneficial or not. Hold a pendulum over a color wheel and ask it to swing toward the most beneficial color.

Muscle test to assess colors. Use muscle testing to ask your body, or that of your client, which colors need to be released and which need to be accentuated or brought into the system. See the section on "Muscle Testing: A Mind-Body Communication Tool" in chapter 15 for how to make use of this applied kinesiology technique.

Apply colored light. You can apply colored light directly to the physical or subtle body by directing a light source (sunlight, a light globe, or light bulb) through some kind of transparent or semi-transparent filter material, such as glass, light fabric, a crystal, or cellophane in a suitable healing color. For example, having determined which color you need, expose an area of your body or energetic anatomy to a beam of sunlight shining through a window covered in cellophane of the selected color. If working with bare skin, expose yourself for no more than fifteen minutes.

Use the grab-bag technique. Assemble a bag of colored glass beads, marbles, or tumbled stones. Holding in your awareness the physical, emotional, or mental healing or balancing you would like, place your hand in the bag, blindly feeling around until your fingers sense or feel the right object—the one with exactly the color you need. Carry the object with you for a few hours or days, as you feel guided to.

Wear your color remedy. Intuitively assess which color(s) will promote the healing or balancing you desire, and dress in the color you need. By wearing the necessary color for a day, you infuse yourself with that color and its healing properties.

Color your world. Surround yourself with the colors that uplift and inspire you and those that calm and soothe you. For example, select the colors of your walls or carpet by considering the vibration that will continually be emitted into the room and, therefore, into you. If you need a specific color for only a little while, you can drape colored cloths over your furniture, choose specifically colored paintings, or simply put colored candles in a room.

Combine color and the healing streams of grace. When calling on the healing streams of grace for yourself or a client, ask the Divine for the appropriate color to be added to the stream. And then trust and know that it has been done.

Create your own color-healing visualizations. Create your own detailed guided meditations involving color healing. The section "Writing Your Own Guided Visualization Scripts" in chapter 15 explains how (and includes tips for *leading* guided visualizations for a client). For instance, if you are working with yellow, you can guide your client to wander through an autumn forest with radiant yellow-golden aspen trees, wearing a yellow poncho and taking in the energy of the yellow sun. The possibilities are endless.

HEALING WITH COLOR:
The Emerald Alignment

JENNIFER WARTERS, a well-respected sound healer in England, has developed a unique energetic-alignment technique involving color.[3] It's called the Emerald Alignment. In this process, when you focus on two rays of the electromagnetic spectrum (the fifth ray, which is emerald, and the second ray, which is blue), energy is channeled from the higher vibrational planes and Spirit down through the spine to every part of the body, realigning our core energetic pattern at the cellular level.

The Emerald Ray links Spirit to matter and realigns our molecular structure to its original form.

The Blue Ray strengthens and protects, sealing the auric field at the end of the exercise.

This exercise is particularly effective for treating panic attacks, insomnia, and attachment issues, and for establishing peaceful environments. It is ideal for use with children and the elderly, because it provides ease and calm. It will also deepen meditative processes and assist with therapeutic healing. Warters recommends using it before and after surgery as well.

THE EMERALD ALIGNMENT PROCESS

1. Sit or stand comfortably. Allow your body to relax. Become aware of your crown chakra's entry point at the top of your head. Breathe comfortably and flow energy downward through your body, from the crown through your spine and legs to your feet, releasing any sense of heaviness or discomfort. End with moving your energy through and away from your toes.

2. Return your focus to your crown and then shift your conscious awareness to the top of your spine. Let your energy travel out across your shoulders and down your arms, through your elbows and wrists, to flow out your fingers and thumbs and away from the body.

3. Breathe energy back up from your feet and flow it back upward to the crown of your head, following your spine.

4. Breathe energy back into your body through your fingertips, flowing it up your arms, across your shoulders to the top of your spine, finally landing on the crown of your head.

5. Now imagine that the Divine or a higher guide is placing a glowing emerald at the crown of your head. From it emerges a beam of emerald light.

6. Draw this beam of emerald light straight down the center of your body through your spine to the place between your heels. Feel your body straighten in response.

7. Now imagine that the Divine or a higher guide places an emerald at the tip of each shoulder. Beams of emerald light emanate from the shoulders' emeralds and flow down into your arms to the palms of your hands.

8. Envision a blue energy outlining your entire body, extending about an arm's length around it in all directions. Notice this blue energy sealing and protecting you within its circular warmth.

9. Breathe slowly and return to a comfortable place in the center of your body.

AYURVEDIC HEALING WITH COLOR, GEMS, AND PLANETS

In the Vedic scriptures, all creation is said to begin from the divine light that emanates from the Supreme Being. The seven colors of the rainbow—the components of visible light—are believed to be among the *rays* that form the body of the universe. The powers of these rays are identical to the powers and qualities of the Divine.

In Ayurvedic texts, the color rays within creation are joined with the five great elements of earth, water, fire, air, and ether. The ancient Vedic healers and scholars concluded that earth is the condensed green color, water is orange and indigo, fire is red and yellow, air is violet, and ether is blue.

Each of the doshas (the constitutional body types in Ayurveda, discussed in chapter 19) is connected to a different element or elements and, thus, is the product of different colors. The vayu or vata dosha combines air and ether, thus originating from blue and violet. The pitta dosha is of and from fire and derived from the colors red and yellow. The kapha dosha is a combination of earth and water, coming from orange, indigo, and green. In Vedic healing philosophy, subtle and gross material creations become animated and able to function on the physical, emotional, and mental levels due to the presence of these cosmic colors. To remain healthy or to regain health, the rays within the cells should be in a state of equilibrium.

The Vedic healers observed that specific precious gemstones hold within them the strongest concentration of the light rays found on the planet. In Vedic astrology (the *jyotish* astrological system), the following seven gemstones are among the most potent healing tools available. Each is linked to not only one of the rays, but also one of seven planetary bodies.

Ruby emits the same ray as the sun—red.
Red coral emits the same ray as Mars—yellow.
Yellow sapphire emits the same ray as Jupiter—blue.
Pearl emits the same ray as the moon—orange.
Emerald emits the same ray as Mercury—green.
Diamond emits the same ray as Venus—indigo.
Blue sapphire emits the same ray as Saturn—violet.

In your self-healing sessions and client sessions, you can work with these combinations of gemstones, planets, and colors using the intuitive-assessment techniques outlined in this chapter. Whether you use the actual gemstones or invoke their healing properties (as done with spirit plant medicine, described in chapter 20), you can use this ancient knowledge for healing on every level in present time.

Thanks to the Vedic Cultural Fellowship for inspiring this resource.[4]

23

VIBRATIONAL SYMBOLS AND ORACLES

> I found I could say things with color
> and shapes that I couldn't say any
> other way—things I had no words for.
>
> GEORGIA O'KEEFFE

All subtle energy healing, distilled to its bare essence, involves changing vibrational frequencies through field dynamics. In quantum physics, it is known that a simple change can alter the vibrational qualities of an object and, therefore, its effects. In this chapter, we will explore the vibrational transformation that takes place when we call upon some of the oldest tools known to subtle energy healers: shapes, symbols, and numbers. We will also review the key oracles that human beings have relied on for eons to uncover and understand patterns and life cycles.

THE POWER OF SHAPES: THE PRIMORDIAL SYMBOLS OF LIFE

In my 2011 book *Energetic Boundaries*, I discussed the power of shapes and their impact on our energy boundaries:

> *Research conducted by Egyptian architect Dr. Ibrahim Karim over a period of thirty years has demonstrated the amazing effects of geometrical shapes. One study, led by the Egyptian National Research Centre, showed that simple shapes could stop the replication of bacteria. Most frequently, he surrounded*

the subjects of his experiments with materials formed into various shapes, such as triangles, squares, or circles; he has also created an extensive index of thought-provoking shapes that integrate other shapes, such as spirals and lines, each of which promotes different changes, such as the healing of heart disease or the growth of new cells in the body. Another project, which was evaluated by the Egyptian Department of Agriculture, found that chickens grew healthier and faster in an environment that was energy balanced by Karim's method of using shapes, called BioGeometry, than they did when antibiotics and growth hormones were given to the birds. In Holland, Professor Peter Mols of Wageningen Agriculture University discovered that Karim's methods could be used in place of pesticides and artificial fertilizers to grow healthy organic crops.[1]

There are a variety of ways that you can work with shapes. For example, visualizing a shape around your energetic boundaries will strengthen them. You can visualize a separate shape surrounding all of your energetic boundaries or visualize a particular boundary as a specific shape. Using visual intuition, you can look for shapes that might be present in your energy fields or energy bodies and causing problems. Using visualization, you can repair troublesome shapes or insert new shapes that match your healing goals. However you choose to work and play with the subtle energies of these common shapes, I hope you will enjoy discovering how they can be a part of your healing toolkit.

THE PRIMARY SHAPES

There are hundreds of different shapes, but four of the most basic ones—the square, circle, triangle, and cross—are also the most powerful. The essential meanings and the powers of each, described in the following excerpts from *Energetic Boundaries*, represent a multicultural, multidimensional amalgamation of esoteric symbolism:

Square. *A square is the symbol of stability and strength. The corners contain the most active energy and stimulate reactions when they touch something (or someone). If you want to manifest something, visualize a square with the request within it and, outside, the corners touching all parts of that bigger image. . . .*

Inserting a square (or a rectangle) into an energetic center or field will protect, ground, and stabilize you. If, when you psychically examine your field or an energy center, you find a small square lodged within it, see if there is a substance within the shape; whatever you find within the square is something that you are storing, repressing, or hiding. We often conceal feelings, beliefs, memories, others' energies, parts of our soul, and dreams. Repress enough feelings, and we create depression. . . .

Warped squares, or those with broken sides or cut-off corners, signify incomplete protection or boundary violations, or undeveloped abilities, thoughts, or gifts. Repairing these squares will allow each to resume their correct purpose.

Circle. *A circle promotes relationships, harmony, and connection. A circle envisioned between two or more people (or living beings) invites an exchange of energy. Check the energy. If it's bright and loving, the swap is positive. If it's negative or dark, the exchange is hurting you and creating a syndrome [a recurring energy-boundary problem].*

Establishing a circle around ourselves, through any or all of the energetic boundaries, will emphasize wholeness and send an energy of love to others. It will also create a "sacred circle," a protected space that only love can enter. You can psychically draw a circle around a part of you, such as your inner child or a need, and keep it secure.

If you constantly pick up energy from others or the environment, go a step further and imagine a circle (a silver one is best) drawn under your feet and moving everywhere you move. This circle will cleanse the ground you walk on and shimmer upward through your entire field, deflecting negative energies.

A broken circle sandwiched in your energy field or extending between you and someone else indicates a broken relationship and, potentially, betrayal or heartache for you. If you fix the circle, you fix the relationship. But before you do, make sure you want the relationship back; it might be in both your and the other person's best interest to dissolve the circle entirely.

Smaller circles within a field or in the body might be holding your relationship issues, your true feelings about a relationship, or a part of you that you don't want to reveal. If you find a circle within an energy boundary, check to see what substances or energies are inside.

A spiral is a form of a circle. Counterclockwise spirals bring energy out, so they can be used to take energies away from our field. Clockwise spirals bring energy in, so they can be used to attach us to sources of positive energies.[2]

Tip: Another way to utilize circles for healing is to draw a circle around something that you would like to bolster or amplify, such as an idea, a desire, a dream, or even healing energy.

Triangle. *Related to the pyramid, a triangle represents creativity, mental activity, and connection with the Divine. A triangle will intensify or amplify energy, so be careful about what you energetically put into it. It can increase debt or abundance, disease or healing.*

Use a triangle around your body to promote activity and growth. Say you want to write a book or a report. Take the nugget of your idea, insert it in a triangle, and watch your creativity explode.

Triangles can be inserted into any boundary or place within it that needs healing to promote change and transformation. A broken or spotted triangle indicates a misfiring, a place where you're not thinking logically or appropriately. A broken triangle connecting you and someone else, a job, your finances, or a project can indicate that you aren't accurately perceiving what's occurring or that your interactions are off and need to be fixed.[3]

Tip: Adding a triangle to a chakra will empower that chakra, inviting higher perspective, security, and growth.

Cross or X. *An X is a form of a cross, symbolizing the magical properties of a crossroads. When seen in a cross form, such as in a T shape, the cross represents protection. An X also obstructs or blocks. It bars the doorway to negativity and protects from marauders, visible and invisible. Depending on the reason it's present, it can also block wisdom, truth, and love.*

Consider the use of the swastika in Nazi Germany. In ancient Hindu and Buddhist origins, the swastika represented auspiciousness and eternity. By reversing the flow of the cross and making it more of an X than a T, the Nazis erased their followers' free will and inserted a message in their energetic

THE MEANING OF SHAPES

INTUITIVELY ASSESSING THE shapes present in the subtle body is actually a pragmatic method for performing diagnosis and healing. When diagnosing energy issues, you will want to pay attention to areas in the physical body or energy body that include harmful symbols. Knowing the meaning of the broken or misshapen symbol, you can start to work on the related issues. Visualizing or energetically focusing on the spirit-enhancing meanings of the symbols provides energy for fixing the problems.

SPIRIT-ENHANCING SHAPES

Circle	Wholeness
Square	Foundation
Rectangle	Protection
Triangle	Preservation and immortality
Spiral	Creation and cycles
Five-pointed star	Alchemy and movement
Six-pointed star	Resurrection
Cross	Human-divine connection and spiritual protection

HARMFUL SHAPES

Altered circle	Shows areas of hurt, injury, damage, or separation
Altered square	Indicates poor boundaries or damage from negative systems, such as family systems
Altered rectangle	Reveals areas exposed to danger
Altered triangle	Shows areas vulnerable to illness, disease, unbalancing forces, and death
Altered spiral	Indicates abrupt endings and areas out of rhythm or out of appropriate cycles
Altered five-pointed star	Points to areas that are stifled, overcontained, or repressed
Altered six-pointed star	Shows areas of stuckness, despair, and depression; also shows the influence of negative forces
Altered cross	Indicates overreliance on ego, self or other's
An X	Shows vulnerability to evil or negative influences

boundaries. When I see an X on or in someone's energy field or in a chakra, I know that they have an energy marker telling the world to mistreat them in some way. These imprints can keep us from meeting a mate, making money, getting a job, or healing. They often indicate the presence of a syndrome [a recurring energy-boundary problem], because energy markers uphold repetitive energetic patterns. It's important to erase these energy markers to free yourself from old patterns.[4]

THE YANTRAS: CONDUITS OF SUBTLE ENERGY

Each chakra of the human energy body is associated with a distinct vibrational frequency, color, and sound. In Eastern mysticism, the subtle energy field of each of the seven in-body chakras is also associated with a specific geometric shape. These shapes are called *yantras*, and they are used in meditation as centering devices that also liberate the energies and gifts of the chakras. Refer to the table "The Chakra Yantras" for descriptions of the shapes and gifts associated with each chakra.

Focusing on the yantras also allows one to interact with the emotions and qualities of the corresponding chakras. Claude Swanson, PhD, is one of the researchers who has written extensively about this powerful practice in his book *Life Force: The Scientific Basis.*[5]

The following exercise is a simple process for placing your attention on the yantras in order to unblock, clear, activate, and *enliven* each of the chakras. If you are drawn to zero in on one or two specific chakras and corresponding yantras, simply apply the directions accordingly and go right to the information that applies to the chakras you wish to interact with.

Step 1: Preparation. With your journal or a notebook and pen in hand, find a comfortable, quiet place where you can relax and focus. You may want to allot fifteen to twenty minutes for this exercise, if you're focusing on all seven in-body chakras. If you would like, you can enhance the meditative energy of your environment by lighting a candle and playing soft, instrumental music.

Step 2: Symbols. Focus on each of the seven primary chakras, one by one, using the Chakra Yantras table provided after the exercise. With each chakra, envision the associated symbol or shape—the yantra. First read about the lotus flower that is unique to each chakra (in color and number of petals). Then read about the symbol that is traditionally contained within the inner circle of the lotus flower. See that symbol in your mind's eye. If you would like, draw the symbol on the paper you have in front of you.

Step 3: Emotions and gifts. As you focus on the yantra, bring into your awareness the emotions associated with each chakra, as well as the gifts that are particular to each chakra. For this exercise, the emotions are specifically those associated with the developmental stage of each chakra

THE CHAKRA YANTRAS

Chakra	Lotus Flower	Symbol Inside the Lotus (the Yantra)	Emotions Originating in This Chakra	Gifts
First	Four red petals	A square with a downward triangle inside the square	Feelings about self and the world, the right to exist, and primal feelings such as guilt, terror, rage, joy, and shame	Manifesting
Second	Six orange-red petals	A crescent moon in a circle	Subtle feelings, choices about which feelings to feel and which to repress	Creativity and compassion
Third	Ten yellow petals	A downward-pointing triangle	Fears and self-esteem	Administrative abilities and mental acuity
Fourth	Twelve green petals	Two intersecting triangles that create a six-pointed star	Compassion, love, gratitude, and other heart-based emotions	Healing and relating with others
Fifth	Sixteen blue petals	A downward-pointing triangle with a circle inside, symbolizing the full moon	Stored frustrations, pride, disillusionment, and grandeur, and the mature expression of needs and feelings	Communicating, including orating, writing, and musicality
Sixth	Two large purple/indigo petals, one on each side	A downward-pointing triangle	Feelings about the self and self-image, plus feelings about our gender and its capabilities	Visioning and strategy
Seventh	The thousand-petaled lotus	No shape, simply open space—the infinite dwelling place that is sometimes called the void	Confusion about our goals and purpose; all feelings that relate to the sense of belonging and the choices about what groups or systems to join	Creating good out of bad, ministering to others

in early life (see "Chakra Development" in chapter 4). By focusing on the yantras, which amplify these emotions and chakra gifts, you are facilitating the release of any stuck energy and embracing the life-enhancing powers of each chakra.

Step 4: Inspired communication. Write down anything that comes to you as you focus on each of the chakra yantas. It could be one empowering word, an affirming phrase, an action step, or perhaps a new decision. Simply receive the communication that comes to you from your higher guidance.

PENDULUM POWER AND THE CHAKRAS: EVALUATING THE ENERGY BODIES

A pendulum is a weighted object suspended by a chain or string. It's used for divination and dowsing, which are simply methods of obtaining information that the normal physical senses are unable to access on a conscious level. Because it can provide insight or information at the subtle, vibrational level, a pendulum is an excellent tool for detecting imbalances in the chakras and the energy fields.

When held and allowed to swing freely, a pendulum will respond to the electromagnetic frequency from a chakra, back side or front side. When holding a pendulum over the chakra area, you are primarily evaluating the outer wheel of the chakra. If the outer wheel is moving clockwise, the inner wheel is probably doing the same. The inner wheel nearly always runs clockwise, unless there is an extreme crisis, such as birth or death.

You can make a pendulum assessment of a client's chakras, which will usually reflect the movement of the outer wheel. The inner wheel is best analyzed using your intuition but will usually be flowing clockwise. It is the outer wheel that reflects our issues, programs, and cheers and travails and because of this, shifts the most frequently. A pendulum can be used by following these simple steps:

1. Have your client lie flat. Stand over your client, holding the pendulum six inches to a foot over the center of a chakra. To test the chakras below the feet and above the head, as well as the eleventh and twelfth chakras surrounding the body, have your client lie down and hold the pendulum above the appropriate sites.

2. The shape, direction, movement, and speed of the circling pendulum will indicate the openness and spin of each chakra. (See "Chakra Structure" in chapter 4.) For instance, no movement of the pendulum could indicate a client's mistrust in the process or a completely blocked chakra. Small

swings can show that the chakra isn't open enough; irregular, large swings can indicate that the chakra is too open and might be taking in others' energies. Test to see if the back side of the chakra, as well as the chakras just above or below the problem area, are open, closed, vertical, horizontal, or diagonal as compensation. Here is what different swings might indicate:

Swing is mainly vertical: The client is lacking practical insight in this chakra.

Swing is mainly horizontal: The client is lacking a spiritual perspective in this chakra.

Swing veers to the upper right or the feminine side of the client's body: This chakra is missing a masculine energy.

Swings to the upper left or masculine side of the client's body: This chakra is lacking a feminine energy.

Swing is very tight: The chakra is not open enough.

Swing is extremely wide. The chakra is too open.

Swing is counterclockwise. The chakra might be processing or releasing energy; it might also be losing energy.

Swing is clockwise. This chakra is functioning well.

3. Once you have observed a potentially unhealthy pattern, you can address the issue and then retest the chakra swing to see if it is repaired.

You can also use a pendulum to assess stages of chakra development. For example, along with the information you receive from a client about what's taking place in their life right now (through dialogue, observation, intuitive sensing, and other means), you can simultaneously explore whether their primary issue might have started in infancy, childhood, or adulthood.

There are two ways to assess the child-development stage at which an issue was incurred: You can assess which chakra is most damaged and look to the "Chakra Development" section in chapter 4 to see the age at which this chakra developed. You can also use a pendulum over the disturbed chakra. First ask a yes-no question to establish which pendulum movements indicate yes or no. Then go through the childhood stages, asking that the energy of the chakra provide a yes swing when you say the appropriate age.

SACRED GEOMETRY: ATTUNING TO THE MYSTICAL LAWS OF CREATION

Geometry is an important part of energy healing because subtle energies often organize themselves in shape and form. An entire field of study called *cymatics* has proven that different sounds can take different geometric forms or visual shapes. Because of the transformational ability of vibrations to change from one form to another, almost as if by metamorphosis, healers throughout history have invoked healing by visualizing or using sounds that call forth the specific powers of geometric forms and vice versa. They have also constructed healing instruments in various shapes.

The following list showcases the most powerful and universal geometric shapes across time and, when appropriate, shows ways you can use sound or visualization for healing. This section also shares an easy way to construct a healing instrument based on the geometric concept being described.

BASIC GEOMETRIC CONCEPTS AT A GLANCE

Sine waves. Sine waves are used to depict frequency, waves, and vibrations, the underlying measurement of energy. All tones are sound waves, which means that sound healing involves using sine waves for bettering your health and wellbeing.

Sine waves compare to yet another waveform, called the *square wave*. Whereas sine waves are used for regeneration and healing, square waves are used for killing pathogens.

There are several commercial instruments that generate healing tones, as well as music that can be played with headphones. (The Rife machine is a commercial product known for using square waves.) In general most commercial music and products entrain your brain waves. (See chapter 15, "The Subtle Mind," for more about healing with brain waves.)

You can turn your body into its own sine-wave generator. Start by standing with your feet shoulder-width apart. Bend your knees slightly and put your left hand a few inches in front of and below your belly, palm up. Put your right hand a few inches in front of and above your chest, palm down. Now move your hands toward each other until they exchange positions. Repeat this process. By humming, singing, or chanting with the intention of harmonizing your body, mind, and soul while doing this hand movement, you will harmonize the top and bottom halves of your chakra system with each other, integrating your heavenly and earthly selves, and supporting your intention.

The Fibonacci sequence. This is a numerical series in which each number except for the first two is the sum of the preceding two. The most accessible way to access the power of this sequence is to invest in Fibonacci tuning forks. These sound tools balance the nervous system, assist with healing trauma and addictions, bolster your state of consciousness, and increase creativity.

The torus. When a circle rotates around a line in the same plane as the circle but not intersecting it, a donut-shaped geometric surface—a torus—is created. Healer and author Amara Karuna has developed several methods for tapping into the power of the torus shape, believing that this shape can increase vitality, generate a higher and more protective electromagnetic current in your body, discharge blocks, and heal physical pain and chronic illnesses.

You can turn your body into its own torus-based healing instrument by visualizing your body centered within streams of energy, which radiate from your body in a coil-like fashion for about three feet outward. On your in-breath, imagine these lines of energy moving up your feet to the top of your head. As you exhale, watch as these streams of light flow outward to coil around your body. Then watch as these lines spiral inside and around your body with each breath.[6]

The golden section. The golden section is a line segment sectioned into two according to the golden ratio (which is linked to the golden spiral, a continually curved spiral found in nature). One way to tap into the power of the golden section is to work with the "balance frequency," the name for 360 hertz. This frequency is derived from the golden section and enables joy, healing, and a balance to health. It is interesting that NASA astronauts proved long ago that the earth creates a tone of 360 hertz in space.[7] You can use a tuning fork with this ratio or tones at this pitch through headphones.

The Merkaba. Consisting of two oppositely oriented but interpenetrating tetrahedrons, the Merkaba is considered to be a vehicle for soul travel or opening to higher consciousness. By meditating upon the Merkaba or holding or wearing a device in its shape, you can activate both sides of your brain, invite spiritual growth, restore the flow of prana through your pineal gland, and activate telepathic and intuitive abilities. You can also imagine your entire energetic field within its shape while performing journeying, remote viewing, or other visitations to the spiritual worlds. As an extrasensory traveling vehicle, the Merkaba provides protection and intensifies your psychic experiences.

The Platonic solids. The Platonic solids are five three-dimensional, solid shapes—the tetrahedron, cube, octahedron, icosahedron, and dodecahedron—each containing congruent angles and sides. Plato linked these shapes to the four primary elements and heaven. Each of the solids, in printed or 3-D form, can be used as a yantra during meditation. You can gaze at a drawing of the shape, or hold a crystal or some other object that is in your chosen shape. As well, you can imagine yourself surrounded by any of these solids or insert just one into a particular energy field. Finally, you can place objects of these shapes in your home or office to enhance the energy of the space.

Each Platonic solid holds the following properties, in addition to those qualities described earlier in this chapter.

Sphere: completion, infinity, increased self-awareness.

Cube: grounding, decreased volatility; slows down what is moving too fast, such as stressing agents.

Tetrahedron: health, expansion of the mind.

Octahedron: peace, love, and spiritual development; increased self-awareness and an intuitive understanding of life.

Dodecahedron: meditation and focus; links to higher self; helps you understand what is happening in your life and why.

Icosahedron: connects sexuality and emotions; facilitates movement and flow of abundance.[8]

VIBRATIONAL HEALING AND THE NINTH CHAKRA: Soul-to-Body Healing

THE NINTH CHAKRA is the "seat of the soul" and center of "soul genes," which includes shapes, symbols, archetypes, and numbers, all of which I call "zymbols." This chakra is comparable to the energy center called the "transcendent chakra" in many cross-cultural systems, as well as the ninth chakra in the Incan schematic. Accessing symbols and ideas that can shift reality when we tap into their hidden powers is a universal concept.

Essentially, the ninth chakra works just like one of our physical cells. It contains our soul genes, the programs underlying the prebirth choices we have made regarding our physical body, emotional states, and mental beliefs. In the groundbreaking book *Vibrational Medicine*, Richard Gerber, MD, refers to these genes as a template, suggesting that the etheric body is the skeleton for the physical body. He adds, "Energetic changes occur at the etheric level before becoming manifest as physical cellular events."[9]

Healing is supercharged when integrated into our energy system by being locked into the ninth chakra (the portal to our soul body). By healing the soul body, which carries all data from one incarnation to another, we can be assured that we are not just going to repeat our lessons over and over, lifetime after lifetime. Our soul body is the entirety of our soul. When leaving a lifetime at death, we absorb that lifetime's memories, issues, and feelings into our soul etheric, the field of energy surrounding our soul. These energies are then mixed with the memories already present within our soul. When our soul comes into a new life, energies from every lifetime, along with our upcoming soul contract, are downloaded into our ninth chakra. To lock healing into the ninth chakra, you can visualize supportive symbols, shapes, and numbers while breathing deeply, thus applying the power of your diaphragm, the bodily site related to your ninth chakra. By doing this, you send healing into your soul as well as your body.

Metatron's cube. The basis for the Platonic solids, Metatron's cube contains two tetrahedrons, two cubes, and an octahedron, icosahedron, and dodecahedron. It is said to represent the gridwork of our consciousness and the matrix forming our universe. When looking at Metatron's cube, you are seeing all of the Platonic solids simultaneously. You can use the cube as a mandala while setting an intention for what you want to manifest or heal, or you can imagine your entire energy field within the cube while doing the same.

The Flower of Life. A pattern often found within other sacred geometrical figures, the Flower of Life is composed of evenly spaced, overlapping circles that create a flowerlike pattern. It is considered a universal template for healing that contains all the Platonic solids and therefore symbolizes the connection between physicality and spirituality. It is often considered a window into higher perspectives. One of the easiest ways to tap into its power is to use it as a mandala, focusing on its form while concentrating on a question. Let your mind be drawn to the aspect of the Flower that holds fascination for you. Now ask Spirit to reveal, through this part of the Flower, the information that has been previously hidden from your awareness.

THE POWER OF NUMBERS: UNIVERSAL SYMBOLS OF LIFE

Numbers tell a story. As I discussed in *Energetic Boundaries*:

> *The most learned of the ancients believed that numbers presented the fundamental principles of the universe, providing the only true explanations of the enigmas of reality. Today, many scientists are drawing upon the workings of mathematics, frequencies, geometry, and other numerically based approaches to explain healing, create new therapeutic modalities, and solve the puzzles of medicine. This concept is part of an esoteric and mystical lore called numerology, which is the study of numbers for practical application. Cultures throughout time have reduced reality to numerical equations.*[10]

Numbers are the basis of ancient Sumerian thinking, as well as healing modalities among many Hindu, Vedic, Egyptian, Tibetan, Mayan, Siberian, Chinese, Jewish Kabbalah, Christian, and cross-cultural sects. Certain Kabbalists, for example, analyzed the Old Testament book of Ezekiel and the apocryphal books of Enoch and IV Ezra (the fourth book of Ezra, part of 2 Esdras the Apocrypha) to speculate on the hidden meanings of numbers and letters. In Hindu scripture, numbers are often correlated with astrological bodies and their supposed traits. Ayurveda, the East Indian healing system, often relies upon a person's number (determined by one's birth date and a formula based on his or her name) to diagnose illness and present holistic solutions. Pythagoras, the great Greek philosopher and mathematician, believed that the universe was orderly and ever evolving, subject to progressive cycles that could be measured with the numbers one through nine.

The meanings of numbers as outlined here are drawn from Egyptian, Chaldean, and Pythagorean philosophy and cover two ways to apply the energy of numbers: (1) The essential energies of numbers for overall wellbeing and wholeness, and (2) the power of numbers for strengthening energetic boundaries. Like shapes, numbers can be visualized, meditated upon, or even drawn on the skin in order to provide vibrational support.

NUMBERS AND THEIR ESSENTIAL ENERGY

Following are the essential meanings of the numbers 1 through 10, plus a few select numbers above 10 that are particularly powerful.

1: Initiates and begins; invokes the Creator; brings your needs to a conclusion and puts yourself first.

2: Represents pairing and duality. Balances relationships, creates healthy liaisons, shares power.

3: Reflects optimism; the number of creation, it brings a beginning and end together; ends chaos.

4: Signifies foundation and stability; provides grounding; achieves balance.

5: Promotes and progresses; creates a space for decision-making; provides the ability to go in any direction at will.

6: The number of service; indicates the presence of light and dark, good and evil, and the choices made between these.

7: Represents the divine principle; opens us for love and grace, erasing doubts about the divine path.

8: The symbol of power and infinity; establishes recurring patterns and illuminates karma. Can be used to erase old and entrenched patterns or syndromes.

9: Represents change and harmony; eliminates the old and opens us to a new cycle. Can erase evil.

10: Signifies building and starting over. The number of physical matter, it can create heaven on earth.

11: Represents inspiration; releases personal mythology; opens us to divine powers; erases self-esteem issues.

12: Signifies mastery over human drama; accesses own divine self, but still encompasses humanity. Excellent for forgiveness.

22: For success in anything you do through partnership with the Divine.

33: For teaching and accepting our own wisdom. Invokes bravery and discipline.[10]

NUMBERS AND ENERGETIC BOUNDARIES

Although I love working with numbers in relation to diagnosis and healing, I am especially enthusiastic about their ability to strengthen and enliven energetic boundaries.

You can intuitively visualize a chosen number superimposed on the outside of a weak or distorted boundary or in the area of the physical body (e.g., the heart, the lower back, the blood) or energy body (e.g., a chakra, a meridian) most affected by the boundary problem. The frequency of the number will permeate your entire energetic biofield, one of four energetic boundaries described in chapter 7, or a specific auric field, and effect a change. For instance, if you easily absorb others' feelings, visualizing the number 1 on your second auric field or your emotional boundary will decrease your reliance on or absorption of others' feelings and reconnect you with your own.

Here is how numbers can transform many of the common energetic boundary problems that can deplete our life force.

1: Helps with victim issues that cause us to put others first or take on their energy.

2: Enables us to partner with someone without giving away our power.

3: Establishes healthy boundaries, especially for those who are susceptible to psychic or environmental invasions.

4: Grounds and stabilizes us, especially if others are frequently pulling on us energetically, mentally, or emotionally.

5: Keeps us from taking on everyone else's issues and thus becoming overburdened. Also breaks repetitive patterns.

6: Defends against evil forces, such as psychic invasions, and enables us to maintain our integrity by maintaining healthy energetic boundaries. Also helps us release the unconscious benefits of a repetitive pattern and embrace more joyful ways of responding to life.

7: Invokes divine assistance, which helps with any boundary problem.

8: Breaks or erases cycles or relationships that hold us hostage or keep us bound by unhealthy patterns.

9: Signals the end of a boundary problem or detrimental pattern, and confirms that we are ready to move forward and embrace new possibilities.

10: Boosts intentions or the energy of a new direction.

11: Provides access to spiritual guidance and transforms the storyline that established our boundary problems.

12: Supports forgiveness in the spiritual boundary (see chapter 7).

22: Helps us achieve success.

33: Opens us to our own wisdom.

24

THE ENERGETIC ENVIRONMENT

It is not the bacteria, it is the terrain.

LOUIS PASTEUR (ON HIS DEATHBED)

We are made of energy, and so is everything in our environment. Although invisible to the eye, this energy is continuously interacting with us—and us with it. Our health and wellbeing are strongly affected by our subtle surroundings, and there is much we can do to bring greater harmony and balance to the places we typically inhabit on a daily basis.

Largely based on chapter 2's information on energetic fields, this chapter addresses some of the basics of creating a healthy personal and professional environment. Included are discussions about electrical and magnetic dangers in your home and around you, as well as tips for solving these energetic disturbances; methods for healing with magnets; and using the ancient system of feng shui for creating sacred space.

ELECTRICAL AND MAGNETIC DANGERS: IN THE HOME AND AROUND YOU

Holistic practitioners are paying increasing attention to the effects of the energy around us, including human-made electromagnetic fields, which primarily affect us at work and at home. This electromagnetic radiation (EMR) creates electropollution. Our homes are petri dishes of EMR, which is proving to do everything from magnifying major illnesses to increasing daily stress. EMR exists around power lines, power tools, electric stoves, microwaves, heaters, boilers, freezers, and television sets, extending several feet or yards around an appliance even when it's turned off. Long-term exposure may aggravate the conditions listed in chapter 2.

Earth-based magnetic energies can also have a negative impact on our moods and bodies, known as geopathic stress (see chapter 2). Because of irregularities in the earth's fields, we might experience sleep challenges, increased stress levels, mood disorders, and behavioral problems, along with many other problematic symptoms.

Our energetic system responds negatively to both EMR and geopathic stress; in turn, the functioning of our energetic fields, channels, and centers improves when we shift our environment and decrease the amount or effects of these factors in our lives. Here are tips for bolstering our subtle systems by changing the world around us.

DECREASING EMR IN THE HOME (OR OFFICE)

- Save on electricity. Do things manually whenever possible.
- Unplug all appliances except your refrigerator when you're not using them.
- Strengthen your immune system with a nutrient-rich, organic diet.
- Replace home- and personal-care products with chemical-free versions.
- Walk barefoot. It releases EMR into the earth.
- Steer clear of electrical appliances in your bedroom. Use a battery-operated alarm clock, not an electrical one.
- Avoid low-voltage halogen and fluorescent lighting.
- Make sure cell phones and computers are turned off when not in use.
- Avoid electric blankets.
- Sleep in a bed with no metal parts.
- Protect yourself from radiation with the homeopathic remedies Fucus vesiculosus, Sodium alginate, Phosphorus, and Strontium. (See "Homeopathy: Vibratory Medicine from the Kingdoms of Nature" in chapter 20.)
- Clear your auric field of EMR using the techniques in the "Aura Clearing" section of chapter 11, "Healing the Auric Field."
- Use magnetic field therapy, described in the sidebar "Magnetic Field Therapy," to help clear the auric field.

ALLEVIATING GEOPATHIC STRESS

Geopathic stress often occurs in areas where a break has been created in the earth's natural energy flow. These breaks can be caused by natural phenomena, such as cliffs, ravines, streams, and fault lines, or manufactured phenomena, such as property lines, walls, fences, the ridge lines on roofs, and electrical, phone, and cable lines. The blocked or diverted energy from these breaks creates what are known as stress lines.

The most common method for alleviating geopathic stress is to check your surroundings for stress lines and to then ground them so they no longer penetrate your location.

Dowsing, a type of divination used to evaluate natural conditions or locate specific natural phenomena, can be used to check for geographic stress lines. Two of the easiest dowsing methods use a compass and a pendulum.

> **Dowsing with a compass.** Turn the compass until the needle is directly north and move it slowly over the area you are testing. If it passes over an energetic disturbance, the needle will swing away from due north.

> **Dowsing with a pendulum.** You can easily make a pendulum with a metal necklace and a hanging gem or other item. After grounding and centering yourself, establish which movement of the pendulum indicates yes and which indicates no. Then, walking around a specific location, ask yes-no questions, such as, "Is this area causing geopathic stress?"

Having pinpointed the stress lines, you can now ground the line with one of the following techniques:

- Insert a copper or brass staple, a copper ring, or a steel stake in the stress line.
- Block the line with a cork barrier. You can put cork tiles or a cork bath mat under your bed if the stress line affects you when sleeping or near the stress line if it affects you elsewhere. Cork is made from oak trees, which have evolved to have their own defense against geopathic stress.
- Neutralize the line with one of the many electronic-cancellation devices on the market. A few reputable products include the Powerhouse double Lakhovsky coil device and other instruments available through the Energy Store. There are also pendants, available through the organization BioGeometry or the Vesica Institute, for assisting with EMR as well as personal healing needs.[1]

- Nullify the line with crystals, which can be buried or put in the corners of rooms. See the section "Gemstones: Stones of Light" in chapter 20 to select an appropriate gemstone.

Within your home, you can also simply rearrange your furniture, moving your bed, couches, or desk off and away from the stress line.

MAGNETIC FIELD THERAPY

Magnetic field therapy diagnoses and treats both physical and emotional pain and relieves symptoms and causes of disease. Magnets and electromagnetic devices are now widely used to soothe pain, assist with the healing of broken bones, and alleviate stress.

Research by Albert Roy Davis, PhD, found that negative magnetic fields are beneficial to living organisms while positive magnetic fields can be stressful. Robert Becker, an orthopedic surgeon, found that weak electrical currents can promote the regrowth of broken bones, and Kyoichi Nakagawa, MD, director of the Isuzu Hospital in Tokyo, discovered a condition called "magnetic field deficiency syndrome," which results from decreased exposure to the natural geomagnetic fields of the earth and can cause headaches, dizziness, stiffness, chest pain, insomnia, and more.[2]

Magnets can support many healing processes and help alleviate EMR and geopathic stress. Magnetic energies move in spirals and can deflect harmful EMR energies. To use magnets and magnetic devices for this purpose, it's important to first understand the basic difference between the north and south poles of a magnet and what they affect. You can tell the difference in the two poles by suspending a magnet by a thread. The pole pointing toward the north is called the north pole or the negative pole, and the side toward the south, the south or positive pole. You can also move a magnet slowly toward the north end of the compass. If the needle keeps pointing north, you have been using the south-pole side of the magnet.

The north pole of a magnet stops the development of growths and infections. You can use north-pole magnets on infections, menstrual discharge, inflamed gums or teeth, inflammation in general, or for calcium deposits in the joints. They can contract tissue, decrease activity, and sedate pain. The south pole stimulates the growth of tissue and living systems, including bacteria. It will encourage muscle strength, help with prostrate problems, and help prevent miscarriages. South-pole magnets are also useful if you have congestion without an infection, and they can increase the activity of any tissue they are placed on. Do not use north-pole magnets if you are pregnant, as they might trigger a miscarriage during the first trimester. Also do not use them if you have congestion, but no infections, or if you are treating muscular weakness.[3] Finally, do not use magnets if you have a pacemaker or an automatic defibrillator, cochlear implants, or an insulin pump. And magnets should never be placed over an open wound.

The other consideration for selecting magnets is the intensity, which is measured in gauss, a unit of measurement that indicates the intensity of the magnetic field. The higher the number, the more intense the magnet.

The most effective magnets for healing purposes are called medical or therapeutic magnets. You can buy either unipolar magnets or bipolar magnets. Unipolar magnets have been artificially created to have the north pole on one side and the south pole on the other. Bipolar magnets are created with both poles on one side. People usually choose to use the unipolar magnet if they want the effects of one of the two poles without interference from the other pole.

Specific magnet-therapy techniques include the following:

- Using magnetic blankets and beds to reduce stress and promote sleep. (These are not recommended for people with bipolar disorder.)
- Placing a negative magnetic field at the top of the head to promote sleep. You can tape a small magnet to your head with a bandage. You can also obtain a magnetic bed pad composed of small negative magnetics and sleep with it near your head or put small negative magnetics together inside of your pillow.
- Using small Japanese *tai-ki* magnets to stimulate acupoints.
- Placing small disc magnets (ceramic neodymium or iron oxide) around the head to potentially alleviate panic, seizures, delusions, and other conditions.
- Using magnetic jewelry or discs on an inflamed area or site of pain.

USING YOUR NORTH-POLE MAGNETS

North-pole magnets are the most frequently used magnets and are usually considered the safest. You can use south-pole magnets, but sparingly, as they promote growth. North-pole magnets are most often used at an intensity of 2,000 to 4,000 gauss. Following is a treatment that can be used for problems such as arthritis or other painful conditions.

1. Select a unipolar magnet, so that the south pole cannot affect the injured living tissue.

2. Place the magnet, north side down, directly over the afflicted area. You can tape the magnet directly on the skin with athletic tape or an adhesive bandage, or insert it in a small cotton bag and tape this on to your skin.

3. Keep the magnet on for up to twelve hours. You can return to magnet therapy after a day or two if it effectively relieved your pain.[4]

For the duration of a magnetic therapy treatment, the rule of thumb is that the longer magnets are applied to an area, the more quickly the healing is performed.

FENG SHUI: THE ART OF SACRED SPACE

Feng shui is a 3,000-year-old Chinese science and art for balancing the energy of a space to support health. There are many schools of feng shui, but they all recommend a few basic actions:

Clear your clutter. Rivaling any electromagnetic pollution or geopathic stress is the clutter that easily piles up in our homes and offices. From our closets to drawers to basements and even computer desktops, clutter causes stagnation of subtle energies and can create low energy, confusion, and irritation. If you feel overwhelmed at the prospect of clutter-clearing, consider taking one closet, one corner, one drawer, or one purse at a time.

Improve your lighting. Throw open the curtains and allow as much natural light as possible into your home and office. Use full-spectrum light bulbs.

Improve your air quality. Open windows, bring air-purifying plants into your environment, and consider adding an air purifier.

Bring in the beauty. Incorporate oxygenating plants, fresh flowers, sacred objects that hold meaning for you, candles, and music into your space. All of these items can subtly (and sometimes dramatically) alter the energetics of any space and help to reduce the impact of EMR pollution and other environmental stressors.

Open to prosperity. Arrange your desk so the wall is behind you and you have a full view of the room and its door. Opportunities expand when your view is expansive. Consider putting up an inspirational poster to motivate yourself. In fact, make sure all your furniture faces the door to assure the movement of chi and a prosperous flow in every area of your life.

Make use of mirrors. Chi can't flow in dead ends. Use mirrors at the end of hallways to create the illusion of endlessness and keep your hallways open so the chi can move freely.

Select colors thoughtfully. In general, serene, neutral colors and smooth textures ensure a peaceful environment. Avoid bright colors except as accents, as they overstimulate the mind and body. (Also see the "Colors of the Five Elements" section in this chapter.)

Let the water flow. Flowing water stimulates creativity and the movement of emotions. Water also represents abundance. Use a small fountain to bring moving water into your space.

Watch your clocks. You can hang clocks in your kitchen, living room, or office, but don't place them in an entryway. You do not want a visitor seeing a clock first thing and thinking that there is a time limit on the visit. Also avoid hanging a large clock in your bedroom. This is the place to listen to your internal clock rather than an artificial one. In general, avoid display clocks made of metal, which can inhibit the health and joy of family members.

BEING YOUR OWN FENG SHUI MASTER

You can use this simple intuitive exercise to determine if there are any changes you can make in your environment to support the wellbeing of all areas of your life.

COLORS OF THE FIVE ELEMENTS

TO CREATE BALANCE in a space, make sure you have at least one color from each of the five feng shui elements in each room.

Fire: Red, orange, shades of pink, purple, and bright yellow. Use in any room where you are seeking recognition and extra energy. Often used in the southerly direction of a house to invoke passion.

Wood: Brown and green. Often placed in the southeast and eastern directions to encourage healing and promote wealth, but can be used anywhere for these reasons.

Water: Blue and black. Will encourage abundance in all areas of life. Will promote calm and renewal, and if used in the north, will also enhance purity and comfort.

Earth: Light yellow and light brown or beige. Will add stability and emphasize nourishment. Especially useful in the southwest and northeast areas of your home.

Metal: Gray, white, and silver. Metal helps you focus and can be used when you need efficiency and precision. Use in the northwest area of your home to emphasize these traits.[5]

You can use almost anything to add color, including pictures, plants, gemstones, candles, cloth, and more.

Using your intuitive senses, tune into each room in your home (and your workspace, if you feel inspired to do so). You can do this meditatively, or you can do a physical walk-through to merge your sensory and subtle faculties. How is the energy of your space influencing your wellbeing? Could you put some extra attention on the part of your home or office representing an area of your life you want to enhance? Would it change the energy of the space to move the furniture or artwork around? Do you need to clean or clear clutter? Is there a spot where you might want to apply a simple feng shui "cure," such as a green plant, a red cloth, a grounding stone, or a bowl of water? Make a list of the impressions and ideas that come to you.

CONCLUSION
FROM SUBTLE BODY TO PRIMARY SELF

> Healing yourself is connected
> with healing others.
>
> YOKO ONO

It's only fitting to conclude your journey through the world of subtle energy with one more exercise, one designed to integrate all three parts of your energetic anatomy while reestablishing your inherent wholeness.

A brilliant researcher of regenerative healing modalities, Grant McFetridge, PhD, developed a hypothesis known as *primary cell theory*. He developed this theory while studying concepts like peak states of consciousness, performance heightening, and spiritual awareness. His driving goal was, and is, to enable individuals to achieve a higher quality of life—an exceptional quality of life, in fact. He believes that the peak state, our optimum way of being, isn't something we acquire or gain; it is something we *regain*. Although temporarily blocked by the distractions and the traumas of human life, our peak state exists as full, awake consciousness within just one cell. In McFetridge's theory, all other cells in the body are extensions of this single primary cell.[1] What this means is that our primary cell contains all the energies, powers, and understandings that we need to become the greatest self we are capable of. Included in this formula are the structures that eventually develop into our chakras, meridians, auric fields, as well as organellas that hold energies representing our mind and soul. Everything is already in place.

Think about the structures within your primary cell or self, the one that is fully loaded for peak expression. Add one more piece of information. This primary cell, which continues to operate within you from conception onward, is linked to the creative source of the universe. Because this divine stream of light pours into our primary cell—and into and through us—at the most real level of reality, we are eternally empowered for wholeness. The awareness of this glorious and empowered wholeness—a fullness of being that cannot be destroyed by any shock, illness, betrayal, or loss—is perhaps one of the greatest tools you could employ as a subtle energy healer. As this awareness grows within you, you recognize the primary nature of others and relate to them from this place of knowing.

To play with this awareness (opening to it and expanding it), we will slip into a light meditative state that you are now well acquainted with.

1. Gently close your eyes and take a slow, deep breath. If you feel any tension in your body or mind, simply breathe into those areas, filling them with the warmth and radiance of your inner light.

2. Acknowledge yourself for having arrived at the final page of this book, for the passion and compassion that fuels your quest for health and healing.

3. Allow your attention to go to that place just above and between your eyebrows, your sixth chakra, the indigo or violet energy center known as your third eye. Envision a luminous bubble of light, perhaps lit with shimmering hues of purple, blue, and pink tinged with gold. Imagine this bubble as your primary cell—the center point of your consciousness, the state of oneness that you remember in your deepest being.

4. Take another slow, deep breath. Now notice what you sense about your primary cell, your primary self. What do you feel? See? Hear? What do you *know* about yourself in your state of peak awareness, peak power, and peak love?

5. Ask your primary self what it wants you to know about your journey as a subtle energy practitioner. Breathe in and allow its message to arrive. It could be a specific message about a field of study to pursue, a new course of action to take. Or it could be a message about your purpose as a subtle energy practitioner. What is important for you to know right now about your work with subtle energy?

6. Allow yourself to see or know the contribution that you make—the contribution that only you can make.

7. With that knowledge, make the journey back from your sixth chakra to the room where you sit. Write down in your journal or on a piece of paper the next step you're going to take on your subtle energy journey.

Now take a few moments to reflect on the commitment you are now making to yourself. Can you sense that through this acknowledgment of yourself, you are recognizing your own powers and aptitudes as a healer? That in embracing a future aimed at healing, you are establishing a healthier pathway?

There is a lovely Cherokee blessing prayer that can encourage you toward this future of even more joy and happiness. May it envelop you in the same spirit that the Greater Spirit already sees you as.

May the Warm Winds of Heaven
blow softly upon your house.
May the Great Spirit
bless all who enter there.
May your moccasins
make happy tracks
in many snows,
and may the Rainbow
always touch your shoulder.

2. FIELDS OF HEALING: THE ENERGY AROUND YOU

1. Catherine Brahic, "Does the Earth's Magnetic Field Cause Suicides?" *New Scientist* (April 24, 2008). Available at newscientist.com/article/dn13769-does-the-earths-magnetic-field-cause-suicides.html.

2. Nigel and Maggie Percy, "The Cause of Cancer? What Doctors Have Said," Sixth Sense Consulting. Online summary available to newsletter subscribers; available at professional-house-clearing.com/cause-of-cancer.html. Elora Gabriel, "Geopathic Stress and Radiation: A Breakthrough in Earth Healing," *Explore!* 9, no. 1 (1999). Article online, available at rubysemporium.org/geo_stress.html.

3. William Bengston, *The Energy Cure* (Boulder, CO: Sounds True, 2010).

4. Judy Jacka, *The Vivaxis Connection: Healing through Earth Energies* (Newburyport, MA: Hampton Roads, 2000).

4. BODIES OF HEALING: THE CHAKRAS

1. See Cyndi Dale, *The Complete Book of Chakra Healing* (Woodbury, MN: Llewellyn Publications, 2009) and *Advanced Chakra Healing* (Berkeley, CA: Crossing Press, 2005).

2. David Furlong, *Working with Earth Energies* (London: Piatkus Books, 2003). Katrina Raphaell, The Crystal Academy of Advanced Healing Arts, webcrystalacademy.com.

6. INTUITION AND TRUST

1. Cyndi Dale, *The Intuition Guidebook* (Minneapolis: Deeper Well Publishing and Brio Press, 2011).

11. HEALING THE AURIC FIELD

1. Stephen Barrett, Chios Energy Healing, chioshealing.com.
2. Leslie Swartz and Elmarie Swartz, Healing Journeys Energy School of Energy Healing, healing-journeys-energy.com.

12. HANDS-ON HEALING

1. Dorothea Hover-Kramer, *Healing Touch: Essential Energy Medicine for Yourself and Others* (Boulder, CO: Sounds True, 2011), 12.
2. Sanjay Pisharodi, "Ten Acupressure Points Lead to a Healthy, Wholesome Life," NaturalNews.com, October 21, 2011. Available at naturalnews.com/033933_accupressure_health.html#ixzz1n44SlWRh.
3. Michael Reed Gach, *Acupressure's Potent Points: A Guide to Self-Care for Common Ailments* (New York, NY: Bantam, 1990).
4. The seven acu-exercises were adapted from those in the following online articles: Melissa Smith, "Acupressure Points for Healing," Livestrong.com, September 2, 2010. Available at livestrong.com/article/213496-acupressure-points-for-healing/#ixzz1n3zAJ5Xs. Sumei FitzGerald, "Anti-Anxiety Acupressure Points," Livestrong.com, August 18, 2011. Available at livestrong.com/article/516869-anti-anxiety-acupressure-points/#ixzz1n4oktXAk. Melissa Smith, "Acupressure Points for Neck Pain," Livestrong.com, September 2, 2012. Available at livestrong.com/article/227586-acupressure-point-for-neck-pain/#ixzz1n4oP3Ezf. Melissa Smith, "Facial Acupressure," Livestrong.com, September 28, 2010. Available at livestrong.com/article/260944-facial-acupressure/#ixzz1n4oAzAMZ. Melissa Smith, "Acupressure Points for Metabolism," Livestrong.com, June 14, 2011. Available at livestrong.com/article/278680-acupressure-points-for-metabolism/#ixzz1n3zm1G7Q. Meg Kramer, "Acupressure Points for Allergies," Livestrong.com, September 9, 2011. Available at livestrong.com/article/539688-acupressure-points-for-allergies/#ixzz1n3zMnH1e.
5. Valerie Lis, MA, certified EFT expert and trainer, Simple EFT, simpleeft.com.

13. MODERN ESOTERIC HEALING

1. Jacka, *The Vivaxis Connection*.
2. Jack Angelo, *Distant Healing: A Complete Guide* (Boulder, CO: Sounds True, 2008).

14. HEALING MOVEMENT

1. Gertrud Hirschi, "Finger Meditations, a.k.a. Mudras," article on the website InnerSelf.com (no date). Available at innerself.com/Meditation/finger_mudras.htm. Article excerpted from Gertrud Hirschi, *Mudras: Yoga for Your Hands* (San Francisco: Weiser, 2000).

15. THE SUBTLE MIND: FROM MEDITATION TO SUBCONSCIOUS REPROGRAMMING

1. Jon Kabat-Zinn, *Full Catastrophe Living: Using the Wisdom of Your Body and Mind to Face Stress* (New York: Delta, 1990).
2. Sue Schmidt, "Brain Wave Therapy," webpage on the website Mind Power for Positive Change (2009). Available at mindpower1.net/brainwaveinfo.html
3. Vianna Stibal, "About Vianna Stibal" webpage on the website ThetaHealing, thetahealing.com.
4. Cyndi Dale, *The Subtle Body: An Encyclopedia of Your Energetic Anatomy* (Boulder, CO: Sounds True, 2009), 106.
5. Franz Bardon, *Initiation into Hermetics*, trans. Dieter Rüggeberg (Salt Lake City, UT: Merkur, 2001). Original German edition, 1956. First English edition, 1962.

17. HEALING WITH THE ANCIENTS

1. Carlos Castaneda, *The Teachings of Don Juan: A Yaqui Way of Knowledge* (Berkeley, CA: University of California Press, 2008). The Yaqui are a native tribal people living in northern Mexico and in Arizona. Although Castenada's books are fiction, they are based on his real-life experiences. I have found the shamanic information they contain is consistent with my own experiences.
2. Jon Whale, "Core Energy: Shifting the Assemblage Point," *Positive Health*, no. 17 (January 1997). Available at positivehealth.com/article/energy-medicine/core-energy-shifting-the-assemblage-point.

18. HEALING BREATH

1. Amir Farid Isahak, "The Ki to Longevity" (May 7, 2007), SuperQiGong.com. Available at superqigong.com/articlesmore.asp?id=123. S. Tsuyoshi Ohnishi and Tomoko Ohnishi, "The Nishino Breathing Method and Ki-energy (Life-energy): A Challenge to Traditional Scientific Thinking," Evidence-Based Complementary and Alternative Medicine 3, no. 2 (June 2006), 191–200. DOI: 10.1093/ecam/nel004.

20. HEALING WITH THE NATURAL WORLD

1. James Mattioda, PhD, DHom (Med), owner of Arcana Empothecary, San Diego, California, ArcanaEmpothecary.com.

2. "Dangerous Essential Oils," online page/list on the website Elaine: Webbed. Available at eethomp.com/AT/dangerous_oils.html.

3. Jodi Baglien, certified clinical aromatherapist, well being + wisdom studio, Osseo, Minnesota, JodiBaglien.com.

4. "The 38 Bach Flower Remedies, in Dr. Bach's Own Words," page of the website The Original Bach Flower Remedies. Available at nelsonsnaturalworld.com/en-us/us/our-brands/bachoriginalflowerremedies/.

5. Tim Simmone, ChargedWater.com.

6. "Liquid Crystals Light Way to Better Data Storage," article online at ScienceDaily, June 24, 2010. Available at sciencedaily.com/releases/2010/06/100622095050.htm.

7. John Matson, "Crystal Memory Allows Efficient Storage of Quantum in Light," June 29, 2010, entry in the blog "Observations," on the website Scientific American. Available at blogs.scientificamerican.com/observations/2010/06/29/crystal-memory-allows-efficient-storage-of-quantum-information-in-light/.

21. SOUND HEALING

1. Kay Grace, CAEH, sound healing practitioner and educator, Minneapolis, Energy Express, energyexpress.com.

2. Ken Cohen, *The Way of Qigong: The Art and Science of Chinese Energy Healing* (New York: Ballantine Books, 1999), 165–166. As cited in Joseph F. Morales, "Six Healing Sounds," Baharna.com, article online, available at baharna.com/chant/six_healing.htm.

3. Michael Baird, "Reiki and the Healing Drum," The International Center for Reiki Training: Reiki Articles (2000), article online, available at reiki.org/reikinews/Reiki%20and%20the%20Healing%20Drum.htm.

4. Susan Govali, Singing from the Center, singingfromthecenter.com.

22. COLOR HEALING

1. "Sunlight Can Prevent Cancer (& Other Illness)," a collection of excerpted articles on the website Healing Cancer Naturally (no date). Available at healingcancernaturally.com/sunlight-prevents-cancer.html. Oliver Gillie, "Article 38: Sunlight Prevents Cancer," article online on the website

Multiple Sclerosis Resource Centre (no date). Available at msrc.co.uk/index.cfm/fuseaction/show/pageid/1089.

2. Joseph Mercola, "Light as a Nutrient," article online on the website International Alliance for Animal Therapy and Healing (IAATH, 2006). Available at iaath.com/light.htm.

3. Jennifer Warters, BSc, MA, sound healer and teacher, United Kingdom, rainbowlightfoundation.net/Jennifer_Warters.html.

4. Howard and Jennifer Beckman, "Healing with Color and Gems," webpage on the website Vedic Cultural Fellowship. Available at vedicworld.org/healing-with-color-and-gems/.

23. VIBRATIONAL SYMBOLS AND ORACLES

1. Abraham Karim, "The Science of BioGeometry" article on the website Rexresearch.com (1997). Available at rexresearch.com/biogeom/biogeom.htm.

2. Cyndi Dale, *Energetic Boundaries: How to Stay Protected and Connected in Work, Love, and Life* (Boulder, CO: Sounds True, 2011), 111–113.

3. Ibid., 113–114.

4. Ibid., 114.

5. Claude Swanson, *Life Force: The Scientific Basis: Volume 2* (Tucson, AZ: Poseidia Press, 2009).

6. Mary Desaulniers, "The Torus of Life Healing Meditation," article on the website Suite 101 (March 10, 2010). Available at suite101.com/article/the-torus-of-life-healing-meditation-a211628.

7. "Healing With Frequencies," newsletter article on the website Altered States (no date). Available at altered-states.net/barry/newsletter420/.

8. "Platonic Solids," webpage on the online store Crystal Well-Being (no date). Available at crystalwellbeing.co.uk/catalogueplatonicsolids.php. Ilona Anne Hress, "How to Use Platonic Solids for Personal Growth and Evolutionary Development," blog entry at Growing Consciousness: The Center for Evolutionary Activity (January 23, 2010). Available at growingconsciousness.com/?p=47.

9. Richard Gerber, *Vibrational Medicine* (Rochester, VT: Bear & Company, 2001), p. 371.

10. Dale, *Energetic Boundaries*, 115–116.

24. THE ENERGETIC ENVIRONMENT

1. The Energy Store Geopathic and Electro-Stress Balancing (geopathic-stress.info). BioGeometry (biogeometry.com/english). The Vesica Institute (vesica.org).

2. "Magnetic Field Therapy," online article on the website "Alternative Medicine Online" (1998), a student-developed learning project included in ThinkQuest Library. Article available at library.thinkquest.org/24206/magnetic-field-therapy.html.

3. Channary Houle, "How to Use Medical Magnets," webpage on the website Magnetic-Therapy-Living.com (no date). Available at magnetic-therapy-living.com/medical-magnets.html. BiomagScience, "Which Side of a BioMagnet to Use? Because It Matters!" webpage on the website BiomagScience.net (no date). Available at biomagscience.net/magnet-therapy/which-side-biomagnet-use-it-matters.

4. Donn Saylor, "How to Heal With Magnets," article online at eHow.com. Available at ehow.com/how_5533338_heal-magnets.html.

5. Christine Tran, "Transforming White Walls with Feng Shui Colors," article online at GoArticles.com (July 21, 2010). Available at goarticles.com/article/Transforming-White-Walls-with-Feng-Shui-Colors/3131198/.

CONCLUSION: FROM SUBTLE BODY TO PRIMARY SELF

1. Grant McFetridge, PhD, Institute for the Study of Peak States, PeakStates.com.

ACKNOWLEDGMENTS

The making of a book like this is complex. Just as the concepts and techniques in this book feature energy known and unknown, so is there applause for people known and unknown.

Kudos to Debra Evans and Amy Rost, incredible editors who transformed my words into streams of light and sound bites of inspiration. From my deepest—and subtle heart—I thank my business manager, literary agent, and friend, Anthony J.W. Benson, as well as the staff of Sounds True, whose dedication to sharing goodness with the world makes my own and others' works possible. A special thank you to Tami Simon, founder, and Jennifer Brown, acquisitions editor, who have helped so many of us harness stars and help plant them on earth. And how can I not thank my sons, Michael and Gabriel, who have put up with Mom's writing occupying the kitchen table (instead of food) for so many years?

This book also begs another line of thanks—or lineage for which to be grateful, for that matter. Our understanding of the subtle body and its powerful practices is the culmination of the work of thousands, if not millions, of dedicated sages, mystics, shamans, healers, philosophers, and medics. These masters of heart, light, and mystery now lie in the shadows, but their wisdom has been preserved and passed down from generation to generation. Besides thanking these forefathers and foremothers, we must also recognize the subtle energy practitioners, whether professional or lay, who are each furthering and expanding the ancient knowledge of subtle medicine. It is to all of you that I dedicate this book.

INDEX

ABOUT THE AUTHOR

CYNDI DALE is known and respected worldwide as an energy healer and an authority on subtle energy anatomy. Having studied with healers from all parts of the world, including Peru, Belize, Costa Rica, Japan, Iceland, and Mexico, as well as teachers from the Lakota and Hawaiian kahuna healing traditions, she now conducts workshops, training sessions, and college classes across the globe. Her enthusiasm, care, and down-to-earth teaching style make her wisdom and techniques accessible to everyone.

Her bestselling books on energy healing include *New Chakra Healing* (published in more than ten languages and republished and expanded in *The Complete Book of Chakra Healing* in 2009), *Advanced Chakra Healing*, *The Intuition Guidebook*, and the award-winning encyclopedia *The Subtle Body*. She has also created several DVD and CD trainings, including *Advanced Chakra Wisdom*, *Illuminating the Afterlife*, and *Healing Across Space and Time: Guided Journeys to Your Past, Present, and Parallel Lives*; *Healing Across Time*; and *Cyndi Dale's Essential Energy Healing Techniques*.

She lives in Minneapolis, Minnesota, with her two sons, two dogs, and a frog. More information on Cyndi's products, classes, and services is available at cyndidale.com.

ABOUT SOUNDS TRUE

SOUNDS TRUE is a multimedia publisher whose mission is to inspire and support personal transformation and spiritual awakening. Founded in 1985 and located in Boulder, Colorado, we work with many of the leading spiritual teachers, thinkers, healers, and visionary artists of our time. We strive with every title to preserve the essential "living wisdom" of the author or artist. It is our goal to create products that not only provide information to a reader or listener, but that also embody the quality of a wisdom transmission.

For those seeking genuine transformation, Sounds True is your trusted partner. At SoundsTrue.com you will find a wealth of free resources to support your journey, including exclusive weekly audio interviews, free downloads, interactive learning tools, and other special savings on all our titles.

To learn more, please visit SoundsTrue.com/bonus/free_gifts or call us toll free at 800-333-9185.

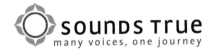

SOUNDS TRUE
many voices, one journey